Inflammatory Bowel Disease

Editor

SIMON LICHTIGER

GASTROINTESTINAL ENDOSCOPY CLINICS OF NORTH AMERICA

www.giendo.theclinics.com

Consulting Editor
CHARLES J. LIGHTDALE

July 2019 • Volume 29 • Number 3

ELSEVIER

1600 John F. Kennedy Boulevard • Suite 1800 • Philadelphia, Pennsylvania, 19103-2899

http://www.theclinics.com

GASTROINTESTINAL ENDOSCOPY CLINICS OF NORTH AMERICA Volume 29, Number 3
July 2019 ISSN 1052-5157, ISBN-13: 978-0-323-67795-0

Editor: Kerry Holland
Developmental Editor: Donald Mumford

Gastrointestinal Endoscopy Clinics of North America (ISSN 1052-5157) is published quarterly by Elsevier Inc., 360 Park Avenue South, New York, NY 10010-1710. Months of issue are January, April, July, and October. Business and Editorial Offices: 1600 John F. Kennedy Blvd., Suite 1800, Philadelphia, PA, 19103-2899. Periodicals postage paid at New York, NY and additional mailing offices. Subscription prices are $359.00 per year for US individuals, $624.00 per year for US institutions, $100.00 per year for US students and residents, $399.00 per year for Canadian individuals, $737.00 per year for Canadian institutions, $476.00 per year for international individuals, $737.00 per year for international institutions, and $245.00 per year for Canadian and international students/residents. To receive student/resident rate, orders must be accompanied by name of affiliated institution, date of term, and the *signature* of program/residency coordinator on institution letterhead. Orders will be billed at individual rate until proof of status is received. Foreign air speed delivery is included in all *Clinics* subscription prices. All prices are subject to change without notice. **POSTMASTER:** Send address change to *Gastrointestinal Endoscopy Clinics of North America*, Elsevier Health Sciences Division, Subscription Customer Service, 3251 Riverport Lane, Maryland Heights, MO 63043. **Customer Service: 1-800-654-2452 (US). From outside the United States, call 1-314-447-8871. Fax: 1-314-447-8029. E-mail: JournalsCustomerService-usa@elsevier.com (for print support) or JournalsOnlineSupport-usa@elsevier.com (for online support).**

Reprints. For copies of 100 or more, of articles in this publication, please contact the Commercial Reprints Department, Elsevier Inc., 360 Park Avenue South, New York, NY 10010-1710. Tel. 212-633-3874; Fax: 212-633-3820; E-mail: reprints@elsevier.com.

Gastrointestinal Endoscopy Clinics of North America is covered in *Excerpta Medica, MEDLINE/PubMed (Index Medicus), and MEDLINE/MEDLARS.*

Contributors

CONSULTING EDITOR

CHARLES J. LIGHTDALE, MD
Professor of Medicine, Division of Digestive and Liver Diseases, Columbia University Medical Center, New York, New York, USA

EDITOR

SIMON LICHTIGER, MD
Professor of Gastroenterology, Columbia University Medical Center, New York, New York, USA

AUTHORS

MARIA T. ABREU, MD
Director, Crohn's & Colitis Center, Martin Kalser Chair in Gastroenterology, Professor of Medicine, Professor of Microbiology and Immunology, University of Miami Miller School of Medicine, Miami, Florida, USA

MANASI AGRAWAL, MD
Division of Gastroenterology, Lenox Hill Hospital, Northwell Health, New York, New York, USA

ASHWIN N. ANANTHAKRISHNAN, MD, MPH
Division of Gastroenterology, Massachusetts General Hospital, Harvard Medical School, MGH Crohn's and Colitis Center, Boston, Massachusetts, USA

JORDAN E. AXELRAD, MD, MPH
Assistant Professor of Medicine, Inflammatory Bowel Disease Center at NYU Langone Health, Division of Gastroenterology, Department of Medicine, New York University School of Medicine, New York, New York, USA

TALAT BESSISSOW, MDCM
Associate Professor, Division of Gastroenterology, McGill University Health Center, Montreal, Canada

ABHIK BHATTACHARYA, MD
Clinical Fellow, Department of Gastroenterology, Hepatology, and Nutrition, Cleveland Clinic Foundation, Cleveland, Ohio, USA

JEAN-FREDERIC COLOMBEL, MD
Professor of Medicine, Director of the Susan and Leonard Feinstein IBD Clinical Center and the Leona M. and Harry B. Helmsley Charitable Trust Inflammatory Bowel Disease Center, Icahn School of Medicine at Mount Sinai, New York, New York, USA

PARAKKAL DEEPAK, MD, MS
Assistant Professor of Medicine, Division of Gastroenterology, Washington University School of Medicine, Washington University Inflammatory Bowel Diseases Center, St Louis, Missouri, USA

SUJAATA DWADASI, MD
Fellow, Section of Gastroenterology, Hepatology and Nutrition, The University of Chicago Medicine, Chicago, Illinois, USA

ROBERT ENNS, MD
Clinical Professor of Medicine, Division of Gastroenterology, Department of Medicine, St Paul's Hospital, University of British Columbia, Vancouver, British Columbia, Canada

JULIA FRITSCH, BS
PhD Candidate, Microbiology and Immunology, Crohn's & Colitis Center, University of Miami Miller School of Medicine, Miami, Florida, USA

AMANDA ISRAEL, MD
Advanced IBD Fellow, Inflammatory Bowel Disease Center, The University of Chicago Medicine, Chicago, Illinois, USA

STEVEN H. ITZKOWITZ, MD, FACP, FACG, AGAF
Professor of Medicine and Oncological Sciences Director, GI Fellowship Program Icahn School of Medicine at Mount Sinai, Mount Sinai Hospital, New York, New York, USA

JENNA L. KOLIANI-PACE, MD
Inflammatory Bowel Disease Center, Section of Gastroenterology and Hepatology, Dartmouth-Hitchcock Medical Center, Lebanon, New Hampshire, USA

GIL Y. MELMED, MD, MS
Co-Director, Inflammatory Bowel Disease Center, Professor of Medicine, Cedars-Sinai Medical Center, Los Angeles, California, USA

GEORGE OU, MD
Division of Gastroenterology, Department of Medicine, St Paul's Hospital, University of British Columbia, Vancouver, British Columbia, Canada

MIGUEL REGUEIRO, MD
Chair, Department of Gastroenterology, Hepatology, and Nutrition, Cleveland Clinic Foundation, Cleveland, Ohio, USA

JASON REINGLAS, MD
Division of Gastroenterology, McGill University Health Center, Montreal, Canada

FEZA H. REMZI, MD, FACS, FTSS (Hon)
Professor, Department of Surgery, NYU School of Medicine, Department of Surgery, Inflammatory Bowel Disease Center, NYU Langone Health, New York, New York, USA

DAVID T. RUBIN, MD
Professor of Medicine, Inflammatory Bowel Disease Center, The University of Chicago Medicine, Chicago, Illinois, USA

MARK S. SALEM, MD
Inflammatory Bowel and Immunobiology Research Institute, Cedars-Sinai Medical Center, Los Angeles, California, USA

DAVID M. SCHWARTZBERG, MD
Department of Surgery, Inflammatory Bowel Disease Center, NYU Langone Health,
Assistant Professor of Surgery, NYU School of Medicine, New York, New York,
USA

SHAILJA C. SHAH, MD
Division of Gastroenterology, Hepatology and Nutrition, Department of Medicine,
Vanderbilt University Medical Center, Nashville, Tennessee, USA

BO SHEN, MD
Section Head, IBD, Department of Gastroenterology, Hepatology, and Nutrition,
The Center for Inflammatory Bowel Diseases, Digestive Disease and Surgery Institute,
Cleveland Clinic Foundation, Cleveland, Ohio, USA

COREY A. SIEGEL, MD, MS
Director, Inflammatory Bowel Disease Center, Section of Gastroenterology and
Hepatology, Dartmouth-Hitchcock Medical Center, Lebanon, New Hampshire, USA

XINYING WANG, MD, PhD
Professor, Department of Gastroenterology, Zhujiang Hospital, Southern Medical
University, Guangzhou, China

Contents

The underlying factors driving the onset and progression of inflammatory bowel disease (IBD) include the interplay between host genetics, microbiota, and mucosal inflammation. The same environmental triggers that are a risk factor for IBD also alter the microbiota, suggesting a link between the microbiome and IBD. Specific IBD-associated genetic polymorphisms change the microbiome linking host genetics to the microbiota. Microbial changes occur at least simultaneously with new onset IBD, and fecal microbial transplant can ameliorate certain types of IBD. A current debate in the field is which comes first, dysbiosis or inflammation? Can restitution of the microbiome "cure" IBD?

Both Crohn's disease and ulcerative colitis are inflammatory bowel diseases (IBD) that can lead to progressive irreversible bowel damage. Selecting the most appropriate therapy for patients is a challenge because not all patients diagnosed with IBD have complications, and the amount of time to develop a complication is different for individuals. Models using patient characteristics, genetics, and immune responses help identify those patients who require early aggressive therapy with a goal to modify their disease course. Future research will help identify the role that the microbiome, metagenomics, metaproteomics, and microRNAs play in a patient prognosis.

The discovery of anti-TNF therapy as a treatment of inflammatory bowel disease (IBD) was a revolution in the management of IBD and has ushered in an era of biological therapies that have changed the natural history of these diseases. By understanding anti-TNF treatments clinicians have learned a tremendous amount about the immune system, immunogenicity, biosilimarity, and therapeutic drug monitoring. The next evolution in these therapies will be defined by advances in our understanding of the pathogenesis of different types of IBD, prediction of response, and sequencing of therapies.

Inflammatory bowel diseases, including Crohn's Disesase (CD) and ulcerative colitis (UC), are chronic, progressive, immune-mediated inflammatory diseases of the gastrointestinal tract. Early therapy using a treat-to-target (T2T) approach, which implies identification of a pre-defined target, followed by optimization of therapy and regular monitoring until the goal is achieved is critical in preventing adverse long-term outcomes. In this review, the authors discuss the T2T guidance developed by the Selecting Therapeutic Targets in Inflammatory Bowel Disease committee, new evidence published on the role of various targets in CD and UC, as well as the real-world applicability of T2T.

Histologic activity in inflammatory bowel disease is associated with an increased risk of clinical relapse, surgery, hospitalizations, and disease-associated dysplasia independent of clinical or endoscopic activity. Several histologic scoring systems exist to capture disease activity. However, none has been validated to assess prognosis or response to therapy and there is no universally accepted definition of histologic healing or remission. Although histologic healing is not a current recommended target for treatment, it may be a more sensitive marker of disease activity. Future studies are needed to determine standardized definitions of disease activity, healing, and evaluating normalization of histology as clinical trial outcomes.

Crohn's disease and ulcerative colitis are chronic inflammatory diseases that lead to progressive bowel damage including the development of stricturing and penetrating complications. Increasingly, cross-sectional imaging with computed tomography or magnetic resonance scans have emerged as leading tools to: (1) assess disease activity; (2) monitor response to therapy or disease recurrence; and (3) identify disease-related complications. Several validated radiological scoring systems have been developed to quantify cross-sectional and longitudinal inflammatory burden in these diseases and to monitor response to treatment. Bowel ultrasound is also a simple and inexpensive tool but is operator dependent in its performance.

Capsule endoscopy (CE) provides visualization of small bowel mucosa for evidence of inflammation. Given its ability to detect subtle mucosal changes, CE is recommended in the diagnostic work-up of small bowel

Crohn's Disesase (CD) and also in monitoring mucosal response to therapy in nonstricturing CD. Patency capsule and cross-sectional imaging can reduce risk of capsule retention in patients with suspected stenotic disease. CE is complementary to magnetic resonance enterography, which can provide extraintestinal information. Device-assisted enteroscopy has limited role in CD.

This article discusses the use of endoscopy in patients with Crohn's Disesase and ulcerative colitis in the postoperative setting. Endoscopy is the most sensitive and validated tool available in the diagnosis of recurrence of Crohn's Disesase in the postoperative setting. It is also the most effective diagnostic modality available for evaluating complications of pouch anatomy in patients with ulcerative colitis. In addition to diagnosis, management postoperatively can be determined through endoscopy.

Perianal diseases, common complications of Crohn's disease, are difficult to diagnose/manage. Patients with perianal Crohn's disease suffer from persistent pain and drainage, recurrent perianal sepsis, impaired quality of life, and financial burden. Conventional medical and surgical therapies carry risk of infection, myelosuppression, incontinence, disease recurrence. Although the phenotype of Crohn's disease has been extensively studied, reported outcomes are inconsistent. Endoanal ultrasonography is also becoming popular because of low cost and ability to acquire images in real time. Emerging management strategies for treatment including laser therapy, local injection of agents, use of hyperbaric oxygen, and stem cell therapy, have demonstrated efficacy.

This article begins with a brief overview of risk factors for colorectal neoplasia in inflammatory bowel disease to concretize the approach to risk stratification. It then provides an up-to-date review of diagnosis and management of dysplasia in inflammatory bowel disease, which integrates new and emerging data in the field. This is particularly relevant in an era of increased attention to cost- and resource-containment from the health systems vantage point, coupled with a heightened prioritization of patient quality of life and shared decision-making. Also provided is a brief discussion of the status of newer therapeutic techniques, such as endoscopic submucosal dissection.

Symptomatic strictures occur more often in Crohn's Disesase than in ulcerative colitis. The mainstay of endoscopic therapy for strictures in inflammatory bowel disease is endoscopic balloon dilation. Serious complications are rare, and risk factors for perforation include active inflammation, use of steroids, and dilation of ileorectal or ileosigmoid anastomotic strictures. This article presents current literature on strictures in inflammatory bowel disease. Focus is placed on the short- and long-term outcomes, complications, and safety of endoscopic balloon dilation for Crohn's Disesase strictures. Adjuvant techniques, such as intralesional injection of steroids and anti–tumor necrosis factor, stricturotomy, and stent insertion, are briefly discussed.

The incidence of inflammatory bowel disease is increasing and despite advances in medical therapy, patients continue to require operations for complications of their disease. Minimally invasive surgical options have impacted postoperative morbidity dramatically with reduction of pain, length of stay and adhesion formation, but additionally, this population of patients are not only concerned with successful operative therapy but also the ability to return to their lifestyle and cosmetics. Laparoscopic and robotic surgery for Crohn's disease has proven to benefit patients with ileocolic or colonic disease, however complicated disease with phlegmon, abscess or fistulae is best served with a hybrid approach. Ulcerative colitis treatment has seen advancements with laparoscopic and robotic platforms, however the benefits of minimally invasive surgery must be balanced with producible and durable outcomes.

GASTROINTESTINAL ENDOSCOPY CLINICS OF NORTH AMERICA

RELATED CLINICS SERIES

Gastroenterology Clinics
Clinics in Liver Disease

THE CLINICS ARE AVAILABLE ONLINE!
Access your subscription at:
www.theclinics.com

Foreword

Management of Inflammatory Bowel Disease: Progress and Promise

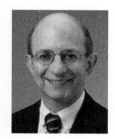

Charles J. Lightdale, MD
Consulting Editor

It is an exhilarating time for clinicians treating patients with inflammatory bowel disease (IBD). The past two decades of anti-TNF therapy have provided true improvement for patients suffering from ulcerative colitis and Crohn's disease. Clinical researchers have honed anti-TNF therapy by using quantitative, personalized, and precision measures to improve safety and outcomes. Gastrointestinal endoscopists have contributed with a new emphasis on treating to target: mucosal healing and histologic improvement based on endoscopic biopsies. There are also new endoscopic approaches to inflammatory and fibrotic strictures. Endoscopic surveillance for dysplasia and cancer has also improved, and endoscopic mucosal resection and endoscopic submucosal dissection for dysplastic colon lesions can offer accurate pathologic diagnosis and potentially minimally invasive management. Laparoscopic approaches have become dominant when surgery is needed, and endoscopy in the postoperative patient has provided new insights into recurrent inflammatory changes and management.

I am extremely pleased that Dr Simon Lichtiger agreed to be the Editor for this issue of *Gastrointestinal Endoscopy Clinics of North America* devoted to IBD. As a leading senior clinical gastroenterologist in IBD, Dr Lichtiger brings a broad and deep perspective to the field and has chosen a cohesive state-of-the-art series of articles authored by a remarkable group of specialist experts. It seems clear that the transformative era of anti-TNF therapy is likely a stepping stone to even further advances, as translational research in the processes of inflammation and the role of the microbiome continues to result in new promising biological and pharmaceutical treatments. Clinicians managing

Gastrointest Endoscopy Clin N Am 29 (2019) xiii–xiv
https://doi.org/10.1016/j.giec.2019.03.003
1052-5157/19/© 2019 Published by Elsevier Inc.

giendo.theclinics.com

IBD should savor this entire issue of *Gastrointestinal Endoscopy Clinics of North America.*

Charles J. Lightdale, MD
Department of Medicine
Columbia University Medical Center
161 Fort Washington Avenue
New York, NY 10032, USA

E-mail address:
CJL18@columbia.edu

Preface

Inflammatory Bowel Disease

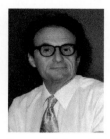

Simon Lichtiger, MD
Editor

It has been an honor to edit this issue of *Gastrointestinal Endoscopy Clinics of North America*, which represents a bridge connecting the past decade to the next one in terms of concepts, tools, and approach to the patient with inflammatory bowel disease (IBD). The future approach incorporates changes in pathogenesis, advances in predicting disease activity and severity, treat to target philosophy, and the prospect of expanding our ability to treat disease with new technical modalities as well as expanding our menu of medication. Each article is a state-of-the-art review on a topic that leads us into the next decade of thought as well as an approach to the patient with IBD. A decade ago, we did not understand the microbiome in IBD, did not think that histology had a role in definition of activity, and did not prognosticate and treat based upon disease severity. We did not treat objective markers, we treated symptoms, nor did we think that laparoscopic surgery would dominate the approach to bowel resection. In the next decade, we may graduate to endoscopic submucosal dissection of dysplastic tissue, use sonography and capsule endoscopy in order to stage disease, and have better medical therapy for stricturing disease so that we may not have to resect bowel in patients with this phenotype of disease.

This issue does not concentrate on medical therapy, yet reflects on the 20 years we have using anti-TNFs, and addresses what we have and have not learned about this revolutionary class of drugs. We still do not have that ability with the newer biologics, as they are still in their infancy. Yet, this issue covers the future of therapy for perianal disease, including stem cell therapy and highlights the approach to the post operative patient. The postoperative patient may be our window to disease, as these postoperative patients are in deep remission and offer us the ability to follow disease progression from its earliest onset.

I thank the authors, each of whom is a recognized expert on their respective topic. Thank you for your time, effort, and commitment necessary in order to publish this issue. It has been my honor and pleasure to coordinate your expertise into a single

Gastrointest Endoscopy Clin N Am 29 (2019) xv–xvi
https://doi.org/10.1016/j.giec.2019.03.002
1052-5157/19/© 2019 Published by Elsevier Inc.

giendo.theclinics.com

issue of *Gastrointestinal Endoscopy Clinics of North America* and to learn from your respective articles. In addition, I thank the junior authors, who sifted through throngs of data, papers, and reviews and contributed so much in the writing and organizing of the articles. You are the next several decades, and I hope that you can continue to contribute to our knowledge of these diseases. And thank you to Don Mumford and Swaminathan Nagarajan, who took isolated articles and made this an issue that will enrich all those who read it.

Simon Lichtiger, MD
Columbia University Medical Center
New York, NY, USA

E-mail address:
slichtiger10@aol.com

The Microbiota and the Immune Response: What Is the Chicken and What Is the Egg?

Julia Fritsch, BS[a], Maria T. Abreu, MD[b],*

KEYWORDS

- Intestinal inflammation • Colitis • Bacterial translocation • Host-microbe interactions
- Crohn's disease • Ulcerative colitis • Innate immunity • Dysbiosis

KEY POINTS

- Although dysbiosis, or an imbalance in the microbiota, has been associated with inflammatory bowel disease, it is not known whether dysbiosis is a cause or consequence of inflammation.
- In patients with inflammatory bowel disease, dysbiosis is associated with a dysregulated immune response, a decrease in antiinflammatory bacteria, and an increase in proinflammatory bacteria.
- Because dysbiosis was found in the stool of newly diagnosed treatment-naïve patients, dysbiosis is at least an early event in inflammation.

Continued

Disclosure Statement: We have read the journal's policy and the authors of this article have the following competing interests: M.T. Abreu has served as a consultant to Prometheus Laboratories, Takeda, UCB Inc., Pfizer, Janssen, Focus Medical Communications and Eli Lilly Pharmaceuticals. M.T. Abreu serves as trainer or lecturer for CME Outfitters and Imedex, Inc. M.T. Abreu serves on the scientific advisory board of AbbVie Laboratories, Celgene Corporation, Shire Pharmaceuticals, Roche Pharmaceuticals, Boehringer Ingelheim Pharmaceuticals, AMGEN, Allergan, SERES, Nestle Health Science, and GILEAD, and on the board of directors for the GI Health Foundation. This does not alter the authors' adherence to the journal's policies on sharing data and materials. All other authors declare no conflict of interest.
This work was supported by grants from the National Institute of Health, National Institute of Diabetes and Digestive and Kidney Diseases R01DK099076, R01DK104844 and T32DK11678; Crohn's and Colitis Foundation Award IBD-0389R; Florida Academic Cancer Center Alliance (FACCA) Award; Pfizer ASPIRE Award; and Takeda Pharmaceuticals Investigator Initiated Research (IIR) Award. Additional funding was provided by The Micky & Madeleine Arison Family Foundation Crohn's & Colitis Discovery Laboratory and Martin Kalser Chair.

[a] Microbiology and Immunology, Center for Crohn's and Colitis, University of Miami Miller School of Medicine, 1011 North West 15th Street (D-149), Gautier Building, Suite 537B, Miami, FL USA; [b] Department of Medicine, Division of Gastroenterology, Crohn's & Colitis Center, University of Miami Miller School of Medicine, 1011 North West 15th Street (D-149), Gautier Building, Suite 510, Miami, FL USA
* Corresponding author.
E-mail address: Mabreu1@med.miami.edu

Gastrointest Endoscopy Clin N Am 29 (2019) 381–393
https://doi.org/10.1016/j.giec.2019.02.005
1052-5157/19/© 2019 Elsevier Inc. All rights reserved.

Continued

- Dysbiosis improves with the reduction of inflammation after anti-tumor necrosis factor or elemental nutritional treatment, suggesting that dysbiosis is a consequence of inflammation.
- Inflammatory bowel disease is more dynamic than just cause and effect; therapies need to target the microbiota and specific characteristics of mucosal immune response.

INTRODUCTION

The mammalian gut is host to 10 to 100 trillion microorganisms, such as bacteria, viruses, yeast, and archaea, that are collectively known as the microbiota. Comprising a 1:1 ratio of human cells to microbial cells, many of these species actually benefit the host.[1] Microbial antigens, which constantly stimulate the intestinal immune system, are compartmentalized from the host by mucus layers and a monolayer of intestinal epithelial cells (**Fig. 1**).

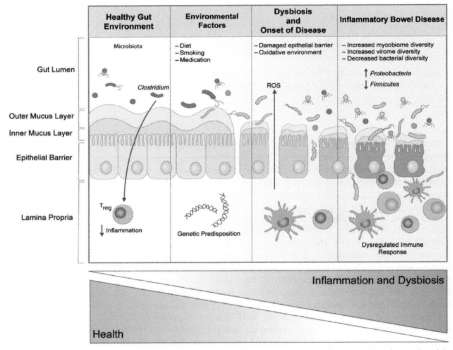

Fig. 1. The microbiota and immune response in inflammatory bowel disease (IBD). In a healthy gut environment, the microbial species are compartmentalized from the host by 2 mucus layers and a monolayer of epithelial cells. The host relies on the microbiota for a variety of important functions, including the induction of T regulatory cells by *Clostridial* species through the generation of short chain fatty acids. Intestinal homeostasis depends on intestinal permeability and bacterial penetration. A disruption of this homeostasis by genetic risk or environmental factors can trigger dysbiosis, inflammation, and an oxidative environment from reactive oxygen species (ROS). The dysregulated immune response further exacerbates intestinal permeability, inflammation and dysbiosis creating a vicious cycle eventually leading to IBD. This results in a decrease in bacterial diversity and an increase in mycobiome/virome diversity.

These intestinal epithelial cells play an important role in regulating intestinal homeostasis because they maintain tolerance to commensal bacteria while still retaining the capability to respond to pathogenic bacteria.[2] The complex interaction of the microbe–host symbiotic relationship is mediated by the recognition of microbial signals via pattern recognition receptors that allows the microbes to communicate with the host.[3] Intestinal homeostasis depends on limiting the amount of bacterial penetration through the epithelial barrier. Innate immune strategies, such as the production of mucus or antimicrobial peptides, are used to prevent the colonization and penetration of bacteria in intestinal epithelial cells.

It is impossible to create a standard "healthy" microbiota because of the high degree of interindividual difference in the microbial community at the species level, likely owing to environmental factors.[4] However, individuals do share a core microbiome at the gene and functional levels.[5,6] These shared set of microbial genes are necessary for host physiologic processes, such as vitamin biosynthesis (vitamins B and K), degradation of xenobiotics, fermentation of indigestible carbohydrates into short chain fatty acids (SCFAs), production of metabolites, immune development, and regulating intestinal homeostasis.[6,7] Indeed, *Clostridial* species caused an induction of T regulatory cells in the colon, potentially by producing the SCFA butyrate, and the supplementation of this bacteria actually caused resistance to colitis in mice.[8] Furthermore, patients with inflammatory bowel disease (IBD) had a decrease in SCFA-producing bacteria (*Firmicutes*) with a decreased concentration of SCFA in the feces.[9,10] These findings support the notion that the microbiota may contribute to health, because the host relies on the microbiota for a variety of important functions. In fact, numerous inflammatory pathologies, such as IBD, obesity, and type 1 diabetes, have been associated with an imbalance of the microbiota, suggesting a link between the microbial community, inflammation, and etiology.[11–15] However, it is unclear if this imbalance of the microbiota, or dysbiosis, is the cause of inflammatory disease, such as IBD, or the consequence of an immune dysfunction that simply exacerbates the disease. It is unclear which comes first, dysbiosis or inflammation.

Studies are ongoing to try and clarify the chicken and egg phenomenon. The Genetic Environmental Microbial (GEM) cohort is a multinational longitudinal study in which first-degree, unaffected relatives of patients with Crohn's disease (CD) are being followed over time for the development of CD. There are some preliminary data that age, gender, genetic polymorphisms, and environmental factors were associated with alterations of the gut microbiota.[16,17] As this cohort matures and unaffected people develop CD, it will be possible to have a sense of whether the dysbiosis preceded the onset of inflammation.

MODIFICATION OF THE MICROBIOME

To understand the order in which dysbiosis and inflammation occurs in IBD, it is crucial to analyze the factors that contribute to the development and maintenance of dysbiosis. The innate and adaptive immune system regulate the microbiota by producing antimicrobial peptides and IgA antibodies after microbial antigens bind to pattern recognition receptors, such as toll-like receptors (TLRs) and NOD-like receptors. Endogenous factors, such as genetic susceptibility, or exogenous factors, such as diet, stress, or medication, have the potential to significantly alter the microbiome.[12,18–22] In fact, environmental risk factors of IBD are also known to cause microbial changes, such as mode of birth, breastfeeding, smoking, infections, antibiotics, diet, stress, hygiene, and sleep patterns, suggesting a link between the microbiome and IBD.[22–27] A transition from a steady microbial state to a dysbiotic state requires extensive environmental and host-related stimuli that eventually lead to an instability in the host–microbe interaction.[28] When this chronic dysbiotic state persists and does not return to the previous state, the host response might become detrimental, contributing to disease.

DYSBIOSIS IN INFLAMMATORY BOWEL DISEASE

Dysbiosis is an alteration in the microbial community that causes an imbalance in the homeostasis of the microbiota, subsequently initiating or propagating disease.[29,30] Indeed, many studies have documented that patients with IBD have a decrease in biodiversity, also called alpha-diversity, and a change in the relative abundance of specific bacterial taxa compared with healthy individuals. Currently, the majority of microbiome studies have focused on stool microbiota owing to the ease of collection. However, accumulating evidence suggests that rectal mucosa-associated microbiota from biopsies may better reflect regional changes in the gut and is a robust predictor of disease.[13,31] Patients with IBD are characterized by changes in the global microbial composition as well as an expansion of potential pathobionts, or commensal microbes that have the potential to act as a pathogenic bacteria and cause disease only under specific conditions.[32] For example, patients with IBD typically have a reduction in abundance of *Firmicutes*, particularly *Faecalibacterium prausnitzii*, and an increase in Proteobacteria.[33–36] In fact, a decreased abundance of *F prausnitzii* correlated with relapse after infliximab withdrawal. Interestingly, CD-associated dysbiosis correlated with the time to relapse after the withdrawal of infliximab, implicating the potential use of bacteria for a predictive marker for relapse.[37] In general, IBD is associated with a decrease in antiinflammatory bacteria and an increase in proinflammatory bacteria compared with healthy individuals (**Table 1**).[38] Dysbiosis in IBD, specifically CD, frequently features an overgrowth of pathobionts, such as the bloom of Enterobacteriaceae (*Escherichia coli* or *Fusobacterium*) or *Mycobacterium paratuberculosis*.[30,39] These expansions in pathobionts have been associated with pathogenesis in patients with CD, but a causal role for a single microbe or microbial milieu has not been identified in humans.[40,41] Although the majority of microbial research has focused on bacterial species, it is important to note that the diversity of the mycobiome (fungal species) and virome (viruses) are significantly increased in patients with CD compared with their first-degree relatives.[42–44] Indeed, it is conceivable that the increase in enteric bacteriophages may contribute to the depletion of the bacterial

Table 1	
IBD is associated with a decrease in anti-inflammatory bacteria and an increase in pro-inflammatory bacteria compared with healthy subjects	
Microbes Decreased in IBD	**Microbes Increased in IBD**
Actinomycetaceae[56]	*Clostridium difficile*[12]
Bacteroidales[12]	Enterobacteriaceae[12]
Bifidobacteriaceae[12]	*Escherichia coli*[41]
Clostridiales[12]	Fusobacteriaceae[12]
Erysipelotrichales[12]	*Mycobacterium avium*[12]
Faecalibacterium[56]	Pasteurellaceae[12]
Firmicutes[56]	Proteobacteria[56]
Roseburia[56]	*Ruminococcus gnavus*[41]
	Serratia marcescens[41]
	Veillonellaceae[12]

microbiota. Therefore, future studies need to also focus on the other microorganisms of the microbiota.

DYSBIOSIS CAUSES INFLAMMATION

To elucidate whether dysbiosis is a cause or consequence of etiology, the pediatric RISK Stratification Study (RISK), which includes pediatric patients with new onset of CD, attempted to address the timing of dysbiosis compared with disease onset.[13] Because dysbiosis was found in stool of newly diagnosed treatment-naive patients, it suggests that dysbiosis is at least coincident with early inflammation.[13,45] It has been shown that ileal exposure to fecal matter after ileal resection in patients with CD triggers an inflammatory response that resembles that of CD.[46] Although this finding provides evidence that bacteria can initiate inflammation in patients with CD, the question of precedence remains to be elucidated. A prospective cohort study investigated the impact of dysbiosis in CD relapse and demonstrated that CD-associated dysbiosis present at baseline was associated with the onset of gut inflammation. Potentially, the loss of antiinflammatory bacteria, such as F prausnitzii, as well as the increase in proinflammatory bacteria, such as E coli, could actually cause inflammation.[37]

However, it is important to note that even though clinical studies have found an association between the microbiome and disease, they have not been able to show causation. Currently, the only possibility to explore the potential causal role of microbiota is to use fecal microbial transplant (FMT) in germ-free mice. IL-2– and IL-10–deficient mice that are prone to develop colitis are protected if raised in germ-free conditions, supporting the notion that the microbiota is required to trigger inflammation.[47] Similarly, mice that do not express both IL-10, an antiinflammatory cytokine, and MyD88, an adaptor protein for TLR4, are also protected from IBD. Because the bacteria are no longer able to signal through the TLR–MyD88 receptor, they are unable to cause colitis, indicating that the microbiota is critical in IBD pathogenesis.[48] These data imply that bacteria are essential for the etiology of IBD in mice. Indeed, the susceptibility to IBD is transmissible through the stool microbiota, demonstrating the existence of disease-associated microbiota. For example, mice that constitutively express TLR4 and are, therefore, more prone to colitis, are able to transmit colitis susceptibility to wild-type mice by cohousing.[49] Furthermore, it has been demonstrated that, once certain conditions are present, such as an altered immune response, the microbiota causes IBD. More specifically, germ-free colitis susceptible mice (IL-10 deficient) and germ-free wild-type mice were colonized with stool from patients with CD and ulcerative colitis (UC). Interestingly, whereas the microbiota isolated from patients with CD-induced colitis in IBD-prone mice activated downstream proinflammatory genes, microbiota isolated from patients with UC did not trigger colitis, even if the mice had a predisposition.[50] It remains unclear why the microbiota from patients with CD and not patients with UC cause colitis. However, these data indicate that CD-associated dysbiosis is transmissible only in IBD-prone mice, implying that dysbiosis is the cause of inflammation only when there are additional host factors. The observation that the microbiome of UC alone could not transmit inflammation, even in genetically susceptible mice, suggests that there are additional factors that may include diet and environment and cannot be reproduced with microbiota alone. These data demonstrate that dysbiosis is not simply a consequence of intestinal inflammation, but can trigger inflammation in a susceptible host. Even in mouse models, the transfer of microbiota from patients with IBD to a normal germ-free mouse does not by itself trigger colitis or ileitis. All of these observations suggest that the microbiome alone, without endogenous host factors, is unlikely to cause IBD. However, the increasing prevalence of IBD globally parallels the industrialization of diet, hygiene, and lifestyle practices,[51] providing evidence that the microbiota initiates the onset of IBD in susceptible humans. As we learn more, these risks should be modifiable.

INFLAMMATION CAUSES DYSBIOSIS

Given the close interaction between the host, microbial antigens, and the environment in the gut, the intestinal epithelial barrier is very susceptible to environmental toxins, and immune activation can easily take place if not properly regulated. The onset of IBD is believed to occur when the homeostasis between the microbiota and intestinal epithelial immune cells are disrupted by genetic and environmental factors, such as diet, stress, and medication. This disruption results in a dysregulated immune response, further exacerbating intestinal permeability and dysbiosis and creating a positive feedback loop. This impaired compartmentalization of the bacteria from the host and loss of intestinal homeostasis cause an overactive immune response in the intestine, which eventually leads to chronic and relapsing inflammation, or IBD.[52–56] Although the microbial diversity varies throughout different regions of the digestive tract, the microbial diversity is relatively uniform throughout the colon.[57] However, in patients with CD there is a decreased biodiversity in the inflamed mucosa compared with the noninflamed mucosa within the same patient, implying that there is an interaction between inflammation and microbial diversity.[58]

An individual's genotype, particularly defects in the innate immune system, is believed to contribute to susceptibility of IBD by causing a disruption in microbe–host homeostasis.[59] In fact, genome-wide association studies analyzing the genetic risk factors for IBD revealed genetic polymorphisms in the pathways for innate immunity, adaptive immune responses, pathogen sensing, maintenance of intestinal epithelial barrier, and response to oxidative stress (glutathione and sulfate transport).[60] For example, NOD2, a gene that mediates the production of antimicrobial peptides, was the first gene identified to increase susceptibility to developing CD.[61] It has also been shown that patients with NOD2 mutations have decreased IL-10. Indeed, IL-10 receptor mutations have been associated with early-onset IBD, and it is also used in mice for a spontaneous model of colitis.[62] Since then, other pattern recognition receptors (ie, NLRP3; TLR1, 2, 4, 6, and 9) have been implicated with the pathogenesis of IBD.[49,63–65] Experimental models of colitis in mice further demonstrated that an abnormal epithelial innate immune response via TLRs, particularly TLR4, were involved in the pathogenesis of colitis, which provides additional support for the link between inflammation, the microbiota, and IBD.[49] Another gene implicated in the pathogenesis of CD is ATG16L1, an autophagy gene that controls the immune response to viruses and bacteria.[66] In fact, the GEM Project linked genetic risk factors associated with dysregulated immune response to the gut microbiota in the pathogenesis of IBD.

Most compellingly, the extent of dysbiosis diminishes with a reduction in inflammation after treatment with anti-tumor necrosis factor or exclusive enteral nutrition.[43] This study also found that the microbiota of patients with CD only became more similar to healthy controls if they were responders to anti-tumor necrosis factor and exclusive enteral nutrition, indicating that dysbiosis is a consequence of inflammation. Furthermore, healthy individuals with high genetic risk variants associated with IBD also have unfavorable alterations in their microbiota, yet they do not have the disease.[59] This finding implies that genetic IBD risk of the gut immune system provides the right environment for the microbiota to unfavorably change.[59] This oxidative environment created by the host selects for and exacerbates dysbiosis. In a healthy individual, an oxygen gradient in the colon exists that selects for a greater abundance of Proteobacteria at high oxygen levels.[67] A disruption in the intestinal epithelial barrier as well as increased inflammation causes more intraluminal oxygen, which leads to an outgrowth of Proteobacteria.[68] Furthermore, facultative anaerobes, such as Enterobacteriaceae, use compounds released during intestinal inflammation as terminal electron acceptors to promote their growth.[68] Inflammation releases more oxygen and compounds that create an oxidative environment that promotes the outgrowth of dysbiotic species. In fact, some aerobic bacteria, such as *Salmonella*, actually create and use an oxidative environment for their survival advantage by depleting *Clostridia* to increase epithelial oxygen levels.[69]

WHICH CAME FIRST, DYSBIOSIS OR INFLAMMATION?

Studies have attempted to elucidate the cause–effect relationship between the microbiota and inflammation in the development of IBD. It remains unclear whether dysbiosis precedes the onset of IBD, causing the dysregulated immune response, or dysbiosis merely reflects the oxidative environment altered by inflammation. Ultimately, a deeper understanding of the mechanism of how microbiota and dysbiosis impact the host is needed to be able to elucidate which factor precedes the other. Furthermore, it is difficult to clarify causation or correlation, because the timing of dysbiosis is difficult to determine in humans. Given the research, it is possible that genetic (also epigenetic) changes in the intestinal immune system create an environment for a more proinflammatory microbiota, increasing susceptibility to IBD. Subsequent microbial alterations owing to secondary environmental triggers could further disrupt the microbe–immune intestinal homeostasis, creating a vicious cycle that eventually leads to IBD (**Fig. 2**). This scenario is most supported by the fact that, in healthy individuals, genetic risk variants associated with IBD altered the gut microbiota.[59] Furthermore, the nature of dysbiosis and how the microbiota behaves is unique to each environmental stressor, as demonstrated by the various metabolic modifications of microbiota in response to intestinal environmental stressors.[43] The pathogenesis of IBD is a complex interplay of genetic risk, environmental factors, inflammation, and the microbiome. Therefore, the relationship between dysbiosis and inflammation in IBD is more dynamic than just cause and effect, the chicken or the egg.

CURRENT AND POTENTIAL FUTURE THERAPIES TO TREAT INFLAMMATORY BOWEL DISEASE

Although it may not be fully elucidated if in fact dysbiosis precedes inflammation, it is well-studied that alterations in the microbiota further exacerbate IBD. Therefore, to obtain the most successful clinical response, it is important to address every factor, both microbial and inflammatory, that contributes to IBD to fully achieve remission. Initially, antibiotics were used in the management of UC, stemming from the observation that germ-free colitis models developed less inflammation compared with conventional mice.[47] However, it is now known that antibiotic use is associated with CD and actually amplifies CD-associated dysbiosis in new-onset CD.[13,43] Antibiotics are also a common trigger for flares of UC, likely because they further decrease diversity.[70] Instead of eliminating all bacteria, clinical trials have switched to amplifying the microbial diversity. For example, prebiotics, which are nondigestible food components that change the composition and activity of intestinal microflora, have been used in clinical trials in an attempt to augment the growth of bacteria by providing a microbial energy source. In a small UC clinical trial, the use of a prebiotic, inulin, did

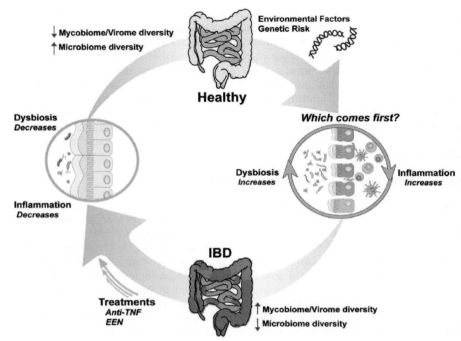

Fig. 2. The cycle of dysbiosis and the immune response. In response to environmental factors, a healthy individual with genetic predispositions, such as NOD2, IL-10R, or ATG16L1 mutations, could either develop dysbiosis or inflammation; however, which comes first remains unclear. The RISK study found dysbiosis in newly diagnosed patients suggesting it is at least coincident with early inflammation. However, dysbiosis was also found in healthy individuals with genetic risk for IBD, suggesting that dysbiosis does not cause inflammation. Once the positive feedback loop of dysbiosis and inflammation begins, overt IBD develops. After treatment with anti-tumor necrosis factor (TNF) or elemental nutrition, inflammation decreases followed by a decrease in dysbiosis, returning to an intestinal homeostasis once again. EEN, exclusive enteral nutrition.

not enhance remission, but it did decrease fecal calprotectin.[71] Furthermore, clinical trials have tested the effects of probiotic interventions including *Lactobacillus* strains (*rhamnosus GG, acidophilus, reuteri* ATCC 55730), *Bifidobacterium* strains (*breve, bifidum, animalis*), *Saccharomyces boulardii, E coli* Nissle 1917, and VSL#3 (*probiotic mix of 4 lactobacilli, 3 bifidobacteria and 1 streptococcus*).[72] Even though the *E coli* Nissle 1917 strain was equivalent to the effectiveness of low-dose mesalamine, an antiinflammatory drug used in IBD treatment, it did not provide complete remission.[73] Furthermore, treatment with VSL#3 was reported effective in causing remission of active UC; however, the sample size was too small, so it could not be recommended as a potential clinical treatment.[74] A metaanalysis of 4 randomized, controlled probiotic trials concluded that conventional therapy with probiotic treatment does not improve overall remission rates in patients with UC. However, a new clinical trial that incorporates both antibiotics to create an ecological niche as well as probiotics (SER-287) to recolonize the gut microbiota has provided promising results in UC. SER-287 consists of purified Firmicute bacterial spores. This study successfully created an ecological niche that cleared the way for reseeding and better engraftment of healthy microbiota with pretreatment by antibiotics. Furthermore, the probiotic

SER-287 obtained a 40% remission rate compared with placebo in a phase Ib trial.[75] Likewise, dietary interventions have attempted to mitigate dysbiosis in IBD, but they have been tried in UC with mixed results. A recent study that used questionnaires to assess the intake of dietary fiber found that patients with CD who consumed high-fiber foods were less likely to have a flare compared with those who did not consume high-fiber foods; however, there was no association between fiber intake and flares in patients with UC.[76,77] Therefore, the current approach of simply altering the microbiota in hopes to achieve a clinical remission have not proven to be sufficient.

Given the detrimental consequences of dysbiosis, therapies have attempted to immediately reconstitute the microbiota by transplanting the microbiota of a healthy donor into patients with IBD. The success of FMT to reverse *Clostridium difficile* gave rise to other clinical trials attempting to treat dysbiosis in other diseases, including IBD. Although FMTs have been successful in mice, clinical trials have a more varied response. Overall, FMT demonstrates the support for a microbiome-based approach in UC; 28% of the donor FMT group achieved clinical remission compared with only 9% in placebo group in the 4 major randomized, controlled trials of FMT.[78] However, FMT does not always have a high success rate, as was the case for patients with CD.[79,80] In fact, another study showed that FMT caused a transient flare-up in patients with UC.[81] More research and clinical trials need to be conducted to determine the duration of treatment, optimum dose, and route of delivery. Furthermore, because dysbiosis has been associated with many disorders, including obesity and depression, it will be necessary to screen the donor pool to avoid any damaging effects from the donor.

SUMMARY

As demonstrated by animal studies, epidemiologic studies, and clinical trials, it is evident that dysbiosis plays a key role in IBD, either in the onset or progression of disease or both. because dysbiosis and inflammation create a vicious feedback loop, IBD therapies need to target both inflammation and the microbiota, not one or the other. Therefore, to successfully force the microbiome back to a healthy steady state and achieve remission of IBD, a multipronged approach that incorporates both reduction of inflammation and restoration of microbiome is necessary. Ideally, personalized approaches that involve an analysis of the microbiota alongside specific characteristics of the mucosal immune response will guide our future therapies.

ACKNOWLEDGMENTS

The authors thank Natasha Kobinger-Wessel for her help preparing the images.

REFERENCES

1. Sender R, Fuchs S, Milo R. Revised estimates for the number of human and bacteria cells in the body. PLoS Biol 2016;14(8):e1002533.
2. Ignacio A, Morales CI, Camara NO, et al. Innate sensing of the gut microbiota: modulation of inflammatory and autoimmune diseases. Front Immunol 2016;7:54.
3. Mogensen TH. Pathogen recognition and inflammatory signaling in innate immune defenses. Clin Microbiol Rev 2009;22(2):240–73. Table of Contents.
4. Structure, function and diversity of the healthy human microbiome. Nature 2012; 486(7402):207–14.
5. Turnbaugh PJ, Hamady M, Yatsunenko T, et al. A core gut microbiome in obese and lean twins. Nature 2009;457(7228):480–4.

6. Qin J, Li R, Raes J, et al. A human gut microbial gene catalogue established by metagenomic sequencing. Nature 2010;464(7285):59–65.
7. Haller D, Bode C, Hammes WP, et al. Non-pathogenic bacteria elicit a differential cytokine response by intestinal epithelial cell/leucocyte co-cultures. Gut 2000; 47(1):79–87.
8. Atarashi K, Tanoue T, Shima T, et al. Induction of colonic regulatory T cells by indigenous Clostridium species. Science 2011;331(6015):337–41.
9. Goncalves P, Araujo JR, Di Santo JP. A cross-talk between microbiota-derived short-chain fatty acids and the host mucosal immune system regulates intestinal homeostasis and inflammatory bowel disease. Inflamm Bowel Dis 2018;24(3): 558–72.
10. Furusawa Y, Obata Y, Fukuda S, et al. Commensal microbe-derived butyrate induces the differentiation of colonic regulatory T cells. Nature 2013;504(7480): 446–50.
11. Swidsinski A, Loening-Baucke V, Verstraelen H, et al. Biostructure of fecal microbiota in healthy subjects and patients with chronic idiopathic diarrhea. Gastroenterology 2008;135(2):568–79.
12. Collins SM. A role for the gut microbiota in IBS. Nat Rev Gastroenterol Hepatol 2014;11(8):497–505.
13. Gevers D, Kugathasan S, Denson LA, et al. The treatment-naive microbiome in new-onset Crohn's disease. Cell Host Microbe 2014;15(3):382–92.
14. Le Chatelier E, Nielsen T, Qin J, et al. Richness of human gut microbiome correlates with metabolic markers. Nature 2013;500(7464):541–6.
15. Kostic AD, Gevers D, Siljander H, et al. The dynamics of the human infant gut microbiome in development and in progression toward type 1 diabetes. Cell Host microbe 2015;17(2):260–73.
16. Turpin W, Espin-Garcia O, Xu W, et al. Association of host genome with intestinal microbial composition in a large healthy cohort. Nat Genet 2016;48(11):1413–7.
17. Turpin W. Association of Environmental Exposures With the Composition and Diversity of the Human Gut Microbiome in Healthy First Degree Relatives (FDR) of Crohn's Patients. Gastroenterology 2016;150(4, Suppl 1):S21–2 [abstract no: 86].
18. Keeney KM, Yurist-Doutsch S, Arrieta MC, et al. Effects of antibiotics on human microbiota and subsequent disease. Annu Rev Microbiol 2014;68:217–35.
19. Vangay P, Ward T, Gerber JS, et al. Antibiotics, pediatric dysbiosis, and disease. Cell Host Microbe 2015;17(5):553–64.
20. Syer SD, Wallace JL. Environmental and NSAID-enteropathy: dysbiosis as a common factor. Curr Gastroenterol Rep 2014;16(3):377.
21. Day AS, Lopez RN. Exclusive enteral nutrition in children with Crohn's disease. World J Gastroenterol 2015;21(22):6809–16.
22. Ananthakrishnan AN. Epidemiology and risk factors for IBD. Nat Rev Gastroenterol Hepatol 2015;12(4):205–17.
23. Kaplan GG, Ng SC. Understanding and preventing the global increase of inflammatory bowel disease. Gastroenterology 2017;152(2):313–21.e2.
24. Jost T, Lacroix C, Braegger CP, et al. Vertical mother-neonate transfer of maternal gut bacteria via breastfeeding. Environ Microbiol 2014;16(9):2891–904.
25. Thaiss CA, Zeevi D, Levy M, et al. Transkingdom control of microbiota diurnal oscillations promotes metabolic homeostasis. Cell 2014;159(3):514–29.
26. David LA, Maurice CF, Carmody RN, et al. Diet rapidly and reproducibly alters the human gut microbiome. Nature 2014;505(7484):559–63.

27. Higuchi LM, Khalili H, Chan AT, et al. A prospective study of cigarette smoking and the risk of inflammatory bowel disease in women. Am J Gastroenterol 2012;107(9):1399–406.
28. Levy M, Kolodziejczyk AA, Thaiss CA, et al. Dysbiosis and the immune system. Nat Rev Immunol 2017;17(4):219–32.
29. Tamboli CP, Neut C, Desreumaux P, et al. Dysbiosis in inflammatory bowel disease. Gut 2004;53(1):1–4.
30. Frank DN, St Amand AL, Feldman RA, et al. Molecular-phylogenetic characterization of microbial community imbalances in human inflammatory bowel diseases. Proc Natl Acad Sci U S A 2007;104(34):13780–5.
31. Eckburg PB, Bik EM, Bernstein CN, et al. Diversity of the human intestinal microbial flora. Science 2005;308(5728):1635–8.
32. Chow J, Tang H, Mazmanian SK. Pathobionts of the gastrointestinal microbiota and inflammatory disease. Curr Opin Immunol 2011;23(4):473–80.
33. Manichanh C, Rigottier-Gois L, Bonnaud E, et al. Reduced diversity of faecal microbiota in Crohn's disease revealed by a metagenomic approach. Gut 2006; 55(2):205–11.
34. Kang S, Denman SE, Morrison M, et al. Dysbiosis of fecal microbiota in Crohn's disease patients as revealed by a custom phylogenetic microarray. Inflamm Bowel Dis 2010;16(12):2034–42.
35. Sokol H, Pigneur B, Watterlot L, et al. Faecalibacterium prausnitzii is an anti-inflammatory commensal bacterium identified by gut microbiota analysis of Crohn disease patients. Proc Natl Acad Sci U S A 2008;105(43):16731–6.
36. Seksik P, Rigottier-Gois L, Gramet G, et al. Alterations of the dominant faecal bacterial groups in patients with Crohn's disease of the colon. Gut 2003;52(2): 237–42.
37. Rajca S, Grondin V, Louis E, et al. Alterations in the intestinal microbiome (dysbiosis) as a predictor of relapse after infliximab withdrawal in Crohn's disease. Inflamm Bowel Dis 2014;20(6):978–86.
38. Plaza-Diaz J, Ruiz-Ojeda FJ, Vilchez-Padial LM, et al. Evidence of the anti-inflammatory effects of probiotics and synbiotics in intestinal Chronic diseases. Nutrients 2017;9(6) [pii:E555].
39. Bernstein CN, Blanchard JF, Rawsthorne P, et al. Population-based case control study of seroprevalence of Mycobacterium paratuberculosis in patients with Crohn's disease and ulcerative colitis. J Clin Microbiol 2004;42(3):1129–35.
40. Hermon-Taylor J, Bull TJ, Sheridan JM, et al. Causation of Crohn's disease by Mycobacterium avium subspecies paratuberculosis. Can J Gastroenterol 2000; 14(6):521–39.
41. Naser SA, Sagramsingh SR, Naser AS, et al. Mycobacterium avium subspecies paratuberculosis causes Crohn's disease in some inflammatory bowel disease patients. World J Gastroenterol 2014;20(23):7403–15.
42. Hoarau G, Mukherjee PK, Gower-Rousseau C, et al. Bacteriome and mycobiome interactions underscore microbial dysbiosis in familial Crohn's disease. MBio 2016;7(5) [pii:e01250-16].
43. Lewis JD, Chen EZ, Baldassano RN, et al. Inflammation, antibiotics, and diet as environmental stressors of the gut microbiome in pediatric Crohn's disease. Cell Host Microbe 2015;18(4):489–500.
44. Li Q, Wang C, Tang C, et al. Dysbiosis of gut fungal microbiota is associated with mucosal inflammation in Crohn's disease. J Clin Gastroenterol 2014;48(6): 513–23.

45. Haberman Y, Tickle TL, Dexheimer PJ, et al. Pediatric Crohn disease patients exhibit specific ileal transcriptome and microbiome signature. J Clin Invest 2014;124(8):3617–33.
46. D'Haens GR, Geboes K, Peeters M, et al. Early lesions of recurrent Crohn's disease caused by infusion of intestinal contents in excluded ileum. Gastroenterology 1998;114(2):262–7.
47. Sellon RK, Tonkonogy S, Schultz M, et al. Resident enteric bacteria are necessary for development of spontaneous colitis and immune system activation in interleukin-10-deficient mice. Infect Immun 1998;66(11):5224–31.
48. Rakoff-Nahoum S, Hao L, Medzhitov R. Role of toll-like receptors in spontaneous commensal-dependent colitis. Immunity 2006;25(2):319–29.
49. Dheer R, Santaolalla R, Davies JM, et al. Intestinal epithelial toll-like receptor 4 signaling affects epithelial function and colonic microbiota and promotes a risk for transmissible colitis. Infect Immun 2016;84(3):798–810.
50. Nagao-Kitamoto H, Shreiner AB, Gillilland MG 3rd, et al. Functional characterization of inflammatory bowel disease-associated gut dysbiosis in gnotobiotic mice. Cell Mol Gastroenterol Hepatol 2016;2(4):468–81.
51. Molodecky NA, Soon IS, Rabi DM, et al. Increasing incidence and prevalence of the inflammatory bowel diseases with time, based on systematic review. Gastroenterology 2012;142(1):46–54.e42 [quiz: e30].
52. Bouma G, Strober W. The immunological and genetic basis of inflammatory bowel disease. Nat Rev Immunol 2003;3(7):521–33.
53. Mowat AM. Anatomical basis of tolerance and immunity to intestinal antigens. Nat Rev Immunol 2003;3(4):331–41.
54. Allez M, Mayer L. Regulatory T cells: peace keepers in the gut. Inflamm Bowel Dis 2004;10(5):666–76.
55. Sartor RB. Microbial influences in inflammatory bowel diseases. Gastroenterology 2008;134(2):577–94.
56. Asquith M, Powrie F. An innately dangerous balancing act: intestinal homeostasis, inflammation, and colitis-associated cancer. J Exp Med 2010;207(8):1573–7.
57. Hillman ET, Lu H, Yao T, et al. Microbial ecology along the gastrointestinal tract. Microbes Environ 2017;32(4):300–13.
58. Sepehri S, Kotlowski R, Bernstein CN, et al. Microbial diversity of inflamed and noninflamed gut biopsy tissues in inflammatory bowel disease. Inflamm Bowel Dis 2007;13(6):675–83.
59. Imhann F, Vich Vila A, Bonder MJ, et al. Interplay of host genetics and gut microbiota underlying the onset and clinical presentation of inflammatory bowel disease. Gut 2018;67(1):108–19.
60. Jostins L, Ripke S, Weersma RK, et al. Host-microbe interactions have shaped the genetic architecture of inflammatory bowel disease. Nature 2012;491(7422):119–24.
61. Ogura Y, Bonen DK, Inohara N, et al. A frameshift mutation in NOD2 associated with susceptibility to Crohn's disease. Nature 2001;411(6837):603–6.
62. Franke A, McGovern DP, Barrett JC, et al. Genome-wide meta-analysis increases to 71 the number of confirmed Crohn's disease susceptibility loci. Nat Genet 2010;42(12):1118–25.
63. Hugot JP, Chamaillard M, Zouali H, et al. Association of NOD2 leucine-rich repeat variants with susceptibility to Crohn's disease. Nature 2001;411(6837):599–603.
64. Pierik M, Joossens S, Van Steen K, et al. Toll-like receptor-1, -2, and -6 polymorphisms influence disease extension in inflammatory bowel diseases. Inflamm Bowel Dis 2006;12(1):1–8.

65. Torok HP, Glas J, Tonenchi L, et al. Crohn's disease is associated with a toll-like receptor-9 polymorphism. Gastroenterology 2004;127(1):365–6.
66. Kuballa P, Huett A, Rioux JD, et al. Impaired autophagy of an intracellular pathogen induced by a Crohn's disease associated ATG16L1 variant. PLoS One 2008;3(10):e3391.
67. Albenberg L, Esipova TV, Judge CP, et al. Correlation between intraluminal oxygen gradient and radial partitioning of intestinal microbiota. Gastroenterology 2014;147(5):1055–63.e8.
68. Winter SE, Baumler AJ. Dysbiosis in the inflamed intestine: chance favors the prepared microbe. Gut Microbes 2014;5(1):71–3.
69. Rivera-Chavez F, Zhang LF, Faber F, et al. Depletion of butyrate-producing clostridia from the gut microbiota drives an aerobic luminal expansion of salmonella. Cell Host Microbe 2016;19(4):443–54.
70. Logan RF. Antibiotics and flare of inflammatory bowel disease: threat or therapy? Nat Clin Pract Gastroenterol Hepatol 2005;2(10):446–7.
71. Casellas F, Borruel N, Torrejon A, et al. Oral oligofructose-enriched inulin supplementation in acute ulcerative colitis is well tolerated and associated with lowered faecal calprotectin. Aliment Pharmacol Ther 2007;25(9):1061–7.
72. Jonkers D, Stockbrugger R. Probiotics and inflammatory bowel disease. J R Soc Med 2003;96(4):167–71.
73. Losurdo G, Iannone A, Contaldo A, et al. Escherichia coli nissle 1917 in ulcerative colitis treatment: systematic review and meta-analysis. J Gastrointestin Liver Dis 2015;24(4):499–505.
74. Derwa Y, Gracie DJ, Hamlin PJ, et al. Systematic review with meta-analysis: the efficacy of probiotics in inflammatory bowel disease. Aliment Pharmacol Ther 2017;46(4):389–400.
75. Bharat M, Curran J, Herfarth HH, et al. SER-287, an Investigational Microbiome Therapeutic, Induces Remission and Endoscopic Improvement in a Placebo-Controlled, Double-Blind Randomized Trial in Patients with Active Mild-to-Moderate Ulcerative Colitis. Gastroenterology 2018;154(6S1): S–25.
76. Ananthakrishnan AN, Khalili H, Konijeti GG, et al. A prospective study of long-term intake of dietary fiber and risk of Crohn's disease and ulcerative colitis. Gastroenterology 2013;145(5):970–7.
77. McGill CR, Fulgoni VL 3rd, Devareddy L. Ten-year trends in fiber and whole grain intakes and food sources for the United States population: National Health and Nutrition Examination Survey 2001-2010. Nutrients 2015;7(2):1119–30.
78. Costello SP, Soo W, Bryant RV, et al. Systematic review with meta-analysis: faecal microbiota transplantation for the induction of remission for active ulcerative colitis. Aliment Pharmacol Ther 2017;46(3):213–24.
79. Vermeire S, Joossens M, Verbeke K, et al. Donor species richness determines faecal microbiota transplantation success in inflammatory bowel disease. J Crohns Colitis 2016;10(4):387–94.
80. Qazi T, Amaratunga T, Barnes EL, et al. The risk of inflammatory bowel disease flares after fecal microbiota transplantation: systematic review and meta-analysis. Gut Microbes 2017;8(6):574–88.
81. De Leon LM, Watson JB, Kelly CR. Transient flare of ulcerative colitis after fecal microbiota transplantation for recurrent Clostridium difficile infection. Clin Gastroenterol Hepatol 2013;11(8):1036–8.

Prognosticating the Course of Inflammatory Bowel Disease

Jenna L. Koliani-Pace, MD[a], Corey A. Siegel, MD, MS[b],*

KEYWORDS

- Crohn's disease • Ulcerative colitis • Inflammatory bowel disease • Prognosis

KEY POINTS

- Patients with Crohn's disease have a variable disease course, and it is important to identify those with a higher risk of complications early, before irreversible bowel damage occurs.
- It is possible to identify which patients with ulcerative colitis are at a higher risk of proximal extension, which in turn predicts a more severe disease course and need for colectomy.
- Genetic and serologic markers play a role in disease prognosis, but the role that the microbiome, metagenomics, metaproteomics, and microRNAs play in a patient's disease course is still under investigation.

INTRODUCTION

Inflammatory bowel disease (IBD) includes both ulcerative colitis (UC) and Crohn's disease. Crohn's disease can have a wide range of clinical symptoms and manifestations, with varying phenotypes, making the development of treatment plans even more challenging.[1] Adding to the complexity of the disease, Crohn's disease can be characterized by discrete periods of acute worsening of clinical symptoms (eg, worsening abdominal pain, diarrhea) and signs (eg, elevated inflammatory markers, endoscopic, or radiologic findings) followed by periods of clinical remission. Even during these periods where patients are asymptomatic, there is often ongoing subclinical

Disclosures: J.L. Koliani-Pace has received travel support from Takeda. C.A. Siegel serves as a consultant/advisory board for Abbvie, Amgen, Celgene, Lilly, Janssen, Sandoz, Pfizer, Prometheus, Sebela, and Takeda and as a speaker for CME activities for Abbvie, Janssen, Pfizer, and Takeda and has received grant support from the Crohn's and Colitis Foundation, AHRQ (1R01HS021747-01), Abbvie, Janssen, Pfizer, and Takeda. Dr C.A. Siegel and Dr Lori Siegel are cofounders of MiTest Health, LLC, that has a patent pending for a System and Method of Communicating Predicted Medical Outcomes.
a Inflammatory Bowel Disease Center, Section of Gastroenterology and Hepatology, Dartmouth-Hitchcock Medical Center, Dartmouth-Hitchcock, 1 Medical Center Drive, Lebanon, NH 03766, USA; b Inflammatory Bowel Disease Center, Section of Gastroenterology and Hepatology, Dartmouth-Hitchcock Medical Center, Lebanon, NH 03756, USA
* Corresponding author.
E-mail address: corey.a.siegel@hitchcock.org

Gastrointest Endoscopy Clin N Am 29 (2019) 395–404
https://doi.org/10.1016/j.giec.2019.02.003
1052-5157/19/© 2019 Elsevier Inc. All rights reserved.

inflammation that leads to irreversible bowel damage and complications of their disease.[2] During these times, clinical symptoms often do not correlate with endoscopic or radiologic findings.[1] Complications of Crohn's disease can be defined as the development of an intestinal stricture; internal penetrating disease, such as fistula or abscess; or the requirement of nonperianal surgery (eg, bowel resection or strictureplasty). The goal of Crohn's disease–directed therapy is to achieve mucosal healing as a means of preventing future complications. There are now studies showing that mucosal healing in the short term leads to increase in clinical remission and decrease in surgeries and hospitalizations.[3–5]

Although the long-term complications of Crohn's disease are well acknowledged, complications of UC tend to be underestimated. Strictures are mostly associated with Crohn's disease, but patients with long-standing UC also can develop benign strictures. Additionally, long-standing disease activity affects the motility of the colon over time. Patients develop anorectal dysfunction and colonic dysmotility manifested as loose stools, tenesmus, and incontinence, even when there is mucosal healing of the colon. The similarity of these symptoms to disease flares can make it even more challenging to appropriately treat patients. Extensive pseudopolyp formation can make colorectal cancer surveillance challenging as well.[6]

When evaluating patients in a clinic, being able to predict their disease course to prevent complications is essential to guiding early effective therapy. As more medications for the treatment of IBD have emerged, research has also led to the discovery that patient characteristics, genetics, and serologic markers can be used to develop prediction tools to help prognosticate the course of IBD. The objective of this article is to evaluate the past, present, and future in predicting the course of IBD (**Table 1**).

CROHN'S DISEASE—THE PAST

In 1932, a landmark article published in the *Journal of the American Medical Association* describing 14 cases of what was initially termed, *regional ileitis*, ultimately taking the name of the first author, Crohn, provides the best first accounts of severe disease.[7] All these patients had been sick for months to years before they sought medical care and were described as having diarrhea, fevers, weight loss leading to emaciation, and progressive anemia. On physical examination, patients were noted to have a palpable mass in the right lower quadrant. Strictures described as the bowel wall becoming "enormously thickened...the lumen of the bowel is greatly encroached on" with the proximal intestine becoming greatly dilated. Fistulas and abscesses were described.[7]

Table 1
Risk factors for a more complicated disease course in Crohn's disease and ulcerative colitis

Crohn's Disease Complications	Proximal Extension of Disease in Ulcerative Colitis	Developing Acute Severe Ulcerative Colitis
• Younger age at diagnosis	• Younger age at diagnosis	• Younger age at diagnosis
• Penetrating/stricturing disease on presentation	• Primary sclerosing cholangitis	• Extensive disease
• Ileal disease location	• >3 flares per year	• Short duration of disease
• Deep/extensive ulcers on colonoscopy	• Need for corticosteroids	
• Bowel damage on MRI	• Need for immunosuppression	
• NOD2 status	• Nonsmoker	
• Immune responses to ASCA, OmpC, CBir1, and pANCA		

Ultimately, these patients developed the complications of Crohn's disease that current therapies are trying to prevent.

It took decades to learn more about the natural history of Crohn's disease. It was not until the epidemiologic studies of Olmsted County, Minnesota; Manitoba, Canada; and Copenhagen, Denmark, among others that helped better understand the natural history of this disease and expose patient characteristics that helped better predict the disease course. A majority of patients, between 56% and 81%, present with nonstricturing or nonpenetrating disease at the time of diagnosis.[8] Not everyone who is diagnosed with Crohn's disease goes on to develop complications. From the population-based cohort from Olmsted County, Minnesota, 51% of patients who presented with an inflammatory phenotype went on to develop a complication within 20 years of diagnosis.[9] These population-based cohorts provide similar data in that approximately half of patients with Crohn's disease require surgical resection within the first 10 years of diagnosis.[10–15] The ability to predict which of these patients will have a more complicated disease course is critical to providing aggressive early therapy in the hope of altering the natural disease progression.

There are several patient characteristics that have repeatedly been associated with increased risk of developing complications. Disease location, in particular isolated ileal disease, and ileocolonic disease in addition to upper tract involvement are more likely to have a complicated disease course. Additionally, younger age at diagnosis and presenting with penetrating or stricturing disease also lead to a more aggressive phenotype.[16] Smoking has been associated with the need for early surgery and increases the need for recurrent surgery after resection.[17,18] Beyond these factors, the initial endoscopic evaluation can be predictive of penetrating disease. Severe endoscopic findings defined as deep and extensive ulcerations encompassing more than 10% of the lumen in at least 1 segment of colon increased the risk of surgery and penetrating disease.[19] Understanding how endoscopic findings correlate with MRI findings is important, because this can help better understand the risk for development of bowel damage. The magnetic resonance index of activity (MaRIA) scores has been validated to quantify the amount of Crohn's disease activity in each segment of the bowel. Additionally, MaRIA has been showed to correlate with the Crohn's Disease Endoscopic Index of Severity.[20,21] Before assessing the need for medical therapy for surgery in Crohn's disease, the amount of irreversible bowel damage present is an important factor, because biologics and small molecules are only effective in treating inflammation. MRI can help distinguish between the amount of inflammation and fibrosis present.[22] The Lémann Index is another MRI scoring system that evaluates disease activity and severity. It has shown to have value in early Crohn's disease, with higher scores associated with an increased risk of surgery and hospitalization.[23]

From patient-related factors, research started examining serologic factors and genetic factors associated with more aggressive phenotypes. A meta-analysis evaluated 10 cohort studies and 14 case-control studies for the association between Crohn's disease and anti–Saccharomyces cerevisiae antibody (ASCA). In both the cohort and case-control studies, there was an increased risk of complicated disease behavior (odds ratio [OR] 2.09; 95% CI, 1.71–2.57 and OR 2.13%; 95% CI, 1.70–2.68, respectively) defined as stricturing or penetrating disease in patients who had an elevated ASCA. Additional work within pediatric patients has shown that there exists variation in immune response to microbial antigens, specifically ASCA, Escherichia coli outer-membrane porin C (OmpC), and anti-CBir1 (anti-flagellin antibody) as well as auto-antigen perinuclear antineutrophil cytoplasmic antibody (pANCA), which may predict more aggressive phenotypes. The number and magnitude of these immune responses were associated with increased risks of internal penetrating or stricturing disease and surgery.[24]

There have been multiple genes associated with Crohn's disease, but the one in particular that has received most of the attention is *NOD2*. A meta-analysis concluded that having 1 mutation in the *NOD2* gene slightly increased the risk of having penetrating or stricturing disease. In patients who have 2 mutations of the gene, however, an increased risk of penetrating or stricturing disease by 41% is seen. Carriers of 1 of the of *NOD2* mutations increased risk of surgery by 58%. The *NOD2* gene mutations have not been associated with increased risk of perianal disease.[25]

CROHN'S DISEASE—THE PRESENT

With all the factors associated with worsening disease course in patients with Crohn's disease, tools have been developed and validated to help predict when complications may develop. Having this glimpse into the future as to what a patient's disease course may look like can help clinicians decide who should be treated with aggressive therapy from the time of diagnosis. One tool called Personalized Risk and Outcome Prediction Tool (PROSPECT) uses multiple variables, including patient and disease characteristics, *NOD2* status, and immune responses to ASCA, CBir1, and pANCA to predict the course of individual disease. PROSPECT provides a visualization for patients to help understand whether they are at low risk, intermediate risk, or high risk of developing complications from their Crohn's disease, including fistula formation or stricturing, that may lead to surgery within 3 years.[26,27] Another model, Korean Crohn's Disease Predication, was developed in Korea using the multicenter longitudinal cohort study called Crohn's Disease Clinical Network and Cohort (CONNECT), which has been validated within this population to predict 5-year and 10-year rates of surgery. Variables included within this model were age at diagnosis, jejunal involvement, initial disease behavior, and perianal disease.[28] Similarly, models have been developed within pediatric cohorts to help predict the risk of complications.[26,29] The pediatric model built from the RISK cohort has a sensitivity of 66% (95% CI, 51–82) and specificity of 63% (95% CI, 55–71) of predicting a disease complication, with a negative predictive value of 95% (95% CI, 94–97).[29] Furthermore, they identified the microbiota Ruminococcus and Veillonella as associated with stricturing complications or penetrating complications, respectively.

CROHN'S DISEASE—THE FUTURE

There are emerging fields of research that hope to advance the knowledge about what causes varying phenotypes of Crohn's disease, including the microbiome, metagenomics, metaproteomics, and microRNAs (miRNA). Microbiome studies have shown that patients with Crohn's disease have a decrease in the diversity of bacteria within their microbiome, specifically within the Firmicutes phylum and increase in Gammaproteobacteria. The lack of diversity of the microbiota has been shown to decrease when inflammation is present in an individual patient.[30] There has been an increase in *E coli* found in tissue samples of patients with ileal Crohn's disease. As a part of the STORI study, which assessed relapse of disease activity after discontinuing infliximab in patients with Crohn's disease who were in remission, the microbiome was noted to be different in healthy controls compared with patients with Crohn's disease. There is a decrease in the amount of *Clostridium coccoides*, *C leptum* (members of the Firmicutes phylum), and *Faecalibacterium prausnitzii* in patients with Crohn's disease. Lower rates of Firmicutes were seen in patients who relapsed after infliximab was withdrawn in comparisons to patients who did not relapse. Furthermore, having lower amounts of *F prausnitzii* and *Bacteroides* predicted relapse.[31] The future hopefully will help in understanding the relationship between fungi and viruses and the development of IBD. More than just the diversity of the bacteria present, the function of those bacteria also may play a role in more severe disease. Metagenomic and metaproteomic studies have shown a decrease in butanoate and propanoate metabolism and overall decrease in the levels of butyrate and other short-chain fatty acids in patients with ileal Crohn's disease, a disease location that has been associated with more severe disease.[30]

miRNAs are noncoding RNAs (RNA molecules that are not translated into a protein) that work at the post-transcription stage to help regulate gene expression.[32] There have been different location-specific miRNAs (ileal vs colon) that have been identified from tissue samples obtained during colonoscopy.[33] The dysregulation of these miRNAs have been seen in NOD-2, tumor necrosis factor, and interleukin-6.[34] How these different miRNAs are expressed has been associated with disease behavior, in particular miRNA-215, which has been associated with fistulizing disease.[34] It is possible that the identification of this miRNA can be used to help predict a more complicated disease course. Beyond the microbiome and the miRNAs that help regulate gene expression, the interactions between these, along with alterations in the immune system and patient characteristics, hopefully can be applied at the time of diagnosis to help guide which patients require early aggressive therapy.

ULCERATIVE COLITIS—THE PAST

Examination of the history of IBD shows that UC was described before the landmark article by Crohn and colleagues.[7] The first case report using the term UC was by Sir Samuel Wilks in 1859, which was followed by a description of several cases by Sir William Hale-White, in 1888. An important year in the history of UC was in 1909 when the Royal Society of Medicine in London held a symposium where more than 300 cases of UC were described. It was during this conference that the first patient characteristics of the disease, such as young age, diarrhea, and hemorrhage, that did not seem infectious in nature were described.[35]

Similar to Crohn's disease, the population cohorts of Olmsted County, Manitoba, and Copenhagen, along with others, have helped clinicians learn about the natural history of the disease and factors associated with more severe disease. Approximately 40% of patients present with left-sided colitis, with approximately 30% of patients presenting with extensive disease and 30% with proctitis. These cohorts have been better able to characterize the rate of disease extension. Patients initially diagnosed with proctitis had their disease extend to include the left colon approximately 30% of the time and progression to more extensive colitis approximately 15% of the time. The rate of progression from left-sided UC to extensive colitis ranged from 21% to 34%. Although a majority of patients have a mild to moderate course from their UC, the rates of hospitalization among patients with UC is measurable. Approximately two-thirds of patients required hospitalization within 10 years of diagnosis. The 5-year and 10-year cumulative rates of hospitalization ranged from 29% to 54% and 39% to 66%.[36] The earliest rates of colectomy suggest that a cumulative 10-year risk of surgery is 45%.[37] A more recent meta-analysis showed, however, that the 10-year rate was significantly lower than initially reported with the risk of surgery of 15%.[38]

These cohort studies helped identify the types of patients with UC who are more likely to have extension of their disease, a more severe disease course, and possibly require surgery for their disease. Patients who were diagnosed at a younger age, had primary sclerosing cholangitis, experienced more than 3 relapses in 1 year, required steroids or immunosuppression, or were nonsmokers were associated with proximal extension of disease.[39,40] It is important to help identify patients who are more likely to have extension of their disease, because progression is associated with a more severe disease course. A single-center case-control study identified that patients who had progression of their disease were more likely to have extraintestinal manifestations; a steroid-refractory course; the need for immunosuppressive medications, including thiopurines, infliximab, and cyclosporine; and surgery.[41] There have not been genetic markers or the immune responses to bacterial antigens identified in Crohn's disease in patients with UC to help to predict the disease course.[42] There is some evidence available that markers, including pANCA and anti-CBir, may be important to understand who is at risk for developing pouchitis after a total colectomy.[43] Multiple studies have examined the effects of C difficile infection on the outcomes of UC. Patients with UC after more likely to present to the emergency department. The risk for colectomy in the short term and long term after infection remains unclear.[44–48]

ULCERATIVE COLITIS—THE PRESENT

Similar to Crohn's disease, tools have been developed to help predict the course of UC. A cohort of patients with UC from the Veterans Affairs identified 699 patients who were followed for a median of 8 years after diagnosis. Two-thirds of the patients were used to help develop the model, and one-third of the patients were used to validate the model. The primary outcome was the use of corticosteroids to treat UC. Variables used in the model to predict corticosteroid use included age, non–African American ethnicity, presence of hypoalbuminemia, iron deficiency anemia at time of diagnosis, endoscopic extent of disease, and severity of disease on index colonoscopy.[49]

Another model looked to predict the risk of acute severe colitis within 3 years of diagnosis. This single-center study created a scoring system from 0 to 3. Patients received 1 point for each of the following: extensive disease, C-reactive protein greater than 10 mg/L, or hemoglobin at the time of diagnosis less than 12 g/dL if the patient was female or less than 14 g/dL if the patient was male. If the patient had all 3 findings at the time of diagnosis, the model predicted a 70% risk of developing severe acute colitis within 3 years.[50]

ULCERATIVE COLITIS—THE FUTURE

The knowledge about the microbiome, metagenomics, metaproteomics, and miRNAs in UC has expanded tremendously and the authors anticipate it will continue to do so. The microbiome in patients with UC has been shown less diverse, with a reduction of Clostridia species and an increase in the Gammaproteobacteria.[51] When comparing biopsies between healthy controls and patients with UC, the overall density of bacteria attached to colonic mucus layer is higher in biopsies obtained from UC patients.[52] This decrease in the biodiversity has been seen in children with UC as well. In particular, children who did not respond to steroids had even less biodiversity than those children who did respond to steroids.[51] A particular species, Fusobacterium, that typically inhabits the oral cavity has been found at higher levels within biopsies of patients with UC. Isolating Fusobacterium varium from humans and then introducing it into mice models via rectal enema has shown to induce colonic mucosal erosions.[30] Twin studies have evaluated how the microbiome differs between a healthy twin and a twin with UC. Patients with UC had a decrease in biodiversity and an increase in Actinobacteria and Proteobacteria in comparison to their twins.[53] The information from the gut microbiome with changes in composition needs further research to help understand the role it may play in predicting more severe disease.

SUMMARY

Both Crohn's disease and UC are progressive inflammatory diseases that ultimately, if left untreated, lead to irreversible damage to the bowels in a high proportion of patients. Initial understanding about disease progression was provided by multiple cohort studies across the world and helped better understand which patient characteristics were associated with a more severe disease course. As the science evolved, it helped better understand the role of genetics and how immune response to microbial antigens can predict the disease course. Models have been developed to help predict which patients are likely to have a more complicated disease course so that these patients can be identified and treated accordingly. The overall goal is to risk stratify patients soon after diagnosis and direct appropriate therapy based not only on their current disease activity but also on how their disease is expected behave over time.

REFERENCES

1. Lichtenstein GR, Loftus EV, Isaacs KL, et al. ACG clinical guideline: management of Crohn's disease in adults. Am J Gastroenterol 2018;113(4):481–517.
2. Pariente B, Cosnes J, Danese S, et al. Development of the Crohn's disease digestive damage score, the Lémann score. Inflamm Bowel Dis 2011;17(6):1415–22.
3. Nuti F, Civitelli F, Bloise S, et al. Prospective evaluation of the achievement of mucosal healing with anti-TNF-α therapy in a paediatric Crohn's disease cohort. J Crohns Colitis 2016;10(1):5–12.
4. Baert F, Moortgat L, Van Assche G, et al. Mucosal healing predicts sustained clinical remission in patients with early-stage Crohn's disease. Gastroenterology 2010;138(2):463–8.
5. Frøslie KF, Jahnsen J, Moum BA, et al. Mucosal healing in inflammatory bowel disease: results from a norwegian population-based cohort. Gastroenterology 2007;133(2):412–22.
6. Torres J, Billioud V, Sachar DB, et al. Ulcerative colitis as a progressive disease: the forgotten evidence. Inflamm Bowel Dis 2012;18(7):1356–63.
7. Crohn BB, Ginzburg L, Oppenheimer GD. Regional ileitis: a pathologic and clinical entity. JAMA 1932;99(16):1323–9.
8. Peyrin-Biroulet L, Loftus EV Jr, Colombel J-F, et al. The natural history of adult Crohn's disease in population-based cohorts. Am J Gastroenterol 2009;105:289.
9. Thia KT, Sandborn WJ, Harmsen WS, et al. Risk factors associated with progression to intestinal complications of Crohn's disease in a population-based cohort. Gastroenterology 2010;139(4):1147–55.
10. Solberg IC, Vatn MH, Høie O, et al. Clinical course in Crohn's disease: results of a Norwegian population-based ten-year follow-up study. Clin Gastroenterol Hepatol 2007;5(12):1430–8.
11. Wolters FL, Russel MG, Sijbrandij J, et al. Disease outcome of inflammatory bowel disease patients: general outline of a Europe-wide population-based 10-year clinical follow-up study. Scand J Gastroenterol Suppl 2006;(243):46–54.
12. Munkholm P, Langholz E, Davidsen M, et al. Disease activity courses in a regional cohort of Crohn's disease patients. Scand J Gastroenterol 1995;30(7):699–706.

13. Binder V, Hendriksen C, Kreiner S. Prognosis in Crohn's disease–based on results from a regional patient group from the county of Copenhagen. Gut 1985;26(2): 146–50.

14. Vind I, Riis L, Jess T, et al. Increasing incidences of inflammatory bowel disease and decreasing surgery rates in Copenhagen City and County, 2003-2005: a population-based study from the Danish Crohn colitis database. Am J Gastroenterol 2006;101(6):1274–82.

15. Gollop JH, Phillips SF, Melton LJ, et al. Epidemiologic aspects of Crohn's disease: a population based study in Olmsted County, Minnesota, 1943-1982. Gut 1988; 29(1):49–56.

16. Torres J, Caprioli F, Katsanos KH, et al. Predicting outcomes to optimize disease management in inflammatory bowel diseases. J Crohns Colitis 2016;10(12): 1385–94.

17. Sands BE, Arsenault JE, Rosen MJ, et al. Risk of early surgery for Crohn's disease: implications for early treatment strategies. Am J Gastroenterol 2003; 98(12):2712–8.

18. Romberg-Camps MJL, Dagnelie PC, Kester ADM, et al. Influence of phenotype at diagnosis and of other potential prognostic factors on the course of inflammatory bowel disease. Am J Gastroenterol 2009;104(2):371–83.

19. Allez M, Lemann M, Bonnet J, et al. Long term outcome of patients with active Crohn's disease exhibiting extensive and deep ulcerations at colonoscopy. Am J Gastroenterol 2002;97(4):947–53.

20. Rimola J, Rodriguez S, García-Bosch O, et al. Magnetic resonance for assessment of disease activity and severity in ileocolonic Crohn's disease. Gut 2009; 58(8):1113–20.

21. Rimola J, Ordás I, Rodriguez S, et al. Magnetic resonance imaging for evaluation of Crohn's diseaseValidation of parameters of severity and quantitative index of activity. Inflamm Bowel Dis 2011;17(8):1759–68.

22. Rimola J, Planell N, Rodríguez S, et al. Characterization of inflammation and fibrosis in Crohn's disease lesions by magnetic resonance imaging. Am J Gastroenterol 2015;110(3):432–40.

23. Fiorino G, Morin M, Bonovas S, et al. Prevalence of bowel damage assessed by cross-sectional imaging in early Crohn's disease and its impact on disease outcome. J Crohns Colitis 2017;11(3):274–80.

24. Dubinsky MC, Kugathasan S, Mei L, et al. Increased immune reactivity predicts aggressive complicating Crohn's disease in children. Clin Gastroenterol Hepatol 2008;6(10):1105–11.

25. Adler J, Rangwalla SC, Dwamena BA, et al. The prognostic power of the NOD2 genotype for complicated Crohn's disease: a meta-analysis. Am J Gastroenterol 2011;106(4):699–712.

26. Siegel CA, Siegel LS, Hyams JS, et al. Real-time tool to display the predicted disease course and treatment response for children with Crohn's disease. Inflamm Bowel Dis 2011;17(1):30–8.

27. Siegel CA, Horton H, Siegel LS, et al. A validated web-based tool to display individualised Crohn's disease predicted outcomes based on clinical, serologic and genetic variables. Aliment Pharmacol Ther 2016;43(2):262–71.

28. Park Y, Cheon JH, Park YL, et al. Development of a novel predictive model for the clinical course of Crohn's disease: results from the connect study. Inflamm Bowel Dis 2017;23(7):1071–9.

29. Kugathasan S, Denson LA, Walters TD, et al. Prediction of complicated disease course for children newly diagnosed with Crohn's disease: a multicentre inception cohort study. Lancet 2017;389(10080):1710–8.

30. Kostic AD, Xavier RJ, Gevers D. The microbiome in inflammatory bowel disease: current status and the future ahead. Gastroenterology 2014;146(6):1489–99.

31. Rajca S, Grondin V, Louis E, et al. Alterations in the intestinal microbiome (dysbiosis) as a predictor of relapse after infliximab withdrawal in crohn's disease. Inflamm Bowel Dis 2014;1. https://doi.org/10.1097/MIB.0000000000000036.

32. Bartel DP. MicroRNAs: target recognition and regulatory functions. Cell 2009; 136(2):215–33.

33. Wu F, Zhang S, Dassopoulos T, et al. Identification of microRNAs associated with ileal and Colonic Crohn's disease. Inflamm Bowel Dis 2010;16(10):1729–38.

34. Peck BCE, Weiser M, Lee SE, et al. MicroRNAs classify different disease behavior phenotypes of Crohn's disease and may have prognostic utility. Inflamm Bowel Dis 2015;21(9):2178–87.

35. Mulder DJ, Noble AJ, Justinich CJ, et al. A tale of two diseases: The history of inflammatory bowel disease. J Crohns Colitis 2014;8(5):341–8.

36. Fumery M, Singh S, Dulai PS, et al. Natural history of adult ulcerative colitis in population-based cohorts: a systematic review. Clin Gastroenterol Hepatol 2018;16(3):343–56.e3.

37. Leijonmarck C-E, Löfberg R, Öst Å, et al. Long-term results of ileorectal anastomosis in ulcerative colitis in Stockholm County. Dis Colon Rectum 1990;33(3): 195–200.

38. Frolkis AD, Dykeman J, Negrón ME, et al. Risk of surgery for inflammatory bowel diseases has decreased over time: a systematic review and meta-analysis of population-based studies. Gastroenterology 2013;145(5):996–1006.

39. Meucci G, Vecchi M, Astegiano M, et al. The natural history of ulcerative proctitis: a multicenter, retrospective study. Am J Gastroenterol 2000;95(2):469–73.

40. Kim B, Park SJ, Hong SP, et al. Proximal disease extension and related predicting factors in ulcerative proctitis. Scand J Gastroenterol 2014;49(2):177–83.

41. Etchevers MJ, Aceituno M, García-Bosch O, et al. Risk factors and characteristics of extent progression in ulcerative colitis. Inflamm Bowel Dis 2009;15(9): 1320–5.

42. Lichtenstein GR, McGovern DPB. Using markers in IBD to predict disease and treatment outcomes: rationale and a review of current status. Am J Gastroenterol Suppl 2016;3(3):17–26.

43. Fleshner P, Ippoliti A, Dubinsky M, et al. Both preoperative perinuclear antineutrophil cytoplasmic antibody and anti-CBir1 expression in ulcerative colitis patients influence pouchitis development after ileal pouch–anal anastomosis. Clin Gastroenterol Hepatol 2008;6(5):561–8.

44. Issa M, Vijayapal A, Graham MB, et al. Impact of clostridium difficile on inflammatory bowel disease. Clin Gastroenterol Hepatol 2007;5(3):345–51.

45. Jodorkovsky D, Young Y, Abreu MT. Clinical outcomes of patients with ulcerative colitis and co-existing clostridium difficile infection. Dig Dis Sci 2010;55(2): 415–20.

46. Kariv R, Navaneethan U, Venkatesh PGK, et al. Impact of Clostridium difficile infection in patients with ulcerative colitis. J Crohns Colitis 2011;5(1):34–40.

47. Navaneethan U, Mukewar S, GK Venkatesh P, et al. Clostridium difficile infection is associated with worse long term outcome in patients with ulcerative colitis. J Crohns Colitis 2012;6(3):330–6.

48. Murthy SK, Steinhart AH, Tinmouth J, et al. Impact of Clostridium difficile colitis on 5-year health outcomes in patients with ulcerative colitis. Aliment Pharmacol Ther 2012;36(11–12):1032–9.
49. Khan N, Patel D, Shah Y, et al. A novel user-friendly model to predict corticosteroid utilization in newly diagnosed patients with ulcerative colitis. Inflamm Bowel Dis 2017;23(6):991–7.
50. Cesarini M, Collins GS, Rönnblom A, et al. Predicting the individual risk of acute severe colitis at diagnosis. J Crohns Colitis 2017;11(3):335–41. Available at: https://academic.oup.com/ecco-jcc/article/11/3/335/2631859. Accessed October 23, 2018.
51. Michail S, Durbin M, Turner D, et al. Alterations in the gut microbiome of children with severe ulcerative colitis. Inflamm Bowel Dis 2012;18(10):1799–808.
52. Swidsinski A, Ladhoff A, Pernthaler A, et al. Mucosal flora in inflammatory bowel disease. Gastroenterology 2002;122(1):44–54.
53. Lepage P, Häsler R, Spehlmann ME, et al. Twin study indicates loss of interaction between microbiota and mucosa of patients with ulcerative colitis. Gastroenterology 2011;141(1):227–36.

The Era of Anti-Tumor Necrosis Factor Is Over. What Do We Know, What Don't We Know, and What Do We Yearn to Know?

Sujaata Dwadasi, MD, Amanda Israel, MD, David T. Rubin, MD*

KEYWORDS

- Anti–tumor necrosis factor therapy • Inflammatory bowel disease
- Therapeutic drug monitoring • Biologics

KEY POINTS

- The discovery of anti-TNF therapy as a treatment for IBD was a revolution in the management of IBD and has ushered in an era of biological therapies that have changed the natural history of these diseases.
- By understanding anti-TNF treatments, clinicians have learned a tremendous amount about the immune system, immunogenicity, biosimilarity, and TDM.
- The next evolution in these therapies will be defined by advances in our understanding of the pathogenesis of different types of IBD, prediction of response, and sequencing of therapies.

The development of the first anti–tumor necrosis factor (TNF) biological therapy (infliximab) marked a revolutionary advance in our treatment of inflammatory bowel disease (IBD), and ushered in an era of biological therapies that changed the face of these diseases. Biological therapies have greatly advanced treatment options for patients with both Crohn's disease (CD) and ulcerative colitis (UC) by increasing disease remission rates, prolonging disease maintenance, and improving overall quality of life. Since the Food and Drug Administration (FDA) approved infliximab for the treatment of moderately to severely active CD in 1998, there have been developed and approved 3 additional anti-TNF therapies, numerous biosimilars to these therapies, and now 2 additional classes of biological therapies that target different components of the immune system. The development of biological therapies in IBD has led to much greater

Inflammatory Bowel Disease Center, University of Chicago Medicine, 5841 S. Maryland Avenue, MC 4076, Chicago, IL 60637, USA
* Corresponding author.
E-mail address: drubin@medicine.bsd.uchicago.edu

Gastrointest Endoscopy Clin N Am 29 (2019) 405–419
https://doi.org/10.1016/j.giec.2019.03.001
1052-5157/19/© 2019 Elsevier Inc. All rights reserved.

understanding of the pharmacokinetics of such treatment strategies, the advent of "precision medicine" approaches to IBD, and, most recently, the challenge of understanding how to choose therapies or sequence them in the care of patients with IBD.

Anti-TNF therapies are believed to act by directly binding to the serum and tissue proinflammatory cytokine, TNF, inhibiting downstream expression of other inflammatory cytokines and, with some of these therapies, induction of apoptosis.[1] Although initially considered as a possible treatment of septicemia, inhibition of TNF did not improve the outcome of such patients, so anti-TNF therapies were then studied for chronic inflammatory conditions. These included rheumatoid arthritis, psoriatic arthritis, and ankylosing spondylitis. Subsequently, anti-TNF therapies became a sensible mechanism to study for the treatment of IBD. In 1998, infliximab became the first anti-TNF therapy approved by the FDA[2] for the treatment of CD, and in fact the first *therapy* approved by the FDA for the treatment of CD. This was followed by the regulatory approval for fistulizing CD, moderately to severely active UC, and similar pediatric IBD indications. There are now 3 more distinct anti-TNF therapies approved by the FDA, namely adalimumab (CD and UC), certolizumab pegol (CD), and golimumab (UC). More recently there has been development and regulatory approval by extrapolation of indication of multiple biosimilars to infliximab and adalimumab. Over time, anti-TNF therapies have been widely adopted in IBD clinical practice thanks to extensive data validating their efficacy and a greater understanding of their safety. In fact, anti-TNF therapies are now frequently used as first-line treatments for IBD to prevent progression of disease and avoid complications.[3]

There are now many new treatment options currently available for the treatment of IBD, and multiple other therapies in development for future regulatory approval. These therapies target different inflammatory mechanisms using monoclonal antibody therapies (vedolizumab, ustekinumab) and small-molecule therapies (tofacitinib). The myriad mechanisms and treatment options now available have led to numerous significant clinical challenges including choice of therapy for individual patients, approach to primary or secondary nonresponse to therapy, and considerations in sequencing these therapies in our patients.

WHAT DO WE KNOW?

When infliximab was initially approved for use in CD, there was much we did not know. In the early days of its use, the need for dose adjustments and maintenance therapy was not fully appreciated and immunogenicity was not understood. Patients receiving episodic dosing (including those in the early clinical trials!) were found to develop anti-infliximab antibodies, which both led to early loss of response of the therapy and an increased risk of immediate and delayed hypersensitivity reactions.[4] The importance of optimizing a sustained response to infliximab was especially critical when infliximab was the only approved therapy for CD, because there were no other options if this failed. Subsequent research was focused on maximizing response and minimizing immunogenicity, and maximizing a sustained response to therapy. As additional anti-TNF therapies received regulatory approval, the next priority area of research was the interpretation of loss of response, and incorporation of measurement of serum drug and antidrug antibody levels that could be used to make management decisions.

DISTINCTIONS AMONG THE ANTI–TUMOR NECROSIS FACTOR THERAPIES
Infliximab

Infliximab is a mouse chimeric immunoglobulin 1 (IgG1) monoclonal antibody against TNF that is approved for moderately to severely active CD, fistulizing CD, and moderately to severely active UC. Infliximab is administered by intravenous (IV) infusions with a loading dose of 5 mg/kg or 10 mg/kg at weeks 0, 2, and 6 and maintenance dosing at 5 mg/kg or 10 mg/kg at an interval of every 4 to 8 weeks.

Infliximab in moderately to severely active Crohn's disease
The efficacy of the induction of infliximab for active CD was first described by Targan and colleagues[5] in a 12-week multicenter, double-blinded, placebo-controlled trial that included 108 moderately to severely active CD patients refractory to steroids. At week 12, 41% of the patients who received a single infusion of 5 mg/kg, 10 mg/kg, or 20 mg/kg of infliximab had a clinical response compared with 12% of the patients in the placebo group.[5]

The ACCENT trials subsequently demonstrated that infliximab was successful in the induction and maintenance of active CD.[5,6] ACCENT I was a randomized, controlled trial with 573 moderately to severely active CD patients (Crohn's Disease Activity Index [CDAI] score >220) who all received a 5 mg/kg infusion of infliximab at week 0. Within 2 weeks, 58% of patients responded to the single infusion.[6] If patients responded, they were then randomized to infusions of placebo at week 2, 6, and every 8 weeks (group I) or 5 mg/kg of infliximab at week 2, 6, and every 8 weeks (group II) or 5 mg/kg of infliximab at weeks 2 and 6, followed by 10 mg/kg of infliximab every 8 weeks (group III). Patients in groups II and III were more likely (39% and 45%, respectively) to have sustained clinical remission (CDAI <150) at week 30 compared with group I patients (21%). Patients in group III had a higher median time (>54 weeks) to develop loss of response compared with groups I (19 weeks) and II (38 weeks). The incidence of serious infections did not vary based on the infusion frequency or dosage of infliximab.[7]

Infliximab in fistulizing Crohn's disease
Infliximab has also been shown to be effective in healing fistulas in patients with CD. Patients with fistulizing disease in the ACCENT II trial had a higher rate of fistula closure at week 54 in the infliximab group (36%) compared with the placebo group (19%).[5] Another study randomized 94 CD patients with fistulas to placebo, 5 mg/kg infliximab, or 10 mg/kg infliximab. Those in the infliximab groups had a reduction of 50% of fistulas from baseline compared with those in the placebo group.[8]

Infliximab in moderately to severely active ulcerative colitis
The ACT 1 and ACT 2 trials were randomized, double-blinded, placebo-controlled studies that demonstrated efficacy in the treatment of moderately to severely active UC (Mayo score of 6–12). In both trials, 364 patients were randomized to placebo or infliximab 5 mg/kg or 10 mg/kg at weeks 0, 2, 6, and every 8 weeks. In the ACT 1 trial, 69% of the patients who received 5 mg/kg infliximab and 61% of the patients who received 10 mg/kg infliximab achieved clinical response at week 8 (a decrease in Mayo score by 3 points and a decrease in rectal bleeding subscore) compared with 37% of patients who received placebo.[9] The ACT 2 trial showed comparable data. Both trials showed that sustained clinical response and mucosal healing were more likely in the infliximab groups than in the placebo group. There was no difference in rate of response in patients who were and were not previously corticosteroid refractory.[7] These studies demonstrate the steroid-sparing, long-term clinical remission rates, and mucosal healing qualities of infliximab in patients with moderately to severely active UC.

A follow-up study of the patients from the ACT 1 and ACT 2 trials showed lower rates of progression to colectomy in the infliximab group (10%) compared with that of the placebo group (17%)[10] and, importantly, that Mayo endoscopic subscores of 0 or 1 were associated with a similar protection against colectomy.

Infliximab in combination with immunomodulators

Before the era of anti-TNF therapy, azathioprine and 6-mercaptopurine were used after first-line therapies (mesalamine, budesonide) failed. Further studies were performed comparing the efficacy of these therapies and anti-TNF therapies.

The SONIC trial was a randomized, double-blind study comparing the efficacy of infliximab, azathioprine, or both in combination in CD patients who were naïve to these therapies. A total of 508 patients were randomized to the following treatment groups: infliximab infusions 5 mg/kg standard induction and maintenance every 8 weeks; azathioprine 2.5 mg/kg plus placebo infusions; or combination of both drugs. At week 26, 56% of the patients on combination therapy were in steroid-free clinical remission (CDAI score <150) compared with infliximab monotherapy (44.4%) and azathioprine monotherapy (30%). Mucosal healing was also higher in patients on combination therapy, while serious infections were actually less in the combination therapy group compared with the other 2 subgroups. There were decreased rates of formation of antibodies to infliximab in the combination group compared with the infliximab monotherapy group.[11] More recently, post hoc analysis of the SONIC trial identified that the infliximab level was more predictive of steroid-free remission than being on concomitant therapy with azathioprine.[12]

The subsequent similarly designed UC-SUCCESS trial to analyze the efficacy of combination therapy with infliximab and azathioprine included 239 UC patients. This study demonstrated that corticosteroid-free clinical remission at week 16 in 39.7% of patients treated with the combination therapy (infliximab 5 mg/kg IV at weeks 0, 2, 6, and 14 and azathioprine 2.5 mg/kg by mouth daily), compared with 22.1% with infliximab monotherapy and 23.7% azathioprine monotherapy. There were fewer patients who developed anti-TNF antibodies in the combination group than in the infliximab monotherapy group.[13]

Another study, the COMMITT trial in immunomodulator- and anti-TNF-naïve CD patients, explored whether methotrexate in combination with infliximab was superior to infliximab and placebo. However, at 16 weeks there was no difference between these 2 arms of the study. One potential explanation for this surprising finding was the possibility that because both arms of the study were treated with prednisone, there was a "ceiling" effect of combined therapy and therefore the presence or absence of methotrexate did not distinguish these groups. In additional analyses, the infliximab and methotrexate arm had higher infliximab serum levels.[14]

Adalimumab

Adalimumab is a human IgG1 monoclonal antibody against TNF that is approved for moderately to severely active CD and UC. Adalimumab is administered subcutaneously (SC) with a loading dose of 160 mg at week 0, 80 mg at week 2, and 40 mg at week 4 followed by maintenance dosing of 40 mg every week or every other week.

Adalimumab in moderately to severely active Crohn's disease

The CLASSIC I and II trials demonstrated the efficacy of adalimumab for induction and maintenance of anti-TNF naïve moderately to severely active CD patients. For induction, 299 patients were randomized to adalimumab (40/20 mg, 80/40 mg, or 160/80 mg) or placebo at weeks 0/2. Adalimumab was superior to placebo for inducing remission (CDAI <150) at week 4, with the 160/80 mg dosing being the most effective. A total of 275 patients from the CLASSIC I trial entered the CLASSIC II trial, and all received adalimumab 40 mg at week 0 and week 2. Patients who continued to be in remission at week 4 were rerandomized to adalimumab 40 mg weekly, 40 mg every other week, or placebo. The patients who received adalimumab every week and every other week had higher clinical remission rates (79% and 83%, respectively) compared with placebo (44%).[15]

The subsequent CHARM trial analyzed 854 moderately to severely active CD patients, including patients who had previous anti-TNF exposure, who then received adalimumab 80 mg/40 mg at week 0/2. The 60% of patients who responded (70-point decrease in CDAI score) at week 4 were rerandomized to adalimumab 40 mg weekly, adalimumab 40 mg every other week, or placebo. Patients receiving adalimumab had higher rates of clinical remission at week 26 and week 54 compared with placebo. There was no significant difference among the patients who achieved clinical remission in regard to their history of previous anti-TNF exposure.[16]

The GAIN trial studied patients who received adalimumab after failure with infliximab (continued symptoms or unable to tolerate). At week 4, 21% of patients who received adalimumab 160 mg at week 0 and 80 mg at week 2 achieved clinical remission, compared with 7% of patients who received placebo.[17]

The EXTEND trial published data in regard to the efficacy of mucosal healing with adalimumab. This study identified an increased incidence of mucosal healing (absence of ulcerations) at week 52 for patients who underwent induction (160 mg/80 mg at weeks 0/2) and maintenance therapy (40 mg every other week) with adalimumab (24%) compared with placebo (0%).[18]

Adalimumab in fistulizing Crohn's disease
Adalimumab has also demonstrated benefit for fistulas in CD patients, but unlike infliximab there was no prospective trial with fistula closure as the primary endpoint. Nonetheless, subset analysis from the CHARM study found that 30% of patients with fistulizing disease achieved complete closure of fistulas in both adalimumab loading dose groups by week 26 compared with 13% of patients in the placebo group.[15] Another study included 117 CD patients with fistulas who were randomized to adalimumab or placebo. At week 16, patients treated with adalimumab had a statistically significant increase in fistula closure compared with those treated with placebo. Previous exposure to anti-TNF therapy (infliximab) did not affect fistula healing.[19]

Adalimumab in moderately to severely active ulcerative colitis
ULTRA I and II are pivotal trials showing efficacy of adalimumab in the induction and maintenance of moderately to severely active UC. The ULTRA I trial studied induction with adalimumab 160/80 mg or adalimumab 80/40 mg or placebo at week 0/2 in UC patients who failed steroids or other immunosuppressants. At week 8, clinical remission (partial Mayo score <2) was achieved in 18.5% of patients in the 160/80 mg group, 10% of patients in the 80/40 mg group, and 9.2% of patients in the placebo group.[20]

The ULTRA II trial studied the induction and maintenance of adalimumab in 494 patients receiving oral steroids or immunosuppressants. The patients were randomly assigned to 160 mg at week 0, 80 mg at week 2, and then 40 mg every other week or placebo. At week 52, 17.3% of adalimumab patients achieved clinical remission compared with 8.5% of placebo patients. This study also demonstrated that 25% of adalimumab patients achieved mucosal healing compared with 15.4% of placebo patients. Overall, there were higher rates of clinical remission in patients who were anti-TNF naïve,[21] an observation that has continued to be noted with all biological therapies in IBD; the first biological therapy has the greatest response and remission rates.

Adalimumab in combination with immunomodulators

Unlike infliximab, there have not been robust studies regarding adalimumab in combination with immunomodulators. There have been retrospective studies, which have shown a higher rate of clinical remission in patients with combination therapy with thiopurine or azathioprine compared with monotherapy.[22]

The REACT trial was a cluster randomization trial designed with early combination therapy with adalimumab in CD patients in comparison with conventional therapy. The study did not show a difference in clinical remission between the 2 groups, but use of adalimumab in combination with azathioprine was associated with lower hospitalizations and surgery notes.[23]

A systematic meta-analysis of 11 randomized controlled trials of anti-TNF agents in patients with luminal or fistulizing CD found that there is no benefit of adalimumab combination therapy compared with monotherapy. Combination therapy was found to be no more effective in inducing 6-month remission, response, partial or complete fistula closure, or maintaining response.[24]

Certolizumab Pegol

Certolizumab pegol is a pegylated humanized Fab' of an anti-TNF monoclonal antibody that inhibits ant-TNF. Certolizumab pegol is an SC injection with induction dosing of 400 mg at weeks 0, 2, and 4 followed by maintenance 400 mg every 4 weeks. Certolizumab pegol is approved for the treatment of moderately to severely active CD.

The PRECISE trial is a double-blind, placebo-controlled study that included 662 moderately to severely active (based on C-reactive protein [CRP] level) CD patients that were randomized to the induction of certolizumab pegol (400 mg at weeks 0, 2, and 4 and then every 4 weeks) or placebo. At week 6, response rates (based on the Inflammatory Bowel Disease Questionnaire) were higher in certolizumab pegol (35%) than with placebo (27%). However, there was no significant difference between the groups in regard to remission rates (CDAI <150).[25]

The PRECISE II trial studied the maintenance therapy of the patients who responded to induction with certolizumab pegol (428 of 668 patients). Clinical remission (CDAI <150) at week 26 was achieved in 48% of the patients in the certolizumab pegol group compared with 29% of the patients in the placebo group.[26]

The WELCOME trial included 539 patients with active CD and secondary failure to infliximab who received certolizumab pegol 400 mg at weeks 0, 2, and 4. At week 6, 62% of certolizumab pegol patients responded (decrease in CDAI score by 100 points) and were randomized to maintenance therapy of 400 mg every 2 weeks or every 4 weeks. There was similar clinical efficacy in the patients who received maintenance dosing every 2 weeks and every 4 weeks.[27]

Golimumab

Golimumab is a human monoclonal antibody against TNF that is approved for moderately to severely active UC. It is an SC injection with induction dosing of 200 mg at week 0 and 100 mg at week 2 followed by maintenance therapy of 100 mg every 4 weeks.

The PURSUIT-SC trial showed the efficacy of induction and maintenance of golimumab in patients with moderately to severely active UC. A total of 1064 patients were randomized to golimumab 200/100 mg or 400/200 mg at weeks 0/2 or placebo.

Clinical remission (partial Mayo score) was achieved at week 6 in 17.8% and 17.9% of the patients in the golimumab groups and 6.4% of patients in the placebo group.[28]

The PURSUIT-M trial evaluated maintenance therapy with golimumab in patients who responded to induction therapy. Patients were randomized to 50 mg of golimumab every 4 weeks, 100 mg of golimumab every 4 weeks, or placebo. Clinical remission and mucosal healing (Mayo endoscopy score) from weeks 30 through 54 were observed in 23.2% and 27.8% of patients in the golimumab groups compared with 15.6% in the placebo group. Steroid-free remission at week 54 was not clinically significant between the groups.[29]

POSTOPERATIVE CROHN'S DISEASE AND ANTI–TUMOR NECROSIS FACTOR THERAPY

During their disease course many CD disease patients may require surgical intervention, the most common of which is an ileocolonic resection. A fascinating and unexplained feature of CD is that the disease recurs at the site of the surgical anastomosis, and there is a great deal of research into monitoring and treatment strategies to prevent such recurrence.

A small randomized trial of infliximab compared with placebo first demonstrated the efficacy of anti-TNF in the prevention of 1-year postoperative recurrence.[30] The subsequent larger PREVENT trial analyzed the efficacy of infliximab on preventing the clinical and endoscopic reoccurrence of CD after ileocolonic resection in 174 patients. Patients were randomized to 5 mg/kg infliximab or placebo. There was no significant difference between the 2 arms of the study in the primary endpoint of clinical remission, but there was a clear and statistical difference in endoscopic recurrence. Only 30% of patients in the infliximab group had endoscopic recurrence (based on Rutgeerts score > i2), compared with 60% of the patients in the placebo group.[31]

In the subsequently performed POCER trial, endoscopic recurrence was studied in postoperative CD patients comparing active care (risk stratification and early colonoscopy with step-up medical therapy with a thiopurine or adalimumab) versus standard care. The active group who received adalimumab had less endoscopic reoccurrence (43%) at 18 months compared with patients who received a thiopurine (61%). These trials demonstrated that anti-TNF therapies are effective in decreasing recurrence of CD postoperatively.[31] The choice of therapy and timing of initiation after surgery remain debated, but it is widely accepted that anti-TNF is an appropriate option for postoperative prevention in high-risk CD patients.

BIOSIMILARS

Cost is one of the greatest barriers of biological therapies, as it highly affects patients' accessibility to these medications in the United States and worldwide. The emergence of biosimilars has provided a less expensive treatment option. Biosimilars are medicines that are very similar to an existing reference biologic, possessing the same activity, efficacy, safety, and immunogenicity. Biosimilars undergo an abbreviated regulatory process that does not require phase 1 or 2 studies and only requires 2 phase 3 studies in any of the approved indications of the originator drugs. When a biosimilar receives FDA approval, it is based on evidence proving there is no clinical difference from its original reference biological medication. In addition, the FDA provides extrapolation of data across clinical indications. All of the biosimilars approved for IBD were extrapolated by clinical trials for rheumatologic conditions. No biosimilar has yet received the "interchangeable" designation by the FDA. Interchangeability would allow substitution without notification of patient or provider.[32]

There have been several studies analyzing the biosimilar for infliximab, CT-P13, in CD and UC patients. NOR-SWITCH was a randomized switch trial demonstrating the comparable efficacy of CT-P13 to infliximab, as well as increased loss of response or increased immunogenicity after the switch. Another trial, the SECURE study, demonstrated that CD and UC patients who switched from infliximab to CT-P13 did not have significant changes in their drug levels at week 16. A study performed in Israel showed that antibodies against infliximab also recognize and inhibit CT-P13. Therefore, patients who develop antidrug antibodies to the biosimilar or the originator should not switch to the other, because the hypersensitivity reaction would still occur.[32]

Since CT-P13, there have been 5 other biosimilars to infliximab and adalimumab approved by the FDA.[32] It is safe and effective in select patients to switch to a biosimilar or start a biosimilar for their treatment of CD or UC. It is important for the physician to have a clear discussion with these patients regarding data available to support the use of biosimilars.[32] The Crohn's and Colitis Foundation has developed a position statement related to the use of biosimilars in IBD.[33]

SAFETY OF ANTI–TUMOR NECROSIS FACTOR THERAPY

Early in the anti-TNF therapy trials it was identified that this mechanism of treatment is associated with a variety of infections, including opportunistic infections with bacteria, fungi and, importantly, reactivation of latent tuberculosis or chronic hepatitis B. Through clinical trials and observational cohort registries such as the large postmarketing TREAT registry, there are extensive data regarding the safety of anti-TNF therapies. Infections are one of the most closely linked adverse effects with anti-TNF therapies. From these studies, many bacterial infections are minor and can be easily treated with antibiotics. However, patients are also at a risk of developing serious bacterial, viral, or opportunistic infections. If patients develop serious infections, withdrawal of the anti-TNF is required. Vigilance with these patients is extremely important to carefully monitor for infectious symptoms and also obtain age-appropriate vaccinations to prevent vaccine-preventable infections.[34]

A drug-induced lupoid reaction is another documented, though rarely occurring, adverse effect of anti-TNF therapy and is thought to be related to apoptosis and exposure of the adaptive immune system to nuclear proteins. Symptoms can be debilitating and sudden, but they are easily treatable with withdrawal of the anti-TNF therapy and use of limited dosing of corticosteroids. In addition, developing anti-TNF-induced lupus does not preclude these patients from restarting another anti-TNF after resolution of symptoms.[34]

Anti-TNF therapies are not associated with solid organ malignancies, with the exception of possibly melanoma, although the data supporting this association are limited. There have been conflicting data regarding increased risk of lymphoproliferative disorders with anti-TNF therapies. Although there has been a clear association between thiopurines and non-Hodgkin lymphoma (NHL), there are no conclusive data regarding anti-TNF therapy and the risk of NHL.[34] A large multicenter inception cohort study of pediatric IBD identified no malignancies in the children receiving anti-TNF monotherapy or anti-TNF therapy in combination with methotrexate, but confirmed an increased risk of lymphoma in children treated with thiopurines with or without anti-TNF therapy.[35] By contrast, a recent nationwide cohort study in France reported an increased risk of NHL in patients receiving anti-TNF therapy as monotherapy or in combination with immunomodulators.[36]

PHARMACOKINETICS OF ANTI–TUMOR NECROSIS FACTOR THERAPY AND APPROACH TO LOSS OF RESPONSE

Clinicians have learned a great deal about the pharmacokinetics of anti-TNF therapy, in part because of the necessity of maintaining and optimizing response in our patients. Monoclonal antibody biological therapies require parenteral delivery for 2 principal reasons: first, to bypass the stomach where these protein-based therapies might be denatured or "digested" and second, because the molecules are too large to allow for passive or active small-intestinal absorption. Infliximab is administered by an IV infusion, which allows a large volume of drug to be administered with rapid absorption rates. Adalimumab, certolizumab pegol, and golimumab are administered SC, whereby only small volumes can be administered with slower absorption rates. For example, adalimumab will have a peak concentration 5 days after the injection with a 64% bioavailability, compared with infliximab with 100% bioavailability and a peak serum concentration almost immediately after infusion. Therefore, compared with intravenous medications, SC medications require more frequent dosing.[37]

There are several factors that influence clearance of medications and some additional factors that are unique to monoclonal antibodies. Understanding the factors associated with decreased or increased clearance provides insight into how patients may lose response to therapy and has implications for how we can prevent such occurrences and optimize response rates. We now know that increased body mass index, male sex, elevated CRP, and low albumin are all associated with increased clearance of monoclonal antibodies and, therefore, increased risk for loss of response to therapy. One of the unique features of IBD that distinguishes it from other immune conditions in which monoclonal antibodies are used is that even moderate inflammation of the bowel may result in considerable intestinal protein loss and, therefore, increased clearance of monoclonal antibodies[3] (**Table 1**).

One of the earliest lessons of anti-TNF therapy use in IBD was the risk of immunogenicity and subsequent hypersensitivity reactions or loss of response. The AGA Guidelines on Therapeutic Drug Monitoring (TDM) in IBD have identified "target" troughs to be: infliximab ≥ 5 μg/mL, adalimumab ≥ 7 μg/mL, and certolizumab pegol ≥ 20 μg/mL.[38] There is insufficient evidence to establish a target trough for

Table 1 Factors affecting the pharmacokinetics of monoclonal antibodies		
	Impact on Pharmacokinetics	**Drug Level/Exposure**
Presence of antidrug antibodies	Decreases monoclonal antibodies Worsens clinical outcomes	Decreased
Concomitant immunomodulators	Increase monoclonal antibody levels Decrease clearance Improve clinical outcomes	Increased
Low albumin	Increases clearance Worsens clinical outcomes	Decreased
High baseline CRP	Increases clearance	Decreased
Increased body mass index	Increases clearance Worsens clinical outcomes	Decreased
Male sex	Increases clearance	Decreased

Adapted from Ordás I, Mould DR, Feagan BG, et al. Anti-TNF monoclonal antibodies in inflammatory bowel disease: pharmacokinetics-based dosing paradigms. Clin Pharmacol Ther 2012;91(4):635–646; with permission.

golimumab. Development of antidrug antibodies occurs when an immune reaction against this non-self protein takes place that can block drug activity and cause faster elimination of drug.[39] In the SONIC post hoc analysis, twice as many patients achieved steroid-free remission at week 26 with higher levels of infliximab on monotherapy compared with those on combination therapy with low infliximab levels.[40] This exemplifies the point that the ability to achieve target circulating drug levels is the key benefit of the combination therapy.

The annual risk of loss of response to infliximab and adalimumab, known as secondary nonresponse, has been reported as 17% and 24%, respectively.[41,42] This can be secondary to the development of immunogenicity or suboptimal dosing. The establishment of assays to detect drug levels and presence of antidrug antibodies for anti-TNF therapies has been so significant in the management of IBD that this concept is now widely accepted in standard of care.[43] Because of our understanding of the basic pharmacokinetics of anti-TNF therapies, there has been a great deal of clinical research in the area of TDM. This has mostly been helpful in the relationship of loss of response to anti-TNF therapy, whereby the measurement of serum drug level and the presence or absence of antibodies to drug inform decisions to dose intensify the existing drug, cycle to another drug within the same class of anti-TNF, or swap to a different mechanism of action (such as anti-integrin, small molecules, or even surgery).[44] Vande Casteele and colleagues[45] describe 4 possible combinations of anti-TNF drug concentrations and antidrug antibodies in secondary nonresponders and interpretations to help guide therapeutic decision making (**Fig. 1**).

Less clearly defined is the use of serum drug levels proactively to adjust therapy and prevent loss of response or enhance clinical response. There have been 2 prospective trials that attempted to demonstrate the utility of such an approach, both of which were negative in their short-term results.[46,47]

Proactive TDM is increasingly valuable to study for its potential drug and cost-effectiveness. In a single study of 285 patients with UC on infliximab, trough concentrations at week 14 were associated with significantly increased relapse-free survival and colectomy-free survival[48]; therefore, some clinicians recommend checking post-induction levels. The TAXIT study randomized patients induced with infliximab to maintenance phase dosing either based on drug concentration or by clinical activity.

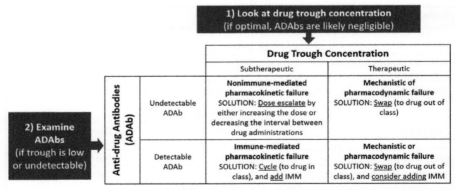

Fig. 1. Therapeutic drug monitoring in secondary loss of response with management strategies. (*Adapted from* Vande Casteele N, Herfarth H, Katz J, et al. American Gastroenterological Association institute technical review on the role of therapeutic drug monitoring in the management of inflammatory bowel diseases. Gastroenterology 2017;153(3):835–57; with permission.)

Dose escalation based on concentration led to better clinical and biochemical outcomes. In addition, this approach did not affect disease activity and reduced drug cost by 28%.[46] There is currently no consensus on proactive TDM although there are several ongoing studies to evaluate where this may fit into standard practice.

The reason this is more complicated is that serum drug levels only measure one component of the pharmacodynamic relationship. Missing from this assessment is measurement of tissue drug levels, stool drug levels and serum, and tissue or stool measurements of the target substrate (TNF). Until this complex relationship is fully understood reliable measures of this are available for clinical practice, the full interpretation and utility of proactive TDM will be subject to some debate and uncertainty.

WHAT WE DON'T KNOW AND YEARN TO KNOW

Although anti-TNF therapies have been tools in our IBD therapeutic armamentarium for more than 20 years, there are still many unanswered questions surrounding their use.

While we do know that patients with shorter disease duration are more likely to respond to anti-TNF therapy (as in the SONIC study and other studies such as REACH in pediatric CD[49]), we are in desperate need of better predictors of which patients will respond to anti-TNF therapy. This has become even more important now that there are other therapies with different mechanisms available and being developed for IBD. Attempts to develop genetic or serologic markers that are predictive of response or loss of response to anti-TNF have so far been limited in their clinical utility.[50] Better measures and clarification of serum, tissue, and stool levels of drug will be needed to understand the complete pharmacokinetic and pharmacodynamic properties of these biological therapies. The sequencing of therapies is a critically important issue and the most frequently asked question by our colleagues. Which anti-TNF treatment (IV or SC) should be used first? If a patient is a primary nonresponder to an injectable anti-TNF (adalimumab, certolizumab pegol, or golimumab), is there utility in providing the IV anti-TNF (infliximab)? Does exposure to an anti-TNF therapy in the first line change the physiology of the disease such that subsequent mechanisms of treatment are less likely to be effective, or is this just a function of "selecting" patients who are more refractory to the disease by the time they get to another treatment mechanism?

Second, we need to understand further the role of combination therapy with anti-TNF treatments. This should include more studies on the use of TDM to predict safe withdrawal of concomitant immunomodulators and additional studies evaluating the combination of other biologics or small-molecule therapies with anti-TNF treatments. The novel small-molecule therapies in development will offer new possibilities of multimechanism control of IBD.

Third, we need to understand the possibilities of proactive escalation or de-escalation of therapy. The general principles of proactive TDM make some sense but have not yet been proved. Given the earlier use of anti-TNF therapies in some treatment strategies now, it is possible to consider that after early aggressive control of the disease is achieved, a step-down or de-escalation strategy may have both physiologic and safety benefits. It is important to define how this might be done safely and appropriately, and how patients might be monitored after such an adjustment to their treatment is made.

Fourth, we should continue to explore the possibilities of restarting anti-TNF after drug holidays. This is important in the patient who has an intentional or unintentional interruption of therapy, and has been shown to be possible, with the use of TDM as a means to predict response and immunogenicity.[51] It is also of interest in patients who have lost response to their anti-TNF therapy, have been treated with other mechanisms of management (such as anti-integrin therapy), but have an insufficient response to this other mechanism or now lose response to this therapy. "Pedaling backward" is a concept of going back to the TNF mechanism of treatment and is a concept worth further investigation. Anecdotally this strategy has been effective.

Lastly, more work is needed to understand the real-world safety and tolerability of switching to biosimilars. As cost of therapy will continue to drive treatment availability, it is anticipated that patients will be forced to switch more than once between multiple biosimilar anti-TNF treatments. Although the early investigation of anti-TNF treatments appears safe, it is unclear whether patients will be put at risk for loss of response, immunogenicity, or hypersensitivity reactions with multiple switches and the possible delays in delivery of therapy that might ensue.

The discovery of anti-TNF therapy as a treatment for IBD was a revolution in the management of IBD, and has ushered in an era of biological therapies that have changed the natural history of these diseases. By understanding the anti-TNF treatments, we have learned a tremendous amount about the immune system, immunogenicity, biosilimarity, and TDM. The next evolution in these therapies will be defined by advances in our understanding of the pathogenesis of different types of IBD, prediction of response, and sequencing of therapies.

REFERENCES

1. Sofia MA, Rubin DT. Current approaches for optimizing the benefit of biologic therapy in ulcerative colitis. Therap Adv Gastroenterol 2016;9(4):548–59.
2. Hommes D, Baert F, van Assche G, et al. Management of recent onset Crohn's disease: a controlled, randomized trial comparing step-up and top-down therapy. Gastroenterology 2005;129(1):371.
3. Feldmann M. Development of anti-TNF therapy for rheumatoid arthritis. Nat Rev Immunol 2002;2(5):364–71.
4. Baert F, Noman M, Vermeire S, et al. Influence of immunogenicity on the long-term efficacy of infliximab in Crohn's disease. N Engl J Med 2003;348(7):601–8.
5. Targan SR, Hanauer SB, van Deventer SJ, et al. A short-term study of chimeric monoclonal antibody cA2 to tumor necrosis factor alpha for Crohn's disease. Crohn's Disease cA2 Study Group. N Engl J Med 1997;337(15):1029–35.
6. Hanauer SB, Feagan BG, Lichtenstein GR, et al. Maintenance infliximab for Crohn's disease: the ACCENT I randomised trial. Lancet 2002;359(9317):1541–9.
7. Sands BE, Anderson FH, Bernstein CN, et al. Infliximab maintenance therapy for fistulizing Crohn's disease. N Engl J Med 2004;350(9):876–85.
8. Present DH, Rutgeerts P, Targan S, et al. Infliximab for the treatment of fistulas in patients with Crohn's disease. N Engl J Med 1999;340(18):1398–405.
9. Rutgeerts P, Sandborn WJ, Feagan BG, et al. Infliximab for induction and maintenance therapy for ulcerative colitis. N Engl J Med 2005;353(23):2462–76.
10. Sandborn WJ, Rutgeerts P, Feagan BG, et al. Colectomy rate comparison after treatment of ulcerative colitis with placebo or infliximab. Gastroenterology 2009; 137(4):1250–60.
11. Colombel JF, Sandborn WJ, Reinisch W, et al. Infliximab, azathioprine, or combination therapy for Crohn's disease. N Engl J Med 2010;362(15):1383–95.
12. Colombel JF, Adedokun OJ, Gasink C, et al. Higher levels of infliximab may alleviate the need of azathioprine comedication in the treatment of patients with Crohn's disease: a sonic post HOC analysis. Gastroenterology 2017;152(5): S37–8.

13. Panaccione R, Ghosh S, Middleton S, et al. Combination therapy with infliximab and azathioprine is superior to monotherapy with either agent in ulcerative colitis. Gastroenterology 2014;146(2):392–400.e3.

14. Feagan BG, McDonald JWD, Panaccione R, et al. Methotrexate in combination with infliximab is no more effective than infliximab alone in patients with Crohn's disease. Gastroenterology 2014;146(3):681–8.e1.

15. Hanauer SB, Sandborn WJ, Rutgeerts P, et al. Human anti-tumor necrosis factor monoclonal antibody (adalimumab) in Crohn's disease: the CLASSIC-I Trial. Gastroenterology 2006;130(2):323–33.

16. Colombel J-F, Sandborn WJ, Rutgeerts P, et al. Adalimumab for maintenance of clinical response and remission in patients with Crohn's disease: the CHARM Trial. Gastroenterology 2007;132(1):52–65.

17. Sandborn WJ, Rutgeerts P, Enns R, et al. Adalimumab induction therapy for Crohn disease previously treated with infliximab: a randomized trial. Ann Intern Med 2007;146(12):829–38.

18. Rutgeerts P, Van Assche G, Sandborn WJ, et al. Adalimumab induces and maintains mucosal healing in patients with Crohn's disease: data from the EXTEND trial. Gastroenterology 2012;142(5):1102–11.e2.

19. Colombel J-F, Schwartz DA, Sandborn WJ, et al. Adalimumab for the treatment of fistulas in patients with Crohn's disease. Gut 2009;58(7):940–8.

20. Reinisch W, Sandborn WJ, Hommes DW, et al. Adalimumab for induction of clinical remission in moderately to severely active ulcerative colitis: results of a randomised controlled trial. Gut 2011;60(6):780–7.

21. Sandborn WJ, van Assche G, Reinisch W, et al. Adalimumab induces and maintains clinical remission in patients with moderate-to-severe ulcerative colitis. Gastroenterology 2012;142(2):257–65.e3.

22. Côté-Daigneault J, Bouin M, Lahaie R, et al. Biologics in inflammatory bowel disease: what are the data? United European Gastroenterol J 2015;3(5):419–28.

23. Khanna R, Bressler B, Levesque BG, et al. Early combined immunosuppression for the management of Crohn's disease (REACT): a cluster randomised controlled trial. Lancet 2015;386(10006):1825–34.

24. Jones JL, Kaplan GG, Peyrin-Biroulet L, et al. Effects of concomitant immunomodulator therapy on efficacy and safety of anti-tumor necrosis factor therapy for Crohn's disease: a meta-analysis of placebo-controlled trials. Clin Gastroenterol Hepatol 2015;13(13):2233–40.e1-2.

25. Sandborn WJ, Feagan BG, Stoinov S, et al. Certolizumab pegol for the treatment of Crohn's disease. N Engl J Med 2007;357(3):228–38.

26. Schreiber S, Khaliq-Kareemi M, Lawrance IC, et al. Maintenance therapy with certolizumab pegol for Crohn's disease. N Engl J Med 2007;357(3):239–50.

27. Sandborn WJ, Abreu MT, D'Haens G, et al. Certolizumab pegol in patients with moderate to severe Crohn's disease and secondary failure to infliximab. Clin Gastroenterol Hepatol 2010;8(8):688–95.e2.

28. Sandborn WJ, Feagan BG, Marano C, et al. Subcutaneous golimumab induces clinical response and remission in patients with moderate-to-severe ulcerative colitis. Gastroenterology 2014;146(1):85–95.

29. Sandborn WJ, Feagan BG, Marano C, et al. Subcutaneous golimumab maintains clinical response in patients with moderate-to-severe ulcerative colitis. Gastroenterology 2014;146(1):96–109.e1.

30. Regueiro M, Schraut W, Baidoo L, et al. Infliximab prevents Crohn's disease recurrence after ileal resection. Gastroenterology 2009;136(2):441–50.e1.

31. De Cruz P, Kamm MA, Hamilton AL, et al. Crohn's disease management after intestinal resection: a randomised trial. Lancet 2015;385(9976):1406–17.

32. Raffals LE, Nguyen GC, Rubin DT. Switching between biologics and biosimilars in inflammatory bowel disease. Clin Gastroenterol Hepatol 2018. https://doi.org/10.1016/j.cgh.2018.08.064.

33. Crohn's and Colitis Foundation. Biosimilars position statement. Available at: http://www.crohnscolitisfoundation.org/assets/pdfs/advocacy/biosimilars-statement-needs.pdf. Accessed February 22, 2019.

34. de Silva S, Devlin S, Panaccione R. Optimizing the safety of biologic therapy for IBD. Nat Rev Gastroenterol Hepatol 2010;7(2):93–101.

35. Hyams JS, Dubinsky MC, Baldassano RN, et al. Infliximab is not associated with increased risk of malignancy or hemophagocytic lymphohistiocytosis in pediatric patients with inflammatory bowel disease. Gastroenterology 2017;152(8):1901–14.e3.

36. Lemaitre M, Kirchgesner J, Rudnichi A, et al. Association between use of thiopurines or tumor necrosis factor antagonists alone or in combination and risk of lymphoma in patients with inflammatory bowel disease. JAMA 2017;318(17):1679–86.

37. Vande Casteele N, Gils A. Pharmacokinetics of anti-TNF monoclonal antibodies in inflammatory bowel disease: adding value to current practice. J Clin Pharmacol 2015;55(Suppl 3):S39–50.

38. Feuerstein JD, Nguyen GC, Kupfer SS, et al, American Gastroenterological Association Institute Clinical Guidelines Committee. American Gastroenterological Association institute guideline on therapeutic drug monitoring in inflammatory bowel disease. Gastroenterology 2017;153(3):827–34.

39. van Schouwenburg PA, Rispens T, Wolbink GJ. Immunogenicity of anti-TNF biologic therapies for rheumatoid arthritis. Nat Rev Rheumatol 2013;9(3):164–72.

40. Colombel J-F, Narula N, Peyrin-Biroulet L. Management strategies to improve outcomes of patients with inflammatory bowel diseases. Gastroenterology 2017;152(2):351–61.e5.

41. D'Haens GR, Panaccione R, Higgins PDR, et al. The London position statement of the World Congress of Gastroenterology on biological therapy for IBD with the European Crohn's and Colitis Organization: when to start, when to stop, which drug to choose, and how to predict response? Am J Gastroenterol 2011;106(2):199–212.

42. Gisbert JP, Panés J. Loss of response and requirement of infliximab dose intensification in Crohn's disease: a review. Am J Gastroenterol 2009;104(3):760–7.

43. Sofia MA, Rubin DT. The impact of therapeutic antibodies on the management of digestive diseases: history, current practice, and future directions. Dig Dis Sci 2017;62(4):833–42.

44. Yarur AJ, Rubin DT. Therapeutic drug monitoring of anti-tumor necrosis factor agents in patients with inflammatory bowel diseases. Inflamm Bowel Dis 2015;21(7):1709–18.

45. Vande Casteele N, Herfarth H, Katz J, et al. American Gastroenterological Association Institute technical review on the role of therapeutic drug monitoring in the management of inflammatory bowel diseases. Gastroenterology 2017;153(3):835–57.e6.

46. Vande Casteele N, Ferrante M, Van Assche G, et al. Trough concentrations of infliximab guide dosing for patients with inflammatory bowel disease. Gastroenterology 2015;148(7):1320–9.e3.

47. D'Haens G, Vermeire S, Lambrecht G, et al. Increasing Infliximab dose based on symptoms, biomarkers, and serum drug concentrations does not increase clinical, endoscopic, and corticosteroid-free remission in patients with active luminal Crohn's disease. Gastroenterology 2018;154(5):1343–51.e1.
48. Arias MT, Vande Casteele N, Vermeire S, et al. A panel to predict long-term outcome of infliximab therapy for patients with ulcerative colitis. Clin Gastroenterol Hepatol 2015;13(3):531–8.
49. Hyams J, Crandall W, Kugathasan S, et al. Induction and maintenance infliximab therapy for the treatment of moderate-to-severe Crohn's disease in children. Gastroenterology 2007;132(3):863–73.
50. Dideberg V, Théâtre E, Farnir F, et al. The TNF/ADAM 17 system: implication of an ADAM 17 haplotype in the clinical response to infliximab in Crohn's disease. Pharmacogenet Genomics 2006;16(10):727–34.
51. Baert F, Drobne D, Gils A, et al. Early trough levels and antibodies to infliximab predict safety and success of reinitiation of infliximab therapy. Clin Gastroenterol Hepatol 2014;12(9):1474–81.e2.

Treat-to-Target in Inflammatory Bowel Diseases, What Is the Target and How Do We Treat?

Manasi Agrawal, MD[a],*, Jean-Frederic Colombel, MD[b]

KEYWORDS

- Crohn's disease • Inflammatory bowel diseases • Long-term outcomes
- Treat-to-target • Ulcerative colitis

KEY POINTS

- Inflammatory bowel diseases (IBD), including Crohn's disease (CD) and ulcerative colitis (UC), are chronic, progressive, immune-mediated inflammatory diseases of the gastrointestinal tract.
- Unless adequate and timely treatment is instituted, IBD can lead to accumulative intestinal injury, complications, and disability.
- Early therapy using a treat-to-target (T2T) approach, which implies identification of a predefined target, followed by optimization of therapy and regular monitoring until the goal is achieved, is critical in preventing adverse long-term outcomes.
- In this review, the authors discuss the T2T guidance developed by the Selecting Therapeutic Targets in Inflammatory Bowel Disease committee, new evidence published on the role of various targets in CD and UC, as well as the real-world applicability of T2T.

INTRODUCTION

Inflammatory bowel diseases (IBD), including Crohn's disease (CD) and ulcerative colitis (UC), are relapsing and remitting immune-mediated inflammatory diseases that primarily affect the gastrointestinal tract.[1,2] In the absence of timely and effective treatment, progressive and accumulative intestinal injury can lead to complications such as strictures, fistulae, loss of bowel function, surgery and cancer, and resultant disability.[1,2] Approximately half of all patients with CD require surgery within 10 years and one-third require multiple surgeries.[3] Symptomatic CD recurs in half of the

[a] Division of Gastroenterology, Lenox Hill Hospital, Northwell Health, 100 East 77th Street, New York, NY 10075, USA; [b] Division of Gastroenterology, Icahn School of Medicine at Mount Sinai, 1428 Madison Avenue, New York, NY 10029, USA
* Corresponding author.
E-mail address: magrawal1@northwell.edu

Gastrointest Endoscopy Clin N Am 29 (2019) 421–436
https://doi.org/10.1016/j.giec.2019.02.004
1052-5157/19/© 2019 Elsevier Inc. All rights reserved.

patients after surgery.[4] Perianal disease, which occurs in nearly one-fourth of patients with CD, carries a higher risk of hospitalization and surgery.[5] Similarly, almost half of all patients with UC will require hospitalization during the disease course and 10% to 15% will require surgery within the first decade of diagnosis.[6] Even after colectomy, complications occur in one-third of patients with UC.[7] Postcolectomy CD can occur as well. In a retrospective study of 238 patients, postcolectomy CD was diagnosed in up to 7% of patients.[8] The goals of therapy have thus evolved from mere control of symptoms and improved quality of life (QoL) toward prevention of disease progression, bowel damage, surgery, and disability. In order to reach these goals therapeutic strategies have evolved with the three pillars of optimal care being early intervention, treat-to-target (T2T), and tight control.

WHAT IS TREAT-TO-TARGET ?

The T2T concept in IBD was developed by the Selecting Therapeutic Targets in Inflammatory Bowel Disease (STRIDE) committee, a group of international IBD experts established by the International Organization for the Study of Inflammatory Bowel Diseases in April 2015.[9] T2T implies identification of a predefined goal, or target, to be achieved with therapy, followed by optimization of therapy and regular monitoring until the goal is achieved, in consultation with the patient and in the context of the patient's individual needs (**Fig. 1**). This concept is modeled after T2T in rheumatoid arthritis and diabetes, in which predefined end points are targeted with therapeutic algorithms and reassessed at predefined intervals along with adjustment of therapy based on response for improved patient outcomes.[10–12]

STRIDE RECOMMENDATIONS

The guidance developed by STRIDE is a major landmark in IBD therapy.[9] It represents a paradigm shift in our understanding of IBD and prioritizes prevention of adverse long-term outcomes over symptomatic relief alone. The STRIDE recommendations for CD and UC are summarized in **Fig. 2**A, B, respectively.

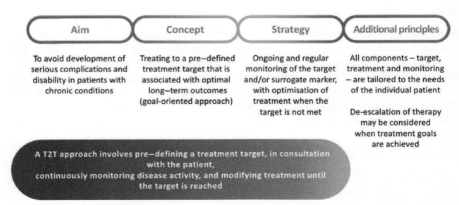

Fig. 1. The concept of T2T in IBD. (*Adapted from* Bouguen G, Levesque BG, Feagan BG, et al. Treat to target: a proposed new paradigm for the management of Crohn's disease. Clin Gastroenterol Hepatol 2015;13:1042–50; and McCloskey EV, Suarez-Almazor ME. Improving treatment adherence in patients with rheumatoid arthritis: what are the options? Int J Clin Rheumatol 2015;10:1–4; with permission.)

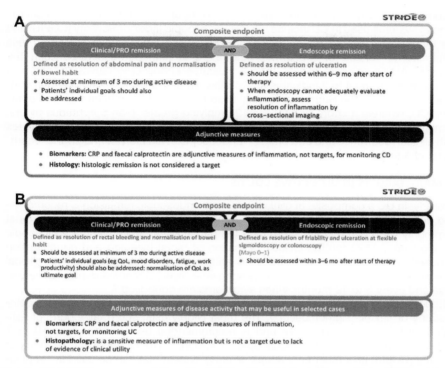

Fig. 2. (*A*) STRIDE recommendations for T2T in CD. CRP, C-reactive protein; PRO, patient-reported outcome. (*B*) STRIDE recommendations for T2T in ulcerative colitis. CRP, C-reactive protein;PRO, patient-reported outcome. (*Adapted from* Peyrin-Biroulet L, Sandborn W, Sands BE, et al. Selecting therapeutic targets in inflammatory bowel disease (STRIDE): determining therapeutic goals for treat-to-target. Am J Gastroenterol 2015;110(9):1324–38; with permission.)

PRIMARY TARGETS IN CROHN'S DISEASE

CD targets include a composite end point of clinical and endoscopic remission and restoration of QoL. In addition, given the diversity of CD symptoms, individual needs of each patient should be evaluated and appropriately targeted. Clinical remission can be evaluated using the CD activity index (CDAI), a validated tool widely used in IBD trials.[13,14] Other tools with high uptake in clinical practice include the Harvey-Bradshaw index and in children, the pediatric CDAI.[15–17] Patient-reported outcomes (PROs) are a set of symptoms derived from qualitative patient interviews, deemed reliable and responsive to change, and recognized by the Food and Drug Administration (FDA) as important clinical trial end points.[18] Abdominal pain and bowel frequency are PROs derived from the CDAI, in accordance with FDA guidance, and are increasingly being used as end-points in clinical trials.[19] Therefore, resolution of abdominal pain and normalization of bowel movements are recommended as clinical/PRO targets in CD. Symptom assessment is recommended every 3 months during active disease and every 6 to 12 months after symptom resolution.[9]

Endoscopic remission was defined by the STRIDE committee as resolution of ulceration.[9] For lesions that cannot be assessed adequately via ileocolonoscopy or other endoscopic procedures, or for perianal disease, cross-sectional imaging is recommended to determine the severity and extent of inflammation. The endoscopic scoring systems used in CD include the CD Endoscopic Index of Severity (CDEIS) and the Simple Endoscopic Score for CD (SES-CD); the latter is a simpler and less cumbersome version of the former and there is high correlation between the two.[20,21] A CDEIS score of less than 3 indicates endoscopic remission, score of greater than or equal to 3 indicates active disease, and decrease by more than 5 indicates response. The Rutgeerts score is used to evaluate the patient with postoperative CD, wherein a score greater than 2, implying greater than 5 aphthous ulcers, demonstrates CD recurrence.[22] Although this score is not validated, it correlates with clinical recurrence and outcomes.[23] Endoscopic evaluation (or imaging) is recommended 6 to 9 months after starting therapy.[9]

PRIMARY TARGETS IN ULCERATIVE COLITIS

Similarly, in UC a composite of clinical/PRO and endoscopic remission is recommended, followed by normalization of QoL.[9] Although the clinical assessment tool most commonly used is the Mayo score (and the partial Mayo score without endoscopic component),[24] PRO targets include cessation of rectal bleeding and normalization of bowel movements. Similar to CD, PRO end points are recommended over clinical assessment tools. Clinical evaluation is suggested every 3 months during active disease and every 6 to 12 months when symptoms are controlled.[9]

Endoscopic remission implies resolution of mucosal friability or ulceration on colonoscopy or flexible sigmoidoscopy. The most widely used score, although not validated, is the Mayo clinic score and is recommended by STRIDE.[9] Mayo 0 or 1 disease is considered to be endoscopic remission.[24] The UC endoscopic index of severity (UCEIS) is another endoscopic scoring system that can be used in conjunction with the Mayo score.[25] Endoscopic remission should be assessed in 3 to 6 months after initiation of therapy.[9]

For both CD and UC, therapy should be tailored to the individual patient to ensure that it is in keeping with the patients' goals. In early disease, the goal of therapy is to ensure complete resolution of symptoms, restoration of QoL as well as prevention of disease progression, complications, and disability. In advanced disease, when injury and disease progression have occurred, control of symptoms and minimization of disability are the primary goals.[9]

ADJUNCTIVE TARGETS

Biochemical targets (C-reactive protein [CRP] or fecal calprotectin [FC]) were not recommended by STRIDE as primary T2T end points due to lack of sufficient evidence in support of their use at the time the guidance was developed.[9] Rather, their use is recommended in both CD and UC to monitor disease course; persistent elevation of CRP or FC warrants further workup, regardless of symptoms.[9]

Histologic remission is not recommended as a target in CD due to lack of data on outcomes and validated histologic scoring system, as well as concerns of sampling error.[9] In UC, although there are more data on outcomes associated with histologic remission, these were not sufficient to demonstrate its clinical utility and it was not recommended by STRIDE as a target.[9]

Imaging targets are considered complementary to endoscopy in CD evaluation, especially if the diseased segment cannot be accessed, but not as primary targets.[9] Ultrasonography (US), computed tomography enterography (CTE), and magnetic resonance imaging (MRI) are equivalent with accuracy of greater than 80%.[26] Magnetic resonance index of activity (MaRIA) is the most established scoring system to determine temporal changes in CD activity.[26] Imaging modalities are not recommended for T2T in UC.[9]

THE PATH FORWARD

The STRIDE guidelines are a consensus of international IBD experts and have transformed the approach to a patient with IBD. However, the supporting evidence is from retrospective research and post-hoc analyses of randomized clinical trials.[27–32] Emerging prospective and trial data on long-term outcomes with T2T will enhance our understanding of T2T implications and help adjust the applicability of various targets in clinical practice. Key data that were published since the STRIDE guidelines are summarized in **Table 1**.

CROHN'S DISEASE
Clinical Targets

Although symptoms can be disparate depending on CD location, severity, and phenotype, abdominal pain and bowel habit continue to be the most significant and treatment-responsive PROs. Newer PRO tools, incorporating more clinical variables in accordance with FDA guidance, have been developed.[33,34] Their applicability and uptake in clinical care as well as clinical trials remain to be determined.

Restoration of QoL is recommended as the ultimate outcome; however, QoL is a subjective parameter and affected by several non-IBD factors. Disability, conversely, is an objective measure of loss of function, and it takes into account the impact of personal and contextual factors. The IBD disability index (IBD-DI) is a validated IBD-specific tool to measure disability, developed in accordance with the WHO International Classification of Functioning, and correlates with disease activity.[35] Future studies determine the impact of T2T on long-term disability and the role of IBD-DI as a target.

Fatigue is a highly prevalent symptom among patients with IBD, which correlates with disease activity, and has negative impact on QoL.[36,37] Validated objective tools to evaluate fatigue in IBD are needed in order to incorporate it as a PRO target.

The T2T model has been suggested in the management of iron deficiency in patients with IBD to improve outcomes, with normalization of ferritin and transferrin saturation as recommended targets.[38] The long-term impact of such a strategy is yet to be determined.

Endoscopic Targets

The most recent studies support the STRIDE recommendation to target endoscopic remission for improved long-term outcomes. In a systematic review and meta-analysis of 12 prospective cohorts of active patients with CD, endoscopic remission (or mucosal healing) on the first posttreatment endoscopy was associated with a higher likelihood of long-term clinical remission (pooled odds ratio [OR] 2.80, 95% confidence interval [CI], 1.91–4.10), maintenance of mucosal healing (14.30, 95% CI, 5.57–36.74), and lower risk of CD-related surgery (2.22, 95% CI, 0.86–5.69).[39] In a small cohort of children with newly diagnosed CD (n = 54), those who achieved complete mucosal healing (SES-CD 0) were more likely to have sustained remission for up to 3 years compared with those who had any evidence of active disease (8/16 [50%] versus 1/19 [6%], P = .005).[40] In the Randomized Evaluation of an Algorithm for Crohn's Treatment (REACT) study, although there was no difference in the primary outcome of steroid-free remission between the 2 groups that received early combined immunosuppression (ECI) (n = 22) and conventional therapy (n = 19), adverse

Table 1
Potential future targets for inflammatory bowel disease therapy

Target	Crohn's Disease	Ulcerative Colitis
Clinical	MIAH-CD CD-PRO/SS IBD-DI, validated fatigue tool	MIAH-UC UC-PRO/SS IBD-DI, validated fatigue tool
Endoscopic	Endoscopic index using pan-enteric capsule endoscopy, intestinal permeability index using confocal laser endomicroscopy	Endoscopic Mayo score and UCEIS of 0 (rather than ≤1), intestinal permeability index using confocal laser endomicroscopy
Histologic	Validated histologic index	Nancy index, RHI, intramucosal calprotectin
Biochemical	CRP, FC, ferritin, transferrin saturation, S100A12, high-mobility group box 1, neopterin, polymorphonuclear neutrophil elastase, hemoglobin, neopterin, alpha1-antitrypsin, human neutrophil peptides, neutrophil gelatinase-associated lipocalin and chitinase 3-like-1	FC, ferritin, transferrin saturation, S100A12, high-mobility group box 1, neopterin, polymorphonuclear neutrophil elastase, hemoglobin, alpha1-antitrypsin, human neutrophil peptides, neutrophil gelatinase-associated lipocalin and chitinase 3-like-1
Imaging	US indices, MRI index to assess smooth muscle hypertrophy and fibrosis	MaRIA, Nancy score, US indices

Abbreviations: CDEIS, CD endoscopic index of severity; CD-PRO/SS, CD patient-reported outcomes signs and symptoms; FC, fecal calprotectin; IBD-DI, IBD disability index; MIAH, monitor IBD at home questionnaire; RHI, Robarts histopathology index; UCEIS, UC endoscopic index of severity; UC-PRO/SS, ulcerative colitis patient-reported outcomes signs and symptoms; US, ultrasound.

outcomes such as surgery, hospitalization, or serious disease-related complications at 2 years were lower in the ECI group (hazard ratio [HR] 0·73, 95% CI 0·62–0·86, $P = 0·0003$).[41] The average disease duration among patients in this study was greater than 12 years, which is likely past the window of opportunity to prevent disease progression and complications. In addition, the use of clinical parameters, rather than objective markers of inflammation, as outcome measures could have affected the results of this study. The REACT2 study to determine the impact of therapy targeting clinical and endoscopic remission versus conventional therapy targeting clinical remission alone, using objective outcomes, is ongoing and will be crucial in determining the impact of T2T on long-term outcomes (ClinicalTrials.gov NCT01698307).[42]

Newer diagnostic modalities could affect T2T application in future. Accurate disease evaluation through the use of a single, safe test would be useful and minimize the risks and expenditure associated with endoscopies and imaging tests. Pan-enteric capsule endoscopy, which can evaluate the entire intestinal tract mucosa noninvasively in a single test, was studied in a small pediatric CD study (n = 48) and was found to be successful in T2T implementation; the rate of combined clinical and endoscopic remission increased from 21% at the start of the study, to 54% at week 24, and 58% at 52 weeks ($P<.05$ for all time-point comparisons).[43] However, its applicability would be limited to those patients with confirmed absence of strictures to minimize the risk of capsule retention as well as lack of perianal disease. Prospective studies comparing it with standard-of-care will be informative. Advanced endoscopic techniques, such as confocal laser endomicroscopy that measures intestinal permeability, could potentially provide accurate disease assessment and affect T2T strategies.[44]

Histologic Targets

There are very few data to support targeting histologic remission in CD. As described earlier, lack of a standardized and validated histologic scoring system to denote remission and risk of sampling error due to "skip" lesions in CD limit the applicability of histologic remission as a target for therapy. In the only study thus far on the impact of histologic remission on CD outcomes, on retrospective analysis of 101 patients' data, histologic remission was associated with a lower risk of clinical relapse compared with endoscopic remission (HR 1.85, 95% CI 1.00–3.44, P = .050).[45] Prospective research in this domain will provide more insight into the implications of histologic remission over endoscopic remission. Until then, histologic remission is unlikely to have a role as a target of CD therapy.

Biochemical Targets

Use of biomarkers to monitor disease activity has the advantage of being noninvasive and relatively inexpensive. Significant progress has been made since STRIDE recently in this regard. The CALM study is the first randomized trial to demonstrate that in patients with early CD (n = 244), therapy based on biochemical targets (CRP and FC) in addition to clinical targets (tight control) is associated with higher endoscopic remission at 1 year compared with therapy based on clinical targets alone (clinical management) (adjusted risk difference 16·1%, 95% CI 3·9–28·3; P = .010).[46] In addition, fewer CD-related hospitalizations occurred in the tight control arm compared with the clinical management arm (13.2 vs 28.0 events/100 patient-years; P = .021). Subsequent follow-up data on 122 patients for 3 additional years (range 0.05–6.26 years), of whom half were in the tight-control arm, revealed that endoscopic remission (adjusted hazard ratio [aHR] 0.44, 95% CI 0.20–0.96, P = .038) and combined endoscopic and clinical (deep) remission (aHR 0.25, 95% CI 0.09–0.72, P = .01) were significantly associated with lower risk of adverse events such as new internal fistula/abscess, stricture, perianal fistula/abscess, CD hospitalization, or CD surgery after adjusting for age, disease duration, prior surgery, prior stricture, and randomization arm.[47] These data support the STRIDE recommendation of combined endoscopic and clinical remission as the primary goal of therapy and escalation of therapy to ensure normalization of biochemical markers as we work our way toward the goal.

A wide array of additional biomarkers are being investigated in IBD and includes S100A12, high-mobility group box 1, neopterin, polymorphonuclear neutrophil elastase, hemoglobin, alpha1-antitrypsin, human neutrophil peptides, neutrophil gelatinase-associated lipocalin, and chitinase 3-like-1, with high diagnostic accuracy in early studies.[48] Future research will determine their role in T2T.

Imaging Targets

Since the publication of STRIDE guidelines, new retrospective and prospective data on CD outcomes with therapy targeting imaging-based resolution of inflammation have been reported. In a retrospective study of 150 patients observed over a median of 9 years, complete resolution of small bowel CD lesions on CTE or MRE was associated with decrease in hospitalization (HR, 0.28, 95% CI, 0.15–0.50) and surgery (HR, 0.34, 95% CI, 0.18–0.63).[49] Similarly, in a prospective study (n = 214), inactive disease on MRE was associated with lower rates of therapy escalation, hospitalization, and surgery at 1 year (OR 0.27, 95% CI 0.13–0.56, P = .001).[50]

US, although less widely used, is an important tool in assessing CD. In addition to being radiation-free and safe, it is inexpensive and widely available. IBD indices have been developed to assess CD severity incorporating parameters such as bowel wall thickness, Doppler signal, wall layer stratification, compressibility, peristalsis, haustrations, fatty wrapping, contrast enhancement, and strain pattern; improved indices incorporating stringent methodology are needed.[51] Although we await prospective randomized trials to clarify the role of imaging targets, imaging remains complementary to endoscopy for T2T especially when CD lesions cannot be accessed via endoscopy.

Recent data have demonstrated that smooth muscle hyperplasia and hypertrophy, rather than fibrosis, may be a primary pathologic pathway in small bowel strictures.[52] MRI can accurately quantify smooth muscle hypertrophy and distinguish it from predominant fibrosis.[53] This may have further implications in T2T, especially if outcomes associated with muscular hypertrophy versus fibrosis are found to be distinct. Furthermore, MRI may also be useful in determining the likelihood of response. In a prospective study of 30 patients, high wall stiffness before starting biological therapy was associated with lack of response and higher risk of surgery.[54]

ULCERATIVE COLITIS
Clinical Targets

Of the two PROs recommended by STRIDE, rectal bleeding is highly associated with endoscopic disease activity but altered stool frequency can occur among patients in endoscopic remission.[55,56] Conversely, normal stool frequency can be seen among patients with endoscopic evidence of active colitis.[55] Altered stool frequency in the absence of active inflammation can be due to underlying bowel damage or dysmotility in those with long-standing UC or coexisting irritable bowel syndrome.[57,58] The latter can occur in up to 27% of patients with long-standing UC.[57] Newer PRO tools, incorporating more clinical variables such as abdominal pain and urgency, have been developed and future studies will determine their utility in T2T.[33,59] Similar to CD, QoL, disability, fatigue, as well as iron deficiency are important clinical targets to be kept in mind while treating the UC patient.

Endoscopic Targets

Although endoscopic remission is a critical target of UC therapy, the scoring systems and criteria used to define it warrant revision. Updates in the endoscopic Mayo score incorporating disease extent correlate with clinical and endoscopic outcomes and may improve its accuracy and applicability.[60,61] There are new data to suggest that the UCEIS is accurate and responsive to change in ulcer size and depth, parameters that are not captured by the Mayo score.[62,63] These changes could improve the applicability of the Mayo score and UCEIS in endoscopic disease assessment. Although the STRIDE recommendations were to target a Mayo (or UCEIS) score of 1 or lower, a score of 0 is associated with lower risk of clinical relapse compared with a score of 1 (5.0% vs 9.4%, respectively).[62,64–66] Therefore, more stringent criteria to define remission are warranted. Randomized clinical trial data to determine long-term outcomes with endoscopic remission in UC are lacking and would be highly impactful in T2T application. Such data will clarify the benefits as well as risks of stepping up therapy to attain the more rigorous target of complete mucosal normalization.

Histologic Targets

Histologic remission, which implies resolution of inflammation on microscopic examination of colonic mucosa, was not recommended as a target by STRIDE due to lack of supporting evidence. Recent studies suggest that achieving histologic healing may have additional benefit in long-term outcomes over endoscopic remission. In a meta-analysis of 15 studies, the risk of UC exacerbation was lower with histologic remission compared with histologically active disease while in endoscopic and clinical remission (risk ratio = 0.81, 95% CI 0.70–0.94).[67] Presence of neutrophils in the epithelium is the primary histologic marker of active inflammation.[68] Obstacles to applying histologic remission as a target include lack of a uniform, validated histologic scoring system, wide interobserver variability, and microscopic heterogeneity.[69] Of the several scoring systems available to assess histology in UC, the Nancy index and the Robarts Histopathology Index (RHI) have undergone the most validation.[70] These have high concordance with clinical and endoscopic disease activity and fecal calprotectin levels.[68]

Newer diagnostic modalities, such as intramucosal calprotectin, that complement current histologic assessment could further affect the relevance of histologic remission as a target in future.[71]

Biochemical Targets

Similar to CD, data on utilization of biomarkers in T2T application in UC were limited and not recommended as primary targets by STRIDE. New data suggest that FC is highly sensitive for the detection of colonic inflammation, predictive of relapse, as well as response to therapy.[72–76] Among patients in clinical and endoscopic remission, higher FC is associated with risk of clinical relapse as well as histologically active disease.[68,72,73] It is dose-responsive; escalation of mesalamine therapy is associated with decrease in FC and FC greater than 200 mcg/g is associated with higher risk of clinical relapse.[74] It can also be followed longitudinally as it rises as early as 3 months before clinical relapse.[75] In a meta-analysis by Mosli and colleagues,[76] the optimal cut-off for FC was 50 mcg/g. Robust, long-term trials are needed to determine the role of FC in T2T, optimal FC threshold, and the impact of FC-based tight control on long-term outcomes.

As described earlier, additional biomarkers are being studied in monitoring of UC activity and seem to have high accuracy in early studies. Future research will determine their application in UC management.[47]

CRP and erythrocyte sedimentation rate, although historically used in the management of patients with IBD, have limited correlation with clinical, endoscopic, or histologic remission in UC.[77,78]

Imaging Targets

Imaging targets are not recommended by STRIDE in the evaluation and staging of UC, primarily a mucosal disease. With recently developed sensitive indices to evaluate the mucosa, MRI could have a role in UC management. MaRIA, an MRI index studied in patients with CD, has high sensitivity to detect mucosal lesions and could have applicability in UC.[26] The Nancy score, a diffusion-weighted MRI index, was found to be sensitive in assessment of mucosal healing in a small cohort of 29 patients with UC.[79] Similarly, UC activity and severity based on MRI colonography correlated strongly with endoscopic disease activity in a study of 50 patients.[80] Further studies to demonstrate long-term outcomes with therapy guided by MRI targets will determine its role in the management of patients with UC. Certainly, lack of invasiveness and radiation exposure renders MRI a safe and appealing diagnostic option.

Similar to CD, ultrasound indices have been developed for UC but require more stringent development and validation.[51] Progressive injury with long-standing active UC can lead to colonic dysmotility and loss of function.[58] Evaluation of colonic function and structure to assess degree of injury and perhaps fibrosis could become an important treatment variable in future.

REAL-WORLD APPLICABILITY OF TREAT-TO-TARGET

The T2T approach is intended for improved long-term outcomes and prevention of disease progression in patients with IBD, but certain more immediate factors can limit applicability and acceptance in clinical practice. Lack of structured T2T algorithms could impede uptake among community gastroenterologists. Increase in physician visits, laboratory testing, endoscopies as well as a lower threshold for biological therapy could deter both physicians and patients from T2T. In a retrospective study of 246 patients with UC in Southern Australia, only 35% were in combined clinical and endoscopic remission and the uptake of T2T by community gastroenterologists was limited.[81] In the Netherlands, 76% of gastroenterologists who responded to the survey indicated that they would target endoscopic remission.[82]

Regimented periodic testing and endoscopies to objectively evaluate inflammation, and upregulation of therapy if it is present, would involve shared decision-making and patient engagement, especially if they clinically feel well. The risks associated with stepping up biological or immunosuppressive medications are important considerations, especially in conjunction with age, comorbid conditions, and functional status. In the REACT and CALM studies, adverse effects were not greater with early biological therapy compared with conventional therapy.[28,41] One treatment approach does not fit all; personalization of therapy with risk stratification and shared decision-making are crucial. In this regard, randomized trials to demonstrate long-term benefits and safety of the T2T approach are critical to establish it as standard of care at the community level.

Demonstration of long-term cost-effectiveness of T2T will also have major implications in its real-world application. In a cost-effectiveness analysis (CEA) by Ananthakrishnan and colleagues,[83] infliximab therapy targeting endoscopic remission, or mucosal healing, was a cost-effective strategy compared with therapy targeting clinical remission, over a 2-year period. Similarly, a CEA using the CALM data, applied in the United Kingdom, demonstrated that the T2T approach in the tight-control arm was cost-effective compared with clinical management, especially in the long term and taking work productivity into account, and was associated with increase in quality-adjusted life years (QALY) (0.09 higher QALY with tight-control, 95% CI 0.16–0.03).[84] In UC, Saini and colleagues[85] studied the cost utility of mesalamine therapy from the payer's perspective in a Markov model of mild-to-moderate UC and determined that therapy based on inflammatory markers was most cost-effective. Long-term cost-effectiveness data with other biologics, in both CD and UC, and in different health care systems, will be highly instructive.

Mobile health tools in IBD are evolving and have the potential to improve T2T applicability while decreasing costs and improving patient convenience. Home monitoring indices for CD and UC, incorporating PROs and fecal calprotectin, have been developed and validated.[33,86] Such tools could improve wide T2T implementation, patient compliance as well as reduction of direct and indirect costs. Future studies will determine the impact of mobile technologies and telemedicine on T2T strategies.

SUMMARY

In summary, the T2T approach represents a critical change in the goals of and approach to IBD therapy. Although STRIDE guidance is a huge leap toward improved care for patients with IBD, there was limited evidence in its support. Reevaluation of the relative roles of recommended targets and revision of STRIDE guidelines are warranted in light of new prospective long-term data. Data in support of T2T continue to evolve and results from ongoing prospective trials will further clarify its long-term implications. Early, effective, and individualized therapy, T2T and tight control, in collaboration with the patient are critical for managing the patient with IBD and for prevention of long-term complications.

REFERENCES

1. Torres J, Mehandru S, Colombel JF, et al. Crohn's disease. Lancet 2017; 389(10080):1741–55.
2. Ungaro R, Mehandru S, Allen PB, et al. Ulcerative colitis. Lancet 2017; 389(10080):1756–70.
3. Cosnes J, Bourrier A, Nion-Larmurier I, et al. Factors affecting outcomes in Crohn's disease over 15 years. Gut 2012;61(8):1140–5.
4. Buisson A, Chevaux JB, Allen PB, et al. Review article: the natural history of post-operative Crohn's disease recurrence. Aliment Pharmacol Ther 2012;35(6): 625–33.
5. Zhao M, Lo BZS, Vester-Andersen MK, et al. A 10-year follow-up study of the natural history of perianal Crohn's disease in a Danish population-based inception cohort. Inflamm Bowel Dis 2018. [Epub ahead of print].
6. Fumery M, Singh S, Dulai PS, et al. Natural history of adult ulcerative colitis in population-based cohorts: a systematic review. Clin Gastroenterol Hepatol 2018;16(3):343–56.e3.
7. Peyrin-Biroulet L, Germain A, Patel AS, et al. Systematic review: outcomes and post-operative complications following colectomy for ulcerative colitis. Aliment Pharmacol Ther 2016;44(8):807–16.
8. Melmed GY, Fleshner PR, Bardakcioglu O, et al. Family history and serology predict Crohn's disease after ileal pouch-anal anastomosis for ulcerative colitis. Dis Colon Rectum 2008;51(1):100–8.
9. Peyrin-Biroulet L, Sandborn W, Sands BE, et al. Selecting therapeutic targets in inflammatory bowel disease (STRIDE): determining therapeutic goals for treat-to-target. Am J Gastroenterol 2015;110(9):1324–38.
10. Verschueren P, De Cock D, Corluy L, et al. Effectiveness of methotrexate with step-down glucocorticoid remission induction (COBRA Slim) versus other intensive treatment strategies for early rheumatoid arthritis in a treat-to-target approach: 1-year results of CareRA, a randomised pragmatic open-label superiority trial. Ann Rheum Dis 2017;76(3):511–20.
11. Paulshus Sundlisaeter N, Olsen IC, Aga AB, et al. Predictors of sustained remission in patients with early rheumatoid arthritis treated according to an aggressive treat-to-target protocol. Rheumatology (Oxford) 2018;57(11):2022–31.
12. Lingvay I, Perez Manghi F, Garcia-Hernandez P, et al. Effect of insulin glargine up-titration vs insulin degludec/liraglutide on glycated hemoglobin levels in patients with uncontrolled type 2 diabetes: the DUAL V randomized clinical trial. JAMA 2016;315(9):898–907.
13. Best WR, Becktel JM, Singleton JW, et al. Development of a Crohn's disease activity index. National Cooperative Crohn's Disease Study. Gastroenterology 1976; 70(3):439–44.
14. Thia KT, Sandborn WJ, Lewis JD, et al. Defining the optimal response criteria for the Crohn's disease activity index for induction studies in patients with mildly to moderately active Crohn's disease. Am J Gastroenterol 2008;103(12):3123–31.
15. Harvey RF, Bradshaw JM. A simple index of Crohn's-disease activity. Lancet 1980;1(8167):514.

16. Vermeire S, Schreiber S, Sandborn WJ, et al. Correlation between the Crohn's disease activity and Harvey-Bradshaw indices in assessing Crohn's disease severity. Clin Gastroenterol Hepatol 2010;8(4):357–63.

17. Hyams JS, Ferry GD, Mandel FS, et al. Development and validation of a pediatric Crohn's disease activity index. J Pediatr Gastroenterol Nutr 1991;12(4):439–47.

18. Levesque BG, Sandborn WJ, Ruel J, et al. Converging goals of treatment of inflammatory bowel disease from clinical trials and practice. Gastroenterology 2015;148(1):37–51.e1.

19. Khanna R, Zou G, D'Haens G, et al. A retrospective analysis: the development of patient reported outcome measures for the assessment of Crohn's disease activity. Aliment Pharmacol Ther 2015;41(1):77–86.

20. Mary JY, Modigliani R. Development and validation of an endoscopic index of the severity for Crohn's disease: a prospective multicentre study. Groupe d'Etudes Therapeutiques des Affections Inflammatoires du Tube Digestif (GETAID). Gut 1989;30(7):983–9.

21. Daperno M, D'Haens G, Van Assche G, et al. Development and validation of a new, simplified endoscopic activity score for Crohn's disease: the SES-CD. Gastrointest Endosc 2004;60(4):505–12.

22. Ferrante M, de Hertogh G, Hlavaty T, et al. The value of myenteric plexitis to predict early postoperative Crohn's disease recurrence. Gastroenterology 2006; 130(6):1595–606.

23. Rutgeerts P, Geboes K, Vantrappen G, et al. Predictability of the postoperative course of Crohn's disease. Gastroenterology 1990;99(4):956–63.

24. Schroeder KW, Tremaine WJ, Ilstrup DM. Coated oral 5-aminosalicylic acid therapy for mildly to moderately active ulcerative colitis. A randomized study. N Engl J Med 1987;317(26):1625–9.

25. Travis SP, Schnell D, Krzeski P, et al. Developing an instrument to assess the endoscopic severity of ulcerative colitis: the Ulcerative Colitis Endoscopic Index of Severity (UCEIS). Gut 2012;61(4):535–42.

26. Ordas I, Rimola J, Rodriguez S, et al. Accuracy of magnetic resonance enterography in assessing response to therapy and mucosal healing in patients with Crohn's disease. Gastroenterology 2014;146(2):374–82.e1.

27. Baert F, Moortgat L, Van Assche G, et al. Mucosal healing predicts sustained clinical remission in patients with early-stage Crohn's disease. Gastroenterology 2010;138(2):463–8 [quiz: e10–1].

28. Colombel JF, Rutgeerts P, Reinisch W, et al. Early mucosal healing with infliximab is associated with improved long-term clinical outcomes in ulcerative colitis. Gastroenterology 2011;141(4):1194–201.

29. D'Haens G, Baert F, van Assche G, et al. Early combined immunosuppression or conventional management in patients with newly diagnosed Crohn's disease: an open randomised trial. Lancet 2008;371(9613):660–7.

30. Neurath MF, Travis SP. Mucosal healing in inflammatory bowel diseases: a systematic review. Gut 2012;61(11):1619–35.

31. Rutgeerts P, Diamond RH, Bala M, et al. Scheduled maintenance treatment with infliximab is superior to episodic treatment for the healing of mucosal ulceration associated with Crohn's disease. Gastrointest Endosc 2006;63(3):433–42 [quiz: 64].

32. Schnitzler F, Fidder H, Ferrante M, et al. Mucosal healing predicts long-term outcome of maintenance therapy with infliximab in Crohn's disease. Inflamm Bowel Dis 2009;15(9):1295–301.

33. de Jong MJ, Roosen D, Degens J, et al. Development and validation of a patient-reported score to screen for mucosal inflammation in inflammatory bowel disease. J Crohns Colitis 2018. [Epub ahead of print].

34. Higgins PDR, Harding G, Leidy NK, et al. Development and validation of the Crohn's disease patient-reported outcomes signs and symptoms (CD-PRO/SS) diary. J Patient Rep Outcomes 2017;2(1):24.

35. Gower-Rousseau C, Sarter H, Savoye G, et al. Validation of the inflammatory bowel disease disability index in a population-based cohort. Gut 2017;66(4):588–96.

36. Huppertz-Hauss G, Hoivik ML, Jelsness-Jorgensen LP, et al. Fatigue in a population-based cohort of patients with inflammatory bowel disease 20 years after diagnosis: The IBSEN study. Scand J Gastroenterol 2017;52(3):351–8.

37. Cohen BL, Zoega H, Shah SA, et al. Fatigue is highly associated with poor health-related quality of life, disability and depression in newly-diagnosed patients with inflammatory bowel disease, independent of disease activity. Aliment Pharmacol Ther 2014;39(8):811–22.

38. Peyrin-Biroulet L, Lopez A, Cummings JRF, et al. Review article: treating-to-target for inflammatory bowel disease-associated anaemia. Aliment Pharmacol Ther 2018;48(6):610–7.

39. Shah SC, Colombel JF, Sands BE, et al. Systematic review with meta-analysis: mucosal healing is associated with improved long-term outcomes in Crohn's disease. Aliment Pharmacol Ther 2016;43(3):317–33.

40. Grover Z, Burgess C, Muir R, et al. Early mucosal healing with exclusive enteral nutrition is associated with improved outcomes in newly diagnosed children with luminal Crohn's disease. J Crohns Colitis 2016;10(10):1159–64.

41. Khanna R, Bressler B, Levesque BG, et al. Early combined immunosuppression for the management of Crohn's disease (REACT): a cluster randomised controlled trial. Lancet 2015;386(10006):1825–34.

42. Enhanced algorithm for Crohn's treatment incorporating early combination therapy (REACT2). Available at: https://clinicaltrials.gov/ct2/show/NCT01698307. Accessed October 23, 2018.

43. Oliva S, Aloi M, Viola F, et al. A treat to target strategy using panenteric capsule endoscopy in pediatric patients with Crohn's disease. Clin Gastroenterol Hepatol 2018. [Epub ahead of print].

44. Chang J, Leong RW, Wasinger VC, et al. Impaired intestinal permeability contributes to ongoing bowel symptoms in patients with inflammatory bowel disease and mucosal healing. Gastroenterology 2017;153(3):723–31.e1.

45. Christensen B, Erlich J, Gibson PR, et al. 603 - histological healing is associated with decreased clinical relapse in patients with ileal Crohn's disease. Gastroenterology 2018;154(6). S-128–S-129.

46. Colombel J-F, Panaccione R, Bossuyt P, et al. Effect of tight control management on Crohn's disease (CALM): a multicentre, randomised, controlled phase 3 trial. Lancet 2017;390(10114):2779–89.

47. Yzet C, Ungaro R, Bossuyt P, et al. OP35 Endoscopic and deep remission at 1 year prevents disease progression in early Crohn's disease: long-term data from CALM. Journal of Crohn's and Colitis 2019;13 (Supplement):S024–5.

48. Di Ruscio M, Vernia F, Ciccone A, et al. Surrogate fecal biomarkers in inflammatory bowel disease: rivals or complementary tools of fecal calprotectin? Inflamm Bowel Dis 2017;24(1):78–92.

49. Deepak P, Fletcher JG, Fidler JL, et al. Radiological response is associated with better long-term outcomes and is a potential treatment target in patients with small bowel Crohn's disease. Am J Gastroenterol 2016;111(7):997–1006.

50. Fernandes SR, Rodrigues RV, Bernardo S, et al. Transmural healing is associated with improved long-term outcomes of patients with Crohn's disease. Inflamm Bowel Dis 2017;23(8):1403–9.

51. Bots S, Nylund K, Lowenberg M, et al. Ultrasound for assessing disease activity in IBD patients: a systematic review of activity scores. J Crohns Colitis 2018; 12(8):920–9.

52. Chen W, Lu C, Hirota C, et al. Smooth muscle hyperplasia/hypertrophy is the most prominent histological change in Crohn's fibrostenosing bowel strictures: a semi-quantitative analysis by using a novel histological grading scheme. J Crohns Colitis 2017;11(1):92–104.

53. Wagner M, Ko HM, Chatterji M, et al. Magnetic resonance imaging predicts histopathological composition of ileal Crohn's disease. J Crohns Colitis 2018;12(6): 718–29.

54. Orlando S, Fraquelli M, Coletta M, et al. Ultrasound elasticity imaging predicts therapeutic outcomes of patients with Crohn's disease treated with anti-tumour necrosis factor antibodies. J Crohns Colitis 2018;12(1):63–70.

55. Colombel JF, Keir ME, Scherl A, et al. Discrepancies between patient-reported outcomes, and endoscopic and histological appearance in UC. Gut 2017; 66(12):2063–8.

56. Narula N, Alshahrani AA, Yuan Y, et al. Patient-reported outcomes and endoscopic appearance of ulcerative colitis: a systematic review and meta-analysis. Clin Gastroenterol Hepatol 2018;17(3):411–8.e3.

57. Henriksen M, Hoivik ML, Jelsness-Jorgensen LP, et al. Irritable bowel-like symptoms in ulcerative colitis are as common in patients in deep remission as in inflammation: results from a population-based study [the IBSEN Study]. J Crohns Colitis 2018;12(4):389–93.

58. Torres J, Billioud V, Sachar DB, et al. Ulcerative colitis as a progressive disease: the forgotten evidence. Inflamm Bowel Dis 2012;18(7):1356–63.

59. Higgins PDR, Harding G, Revicki DA, et al. Development and validation of the Ulcerative Colitis patient-reported outcomes signs and symptoms (UC-pro/SS) diary. J Patient Rep Outcomes 2017;2(1):26.

60. Lobaton T, Bessissow T, De Hertogh G, et al. The modified mayo endoscopic score (MMES): a new index for the assessment of extension and severity of endoscopic activity in ulcerative colitis patients. J Crohns Colitis 2015;9(10):846–52.

61. Balint A, Farkas K, Szepes Z, et al. How disease extent can be included in the endoscopic activity index of ulcerative colitis: the panMayo score, a promising scoring system. BMC Gastroenterol 2018;18(1):7.

62. Arai M, Naganuma M, Sugimoto S, et al. The ulcerative colitis endoscopic index of severity is useful to predict medium- to long-term prognosis in ulcerative colitis patients with clinical remission. J Crohns Colitis 2016;10(11):1303–9.

63. Ikeya K, Hanai H, Sugimoto K, et al. The ulcerative colitis endoscopic index of severity more accurately reflects clinical outcomes and long-term prognosis than the mayo endoscopic score. J Crohns Colitis 2016;10(3):286–95.

64. Barreiro-de Acosta M, Vallejo N, de la Iglesia D, et al. Evaluation of the risk of relapse in ulcerative colitis according to the degree of mucosal healing (Mayo 0 vs 1): a longitudinal cohort study. J Crohns Colitis 2016;10(1):13–9.

65. Boal Carvalho P, Dias de Castro F, Rosa B, et al. Mucosal healing in ulcerative colitis—when zero is better. J Crohns Colitis 2016;10(1):20–5.

66. Kim JH, Cheon JH, Park Y, et al. Effect of mucosal healing (Mayo 0) on clinical relapse in patients with ulcerative colitis in clinical remission. Scand J Gastroenterol 2016;51(9):1069–74.
67. Park S, Abdi T, Gentry M, et al. Histological disease activity as a predictor of clinical relapse among patients with ulcerative colitis: systematic review and meta-analysis. Am J Gastroenterol 2016;111(12):1692–701.
68. Magro F, Lopes J, Borralho P, et al. Comparison of different histological indexes in the assessment of UC activity and their accuracy regarding endoscopic outcomes and faecal calprotectin levels. Gut 2019;68(4):594–603.
69. Harpaz N, Ballentine S, Colombel JF, et al. Microscopic heterogeneity in ulcerative colitis: implications for microscopic measurement of disease activity. Gut 2019. [Epub ahead of print].
70. Mosli MH, Parker CE, Nelson SA, et al. Histologic scoring indices for evaluation of disease activity in ulcerative colitis. Cochrane Database Syst Rev 2017;(5):CD011256.
71. Guirgis M, Wendt E, Wang LM, et al. Beyond histological remission: intramucosal calprotectin as a potential predictor of outcomes in ulcerative colitis. J Crohns Colitis 2017;11(4):460–7.
72. Theede K, Holck S, Ibsen P, et al. Fecal calprotectin predicts relapse and histological mucosal healing in ulcerative colitis. Inflamm Bowel Dis 2016;22(5):1042–8.
73. Patel A, Panchal H, Dubinsky MC. Fecal calprotectin levels predict histological healing in ulcerative colitis. Inflamm Bowel Dis 2017;23(9):1600–4.
74. Osterman MT, Aberra FN, Cross R, et al. Mesalamine dose escalation reduces fecal calprotectin in patients with quiescent ulcerative colitis. Clin Gastroenterol Hepatol 2014;12(11):1887–93.e3.
75. Zhulina Y, Cao Y, Amcoff K, et al. The prognostic significance of faecal calprotectin in patients with inactive inflammatory bowel disease. Aliment Pharmacol Ther 2016;44(5):495–504.
76. Mosli MH, Zou G, Garg SK, et al. C-reactive protein, fecal calprotectin, and stool lactoferrin for detection of endoscopic activity in symptomatic inflammatory bowel disease patients: a systematic review and meta-analysis. Am J Gastroenterol 2015;110(6):802–19 [quiz: 20].
77. Alper A, Zhang L, Pashankar DS. Correlation of erythrocyte sedimentation rate and C-reactive protein with pediatric inflammatory bowel disease activity. J Pediatr Gastroenterol Nutr 2017;65(2):e25–7.
78. Miranda-Garcia P, Chaparro M, Gisbert JP. Correlation between serological biomarkers and endoscopic activity in patients with inflammatory bowel disease. Gastroenterol Hepatol 2016;39(8):508–15.
79. Laurent V, Naude S, Vuitton L, et al. Accuracy of diffusion-weighted magnetic resonance colonography in assessing mucosal healing and the treatment response in patients with ulcerative colitis. J Crohns Colitis 2017;11(6):716–23.
80. Ordas I, Rimola J, Garcia-Bosch O, et al. Diagnostic accuracy of magnetic resonance colonography for the evaluation of disease activity and severity in ulcerative colitis: a prospective study. Gut 2013;62(11):1566–72.
81. Bryant RV, Costello SP, Schoeman S, et al. Limited uptake of ulcerative colitis "treat-to-target" recommendations in real-world practice. J Gastroenterol Hepatol 2018;33(3):599–607.
82. Romkens TE, Gijsbers K, Kievit W, et al. Treatment targets in inflammatory bowel disease: current status in daily practice. J Gastrointest Liver Dis 2016;25(4):465–71.

83. Ananthakrishnan AN, Korzenik JR, Hur C. Can mucosal healing be a cost-effective endpoint for biologic therapy in Crohn's disease? A decision analysis. Inflamm Bowel Dis 2013;19(1):37–44.
84. Panaccione R, Colombel JF, Bossuyt P, et al. DOP065 Long-term cost-effectiveness of tight control for Crohn's disease with adalimumab-based treatment: economic evaluation beyond 48 weeks of CALM trial. J Crohns Colitis 2018;12(Supplement 1):O74–5.
85. Saini SD, Waljee AK, Higgins PD. Cost utility of inflammation-targeted therapy for patients with ulcerative colitis. Clin Gastroenterol Hepatol 2012;10(10):1143–51.
86. Van Deen WK, van der Meulen-de Jong AE, Parekh NK, et al. Development and validation of an inflammatory bowel diseases monitoring index for use with mobile health technologies. Clin Gastroenterol Hepatol 2016;14(12):1742–50.e7.

The Role of Histology in Determining Disease Activity, Treatment, and Prognosis: Are We There yet?

Mark S. Salem, MD, Gil Y. Melmed, MD, MS*

KEYWORDS

- Ulcerative colitis • Crohn's disease • Inflammatory bowel disease • Histology
- Prognosis

KEY POINTS

- Histologic activity has been associated with increased risk of clinical relapse, dysplasia, and adverse outcomes, irrespective of clinical activity or endoscopic appearance.
- Histology could serve as a sensitive marker of disease activity and response to therapy.
- There are several histologic indices in inflammatory bowel disease, although none has been fully validated and there remains no universally accepted definition for remission or healing.
- Histologic activity will serve as a future clinical trial endpoint and should be recognized in the evaluation of inflammation in patients with inflammatory bowel disease.

INTRODUCTION

Ulcerative colitis (UC) and Crohn's disease (CD) are chronic idiopathic systemic conditions characterized by immune-mediated inflammation of the gastrointestinal tract. Disease activity in both conditions can be assessed using clinical, endoscopic, and histologic indices. Historically, treatment has been focused on achieving clinical remission (CR); however, it has been well-established that underlying inflammation can persist despite symptoms, both endoscopically and histologically.[1]

Consensus guidelines from the Selecting Therapeutic Targets in Inflammatory Bowel Disease (STRIDE) program have been developed for treat-to-target strategies in patients with inflammatory bowel disease (IBD). For UC, the target is clinical/patient-reported outcome remission, defined as a resolution of rectal bleeding and diarrhea,

Disclosure statement: The authors have no relationships with commercial companies that have a direct financial interest in the subject matter.
Inflammatory Bowel Disease Center, Cedars-Sinai Medical Center, 8730 Alden Drive 2 East, Los Angeles, CA 90048, USA
* Corresponding author.
E-mail address: Gil.Melmed@cshs.org

as well as endoscopic remission (ER), defined as Mayo Endoscopic Subscore (MES) of 1 or less. In CD, both patient-reported outcome remission and ER, defined as a resolution of ulceration at ileocolonoscopy as well as resolution of findings on cross-sectional imaging in those that could not be adequately assessed with endoscopy, are considered treatment targets. Histologic remission (HR) is considered an adjunctive goal in UC, but was not recommended in CD as a target for treatment.[2]

Numerous histologic scoring systems have been devised to quantify inflammation from tissue samples taken at the time of ileocolonoscopy and can serve as a tool to determine response to therapy. The first histologic disease activity index used in clinical trials for IBD was the Truelove and Richards' Index, which was developed for UC in 1956 and demonstrated that 37% of patients with normal sigmoidoscopy had persistent histologic inflammation.[3] This observation has stood the test of time as more recent studies have estimated that 14% to 40% of patients will have persistent histologic disease with endoscopically normal mucosa.[4–6] In both conditions, biopsies are routinely used to make the initial diagnosis and screen for dysplasia; however, the role of histology in determining disease activity, treatment response, and prognosis is less clear.

HISTOLOGY IN DETERMINING DISEASE ACTIVITY

The definitions of active inflammation, mucosal healing (MH), histologic healing (HH), and HR are presented.

Active Inflammation

Ulcerative colitis
Histologic changes in UC demonstrate features of chronicity, including evidence of prior crypt destruction, crypt architectural distortion, atrophy in which crypts may not reach the muscularis mucosae, Paneth cell metaplasia, and a mucosal inflammatory infiltrate that is typically diffuse. Severe chronic inflammation in the lamina propria can include basal plasmacytosis, basal lymphoid aggregates, and fibrosis among other features.

Inflammatory changes are characteristically continuous, being maximal distally, although patchy inflammation can occur, especially after treatment. The mucosa is predominantly involved, although occasionally the submucosa can be involved in severe disease. Active disease is reflected by neutrophils within the crypt epithelium and crypt lumen, cryptitis and crypt abscesses, and erosions and ulcers. It can also include increased eosinophils within the lamina propria or eosinophilic infiltration within the crypt epithelium.[7–9]

Crohn's disease
CD is characterized by focal, often discontinuous, chronic active mucosal inflammation that includes a transmural lymphoid infiltrate in the most severe areas of mucosal inflammation. The earliest characteristic lesion found in CD is the aphthous ulcer, which is an endoscopically visible focal lesion typically ranging in size up to 3 mm surrounded by a halo of erythema, which represents immune activity. When located in the small intestine, they may arise over lymphoid aggregates with destruction of the overlying M cells and be associated with lymphoepithelial complexes in the colon. These aphthae are usually surrounded by normal mucosa, although villus blunting may be observed in the surrounding small intestinal mucosa. Histologically, crypt architectural distortion may be similar to UC, but noncaseating granulomas, when present, are virtually pathognomonic of CD. The granulomas associated with CD are characterized by collections of epithelioid histocytes and a mixture of lymphocytes, eosinophils, and

occasionally giant cells. There is no central necrosis involved and acid-fast stains are negative, which distinguish them from those associated with tuberculosis. Features of neuronal hyperplasia, muscular hypertrophy, and pyloric gland metaplasia can also be present.[7,9,10]

Mucosal Healing

As part of the STRIDE recommendations, MH was agreed on as the therapeutic goal in clinical practice for both UC and CD because it has been associated with better long-term outcomes in cohort studies as well as randomized controlled trials.[2] In 2007, the International Organization of Inflammatory Bowel Disease defined MH as the absence of friability, blood, erosions, and ulcers in all visualized segments of the gut mucosa, excluding HH from this definition.[11] In clinical trials assessing the efficacy of biologics in UC, MH has been defined as a MES of 1 or less, excluding HH.[12] Over time, this definition has come to signify ER with more recent emphasis placed on histology in the definition of true MH. In 2016, the US Food and Drug Administration issued draft guidance for endpoints in clinical trials in UC and stated that "a claim of mucosal healing would not be supported through endoscopy that provides only an assessment of the visual appearance of the mucosa. Any claim related to findings on endoscopy, in the absence of validated histologic assessment of the mucosa, would be limited to the endoscopic appearance of the mucosa."[13]

Histologic Healing

There is currently no universally accepted definition of HH and the terms "remission" and "healing" may be used interchangeably, although they are not synonymous. Healing could be defined as normalization of the mucosa, and remission could mean mucosa characterized by a resolution of the crypt architectural distortion and the acute and chronic inflammatory infiltrates with some features of sustained damage. The term "quiescent disease" is in contrast to "active inflammation," and has been used to describe mucosa showing features related to architectural damage and recovery in the absence of features of active inflammation.[8,14] Classic features of chronic quiescent disease include architectural distortion of the glands with occasional dropout of the glands, as well as Paneth cell metaplasia distal to the hepatic flexure where they do not normally reside.

Histologic Remission

Despite more than 60 years of clinical trials in IBD, no definition of HR has been validated. The International Organization of Inflammatory Bowel Disease defines HR as (a) the absence of neutrophils (both in the crypts and lamina propria), (b) the absence of basal plasma cells and ideally a reduction of lamina propria plasma cells to normal, and (c) normal numbers of lamina propria eosinophils.[7] Since the introduction of Truelove and Richards' initial histologic scoring system in patients with UC, several scoring indices have been developed to capture histologic activity and remission in IBD. Current STRIDE guidelines do not recommend HR as a target in CD owing to limitations such as sampling error, the segmental and transmural nature of inflammation, and the relative paucity of data for HH as a therapeutic endpoint. In the same consensus statement, histology was not recommended as a target in UC owing to a lack of evidence for clinical usefulness; however, it was considered important to acknowledge its role in the evaluation of inflammation in patients with UC.[2]

Validated scoring indices are required to capture the degree of histologic inflammation and response in therapy, particularly with gaining interest in the target of HH in clinical trials of IBD. Currently, there are approximately 30 proposed histologic indices in UC and 14 in CD, with no index yet fully validated.[15,16] In UC, the Geboes Score (GS), the Modified Riley Score, the Nancy Histologic Index, and the Roberts Histopathology Index are the most commonly used in clinical trials and have undergone partial validation.[17–21] In CD, the Global Histologic Disease Activity Score and the Naini and Cortina score are the most commonly used however neither has undergone validation.[22,23] A summary of the more common clinical indices is provided in **Table 1**, although a detailed analysis of each index is beyond the scope of this review. In clinical practice, a commonly used method to score disease activity in UC is the Histologic Activity Index, which grades inflammation as inactive/normal/quiescent (no epithelial infiltration by neutrophils), mild (<50% of the mucosa shows evidence of activity), moderate (>50% of mucosa with neutrophil infiltration), or severe (presence of surface erosion or ulceration).[24] Thus, mucosal neutrophils, or more specifically epithelial neutrophils, may be the most appropriate characteristic to use in the assessment of histologic status.

Because approximately 30% of patients with ER and CR have histologic activity, histology can serve as a sensitive marker of disease activity.[25] For histologic activity to serve as a meaningful endpoint in clinical practice, scoring indices will need to be validated that are feasible, reliable, and responsive to changes over time. In a study evaluating disease activity in biopsies collected in a phase II, placebo-controlled trial of ozanimod by 4 blinded pathologists using the GS, Modified Riley Score, Roberts Histopathology Index, and Nancy Histologic Index and a visual analogue scale, it was found that the interrater reliability of the histologic indices was substantial to almost perfect (intraclass correlation coefficients of >0.61). All 4 histologic indices were similarly reliable and responsive based on this dataset.[26] These results were derived from expert pathologists from different institutions, which supports the feasibility of scoring these indices in the context of multicenter research; however, it may limit the generalizability of the reliability and responsiveness in routine practice.

Furthermore, scoring indices will vary depending on the number, quality, and location of samples. This factor is particularly relevant to longitudinal studies looking at histology before and after a therapeutic intervention. In a cross-sectional study evaluating histologic activity in patients with UC with endoscopic and CR, 18 of 59 patients (30.5%) demonstrated active microscopic inflammation in at least 1 segment of the colon despite ER (defined as a MES of ≤1). Of the patients with active histologic inflammation without endoscopic inflammation, one-third (5 of 18) had histologic rectal sparing and active inflammation would have been overlooked without proximal biopsy specimens.[27] Although many clinical trials in UC use 2 samples from the most affected areas, some investigators have advocated for 2 biopsy samples from the rectum, sigmoid colon, descending colon, transverse colon, and right colon, regardless of endoscopic appearance.[28] Additionally, biopsy procurement protocols in CD may be even more prone to sampling error. It has been suggested that samples should be taken from the rectum, left colon, transverse colon, right colon, and terminal ileum with the degree of activity in each segment being assessed by the most involved sample.[29] Given the patchy distribution and potential for sampling error in CD as well as the differential distribution of healing, which may occur within the colon in UC, the optimal number of biopsies and location for biopsy procurement are needed to guide standardized practice.

HISTOLOGY IN DETERMINING TREATMENT RESPONSE

Although endoscopic healing has served as a widely accepted endpoint of therapy in IBD, the benefits of HH compared with ER/CR alone have been associated with lower

Table 1
Histologic scoring indices in IBD

IBD	Scoring System	Reference, Date	Histologic Features	Classification of Activity	HR[a]
UC					
	GS	Geboes et al,[17] 2000	(1) Architectural changes (2) chronic inflammatory infiltrate (3) lamina propria eosinophils (4) lamina propria neutrophils (5) epithelial neutrophils (6) crypt destruction (7) erosions or ulcerations	Six grades subdivided into 4 categories. Scoring from 0 to 5.4	0–1 (structural change only-chronic inflammation)
	RS	Riley et al,[18] 1991	(1) Presence of an acute inflammatory cell infiltrate (2) Crypt abscesses (3) mucin depletion (4) surface epithelial integrity (5) chronic inflammatory cell infiltrate (6) crypt architectural irregularities	Each histologic feature graded 0–3 (none, mild, moderate, severe)	Not defined
	MRS	Feagan etal,[19] 2005	Items derived from original RS responsive to changes in acute inflammation (neutrophils in epithelium, lamina propria neutrophils, erosion/ulcer)	Scores range from 0 (normal/inactive colitis) to 7 (severe acute inflammation)	Not defined
	NHI	Marchal-Bressenot et al,[20] 2017	(1) Chronic inflammatory cell infiltrate (2) acute inflammatory cell infiltrate (3) ulceration	Stepwise index ranging from 0 (no histologic significant disease)to 4 (severely active disease)	Grade 0–1
	RHI	Mosli et al,[21] 2017	Derived from GS; (1) chronic inflammatory cell infiltrate (2) lamina propria neutrophils (3)epithelial neutrophils (4)erosions or ulcerations	Each variable scored independently. The total sum ranges from 0 (no activity) to 33 (severe activity)	Score< 6
Crohn's disease					
	GHAS	D'Haens et al,[22] 1998	(1) Epithelial damage (2) architectural changes (3) infiltration of mononuclear cells in lamina propria (4) infiltration of neutrophils in lamina propria (5) neutrophils in epithelium (6) erosions/ulcers (7) granulomas (8) number of biopsy specimens affected	Each item scored Score ranges from 0–12	≤2
	NCS	Naini et al,[23] 2012	Architectural distortion, increased lymphocytes and plasma cells in lamina propria, neutrophilic inflammation including erosions/ulcers, granulomas	Ileal score ranges from 0–10, colonic score from 0–17. Developed initially to support diagnosis of IBD	Not defined

Abbreviations: GHAS, Global Histologic Disease Activity Score; MRS, Modified Riley Score; NCS, Naini and Cortina Score; NHI, Nancy Histologic Index; RHI, Roberts Histopathology Index; RS, Riley score.
[a] No definition of remission has been fully validated.

rates of relapse, hospitalization, need for surgery, and colorectal cancer.[2,12,30–32] Although disease activity is monitored clinically, ,endoscopically and histologically, these measures are known not to perfectly correlate. Patients in CR often have underlying endoscopic and/or histologic disease, and those with ER may have persistent symptoms.[1,33] Histology may serve as an ideal treatment target because it represents inflammation at the microscopic level. Bryant and colleagues[4] demonstrated the concordance between different definitions of remission in a cohort of 91 patients with UC and revealed that, of the patients in HR, 64% and 89% were in CR and ER, respectively. In those with ER, 54% and 75% were in CR and HR, respectively. In addition, approximately 10% of patients with endoscopically active disease will have no histologic activity on biopsy.[34] These results suggest that histology may be a more sensitive measure of disease activity and correlate better with endoscopic activity compared with clinical symptoms and may be useful for monitoring response to therapy.

One of the earliest studies incorporating histology as a treatment endpoint was by Truelove and Hambling in 1958, which demonstrated that patients with distal UC treated with rectal hydrocortisone demonstrated a significant trend toward "histologic mildness" compared with inert therapy.[35] More recent trials evaluating biologics have incorporated histologic indices as an outcome. In a study evaluating 20 patients with moderate to severe UC receiving infliximab, 45% of patients demonstrated endoscopic MH (MES of $\leq$1) with only 15% reaching HR (defined as a GS of <3.0) at 8 weeks. At week 52, 35% of patients reached HR.[36] Furthermore, in a study evaluating 41 UC patients from the GEMINI study, 55% of patients with endoscopic MH (MES of $\leq$1) also achieved HH (defined as a GS of 0–1).[37] This finding suggests that, despite achieving MH, many patients have persistent histologic abnormalities that may lead to rapid mucosal recurrence if maintenance therapy is not continued.

Studies evaluating HH/HR in CD are sparse as well. In a retrospective analysis of 252 patients (CD = 183, UC = 62, unclassified IBD = 7) receiving maintenance infliximab or adalimumab, 43% of the CD cohort and 62% of the UC cohort were found to be in deep remission (defined as CR and ER). Of the patients in deep remission, 81% were found to have histologically inactive disease, although no formal histologic scoring system was used.[38] In a post hoc analysis of a double-blinded, randomized, controlled trial of induction and maintenance adalimumab for patients with ileocolonic CD, HH (defined as a colonic global histologic disease activity score or ileal global histologic disease activity score of $\leq$2) was found in the colon (28.3%) and the ileum (21.2%) in patients treated with adalimumab versus 8.8% and 2.9% in the respective segments in the placebo-treated groups.[39]

These results suggest that HH/HR is only achieved in a minority of patients with IBD. If HR becomes a treatment target, additional therapies for a substantial number of patients would be needed. The STRIDE guidelines do not recommend HR as a therapeutic endpoint and state that a paradigm shift in clinical thinking is required to consider incorporating histopathology into routine patient management in the future.

HISTOLOGY IN DETERMINING PROGNOSIS

Early studies in UC by Wright and Truelove proposed that persistent histologic inflammation may be a better predictor of future clinical relapse than endoscopic appearances alone.[40] These initial observations remained consistent over time, with multiple studies using various histologic indices finding that persistent histologic activity is implicated with an increased risk of clinical relapse and that the resolution of histologic activity is associated with a reduction of hospitalization and colectomy rates.[7]

A recent metaanalysis evaluating 15 studies demonstrated that UC patients with HR demonstrated a 52% relative risk reduction in clinical relapse compared with those with histologic activity. The study also identified that approximately 30% of patients with CR/ER had persistent histologic activity, demonstrating the potential for histology to predict clinical outcomes.[25] Although different histologic indices were used in the individual studies, when any measure of mucosal neutrophils was assessed in the metaanalysis, an approximately 60 to 70% relative risk reduction in relapse/exacerbation were seen for patients without these histologic findings at baseline as compared with those with these findings.[25]

In a study evaluating the significance of achieving complete histologic normalization in 646 patients with UC, decreased rates of clinical relapse were observed when compared with both patients with histologic quiescent disease (hazard ratio, 4.31; $P = .007$) and those with histologic activity (hazard ratio, 6.69; $P = .001$). This study demonstrated the additive benefit of achieving complete histologic normalization in addition to eliminating mucosal neutrophils, although it should be noted that only 10% of the cohort achieved complete normalization.[41]

Studies evaluating the prognostic implication of histology in CD are less robust than in UC. In a single study including patients with CD, it was found that mucosal inflammation was not associated with more frequent clinical relapse, stricture formation, or surgery, although the cohort had a low prevalence of terminal ileitis and stricturing/fistulizing disease at baseline.[1] In a more recent study evaluating patients with CD in CR undergoing surveillance colonoscopy, histologic disease activity at baseline was more predictive of subsequent clinical flares within 1 to 2 years compared with patients without histologic activity; endoscopic activity was not predictive of subsequent flares. Only 2.4% of patients without histologic activity at baseline had a flare at 12 months in contrast with 25.5% of patients with histologic activity. An increase in eosinophils or neutrophils in the lamina propria and cryptitis were associated with higher flare rates.[42] Furthermore, there are conflicting data regarding the prognostic value of inflammation in surgical resection margins. Recent studies have demonstrated that submucosal and myenteric plexitis may be a predictive factor for postoperative recurrence.[43,44]

In addition to predicting clinical outcomes, histologic activity has been shown to be associated with the development of dysplasia in UC. In 1 case-control study evaluating 68 patients with IBD-associated dysplasia, only histologic activity was predictive of neoplasia in multivariate analysis (odds ratio, 4.69).[45] This was also observed in a cohort study of patients undergoing routine surveillance, where the mean histologic score (based on the Histologic Activity Index) correlated with the development of advanced neoplasia (high-grade dysplasia or colorectal cancer), although it did not reach statistical significance.[24] These findings were also observed in a metaanalysis evaluating 6 studies including 1443 patients and found that the presence of endoscopic or histologic inflammation as well as histologic inflammation alone increased the risk of subsequent colorectal neoplasia.[46]

HR has the potential to improve predictions for clinical outcomes when added to ER or CR. Future studies need to focus on whether altering management in response to histologic activity translates to improved outcomes.

SUMMARY

Histology can help to determine disease activity, treatment efficacy, and prognosis for both CD and UC, although the use of histology to guide clinical decisions is still limited. Histologic activity can be used in clinical practice to identify those who may have a greater risk of clinical relapse if maintenance treatment is decreased or discontinued, or in those where optimization of maintenance treatment is feasible. For example, it has been shown that serum drug concentrations may need to be higher to achieve histologic and endoscopic healing compared with endoscopic healing alone and could be optimized in those with persistent histologic activity.[47,48] To date there have been no randomized, controlled trials performed evaluating the efficacy of treatment optimization based on histologic activity. Prospective studies are needed to determine whether HH provides additional outcome benefits beyond endoscopic or CR and if it is cost effective. Although there are several existing histologic indices for both CD and UC, these will need further validation, because the US Food and Drug Administration has issued guidelines for more stringent definitions of MH in future clinical trials to also include histology.

REFERENCES

1. Baars JE, Nuij VJ, Oldenburg B, et al. Majority of patients with inflammatory bowel disease in clinical remission have mucosal inflammation. Inflamm Bowel Dis 2012;18(9):1634–40.
2. Peyrin-Biroulet L, Sandborn W, Sands BE, et al. Selecting Therapeutic Targets in Inflammatory Bowel Disease (STRIDE): determining therapeutic goals for treat-to-target. Am J Gastroenterol 2015;110(9):1324–38.
3. Truelove S, Richards W. Biopsy studies in ulcerative colitis. Br Med J 1956; 1(4979):1315–8.
4. Bryant RV, Burger DC, Delo J, et al. Beyond endoscopic mucosal healing in UC: histological remission better predicts corticosteroid use and hospitalisation over 6 years of follow-up. Gut 2016;65(3):408–14.
5. Zenlea T, Yee EU, Rosenberg L, et al. Histology grade is independently associated with relapse risk in patients with ulcerative colitis in clinical remission: a prospective study. Am J Gastroenterol 2016;111(5):685–90.
6. Bessissow T, Lemmens B, Ferrante M, et al. Prognostic value of serologic and histologic markers on clinical relapse in ulcerative colitis patients with mucosal healing. Am J Gastroenterol 2012;107(11):1684–92.
7. Bryant RV, Winer S, Travis SP, et al. Systematic review: histological remission in inflammatory bowel disease. Is 'complete' remission the new treatment paradigm? An IOIBD initiative. J Crohns Colitis 2014;8(12):1582–97.
8. Magro F, Langner C, Driessen A, et al. European consensus on the histopathology of inflammatory bowel disease. J Crohns Colitis 2013;7(10):827–51.
9. Patil DT, Moss AC, Odze RD. Role of histologic inflammation in the natural history of ulcerative colitis. Gastrointest Endosc Clin N Am 2016;26(4):629–40.
10. Feldman M, Friedman LS, Brandt LJ. Sleisenger and Fordtran's gastrointestinal and liver disease: pathophysiology, diagnosis, management. Amsterdam, The Netherlands: Elsevier Health Sciences; 2015.
11. D'Haens G, Sandborn WJ, Feagan BG, et al. A review of activity indices and efficacy end points for clinical trials of medical therapy in adults with ulcerative colitis. Gastroenterology 2007;132(2):763–86.
12. Colombel JF, Rutgeerts P, Reinisch W, et al. Early mucosal healing with infliximab is associated with improved long-term clinical outcomes in ulcerative colitis. Gastroenterology 2011;141(4):1194–201.
13. Administration. UFaD. Ulcerative colitis: clinical trial endpoints: guidance for industry 2016. Available at: https://www.fda.gov/downloads/Drugs/GuidanceComplianceRegulatoryInformation/ Guidances/UCM515143.pdf. Accessed October 24, 2018.

14. Marchal Bressenot A. Which evidence for a treat to target strategy in ulcerative colitis? Best Pract Res Clin Gastroenterol 2018;32-33:3–8.
15. Mosli MH, Parker CE, Nelson SA, et al. Histologic scoring indices for evaluation of disease activity in ulcerative colitis. Cochrane Database Syst Rev 2017;(5):CD011256.
16. Novak G, Parker CE, Pai RK, et al. Histologic scoring indices for evaluation of disease activity in Crohn's disease. Cochrane Database Syst Rev 2017;(7):CD012351.
17. Geboes K, Riddell R, Öst A, et al. A reproducible grading scale for histological assessment of inflammation in ulcerative colitis. Gut 2000;47(3):404–9.
18. Riley S, Mani V, Goodman M, et al. Microscopic activity in ulcerative colitis: what does it mean? Gut 1991;32(2):174–8.
19. Feagan BG, Greenberg GR, Wild G, et al. Treatment of ulcerative colitis with a humanized antibody to the α4β7 integrin. N Engl J Med 2005;352(24):2499–507.
20. Marchal-Bressenot A, Salleron J, Boulagnon-Rombi C, et al. Development and validation of the Nancy histological index for UC. Gut 2017;66(1):43–9.
21. Mosli MH, Feagan BG, Zou G, et al. Development and validation of a histological index for UC. Gut 2017;66(1):50–8.
22. D'haens G, Geboes K, Peeters M, et al. Early lesions of recurrent Crohn's disease caused by infusion of intestinal contents in excluded ileum. Gastroenterology 1998;114(2):262–7.
23. Naini BV, Cortina G. A histopathologic scoring system as a tool for standardized reporting of chronic (ileo) colitis and independent risk assessment for inflammatory bowel disease. Hum Pathol 2012;43(12):2187–96.
24. Gupta RB, Harpaz N, Itzkowitz S, et al. Histologic inflammation is a risk factor for progression to colorectal neoplasia in ulcerative colitis: a cohort study. Gastroenterology 2007;133(4):1099–105 [quiz: 1340–1].
25. Park S, Abdi T, Gentry M, et al. Histological disease activity as a predictor of clinical relapse among patients with ulcerative colitis: systematic review and meta-analysis. Am J Gastroenterol 2016;111(12):1692–701.
26. Jairath V, Peyrin-Biroulet L, Zou G, et al. Responsiveness of histological disease activity indices in ulcerative colitis: a post hoc analysis using data from the TOUCHSTONE randomised controlled trial. Gut 2018. [Epub ahead of print]. https://doi.org/10.1136/gutjnl-2018-316702.
27. Guardiola J, Lobaton T, Rodriguez-Alonso L, et al. Fecal level of calprotectin identifies histologic inflammation in patients with ulcerative colitis in clinical and endoscopic remission. Clin Gastroenterol Hepatol 2014;12(11):1865–70.
28. Marchal Bressenot A, Riddell RH, Boulagnon-Rombi C, et al. Review article: the histological assessment of disease activity in ulcerative colitis. Aliment Pharmacol Ther 2015;42(8):957–67.
29. Pai RK, Geboes K. Disease activity and mucosal healing in inflammatory bowel disease: a new role for histopathology? Virchows Arch 2018;472(1):99–110.
30. Baert F, Moortgat L, Van Assche G, et al. Mucosal healing predicts sustained clinical remission in patients with early-stage Crohn's disease. Gastroenterology 2010;138(2):463–8 [quiz: e10–1].
31. Shah SC, Colombel JF, Sands BE, et al. Systematic review with meta-analysis: mucosal healing is associated with improved long-term outcomes in Crohn's disease. Aliment Pharmacol Ther 2016;43(3):317–33.
32. Neurath MF, Travis SP. Mucosal healing in inflammatory bowel diseases: a systematic review. Gut 2012;61(1):1619–35.
33. Colombel JF, Keir ME, Scherl A, et al. Discrepancies between patient-reported outcomes, and endoscopic and histological appearance in UC. Gut 2017; 66(12):2063–8.

34. Kleer CG, Appelman HD. Ulcerative colitis: patterns of involvement in colorectal biopsies and changes with time. Am J Surg Pathol 1998;22(8):983–9.
35. Truelove SC, Hambling MH. Treatment of ulcerative colitis with local hydrocortisone hemisuccinate sodium; a report on a controlled therapeutic trial. Br Med J 1958;2(5104):1072–7.
36. Magro F, Lopes SI, Lopes J, et al. Histological outcomes and predictive value of faecal markers in moderately to severely active ulcerative colitis patients receiving infliximab. J Crohns Colitis 2016;10(12):1407–16.
37. Arijs I, De Hertogh G, Lemmens B, et al. Effect of vedolizumab (anti-alpha4beta7-integrin) therapy on histological healing and mucosal gene expression in patients with UC. Gut 2018;67(1):43–52.
38. Molander P, Sipponen T, Kemppainen H, et al. Achievement of deep remission during scheduled maintenance therapy with TNFalpha-blocking agents in IBD. J Crohns Colitis 2013;7(9):730–5.
39. Reinisch W, Colombel JF, D'Haens G, et al. Characterisation of mucosal healing with adalimumab treatment in patients with moderately to severely active Crohn's disease: results from the EXTEND trial. J Crohns Colitis 2017;11(4):425–34.
40. Wright R, Truelove S. Serial rectal biopsy in ulcerative colitis during the course of a controlled therapeutic trial of various diets. Am J Dig Dis 1966;11(11):847–57.
41. Christensen B, Hanauer SB, Erlich J, et al. Histologic normalization occurs in ulcerative colitis and is associated with improved clinical outcomes. Clin Gastroenterol Hepatol 2017;15(10):1557–64.e1.
42. Brennan GT, Melton SD, Spechler SJ, et al. Clinical implications of histologic abnormalities in ileocolonic biopsies of patients with Crohn's disease in remission. J Clin Gastroenterol 2017;51(1):43–8.
43. Lemmens B, de Buck van Overstraeten A, Arijs I, et al. Submucosal plexitis as a predictive factor for postoperative endoscopic recurrence in patients with Crohn's disease undergoing a resection with ileocolonic anastomosis: results from a prospective single-centre study. J Crohns Colitis 2017;11(2):212–20.
44. Decousus S, Boucher A-L, Joubert J, et al. Myenteric plexitis is a risk factor for endoscopic and clinical postoperative recurrence after ileocolonic resection in Crohn's disease. Dig Liver Dis 2016;48(7):753–8.
45. Rutter M, Saunders B, Wilkinson K, et al. Severity of inflammation is a risk factor for colorectal neoplasia in ulcerative colitis. Gastroenterology 2004;126(2):451–9.
46. Flores BM, O'Connor A, Moss AC. Impact of mucosal inflammation on risk of colorectal neoplasia in patients with ulcerative colitis: a systematic review and meta-analysis. Gastrointest Endosc 2017;86(6):1006–11.
47. Yarur AJ, Jain A, Hauenstein SI, et al. Higher adalimumab levels are associated with histologic and endoscopic remission in patients with Crohn's disease and ulcerative colitis. Inflamm Bowel Dis 2016;22(2):409–15.
48. Papamichael K, Rakowsky S, Rivera C, et al. Infliximab trough concentrations during maintenance therapy are associated with endoscopic and histologic healing in ulcerative colitis. Aliment Pharmacol Ther 2018;47(4):478–84.

The Role of the Radiologist in Determining Disease Severity in Inflammatory Bowel Diseases

Parakkal Deepak, MD, MS[a,1], Jordan E. Axelrad, MD, MPH[b,1],
Ashwin N. Ananthakrishnan, MD, MPH[c,*]

KEYWORDS

- Crohn's disease • Ulcerative colitis • MRE • CTE • Abscess • Fistula
- Inflammation • Strictures

KEY POINTS

- Cross-sectional imaging is an important component of evaluation of activity and severity of Crohn's disease and ulcerative colitis. It is useful in establishing a diagnosis, and is increasingly used to monitor therapeutic response and assess radiologic (and transmural healing).
- MR enterography and CT enterography studies are the most sensitive imaging modalities for detection of active inflammation with similarly high sensitivity and specificity. The former is preferred because of lack of radiation exposure, although the latter offers quicker imaging time and higher-resolution images that are less susceptible to motion artifact.
- Diffuse-weighted imaging (DWI) has emerged as a useful addition to standard MRI by improving the ability to detect active inflammation.
- Bowel ultrasonography evaluation may be useful as a point-of-care tool to detect inflammation and disease complications, but requires operator expertise and has a variable performance.

Disclosure statement: P. Deepak has received consulting fees from Janssen and Pfizer, Speaker fees from Abbvie, and has received research support from Takeda. A.N. Ananthakrishnan has served on scientific advisory boards for Abbvie, Takeda, Gilead, and Merck, and has received research support from Pfizer.

[a] Division of Gastroenterology, John T. Milliken Department of Medicine, Washington University School of Medicine, 600 South Euclid Avenue, Campus Box 8124, St. Louis, MO 63110, USA; [b] Division of Gastroenterology, NYU Langone Health, Inflammatory Bowel Disease Center at NYU Langone Health, 240 East 38th Street, 23rd Floor, New York, NY 10016, USA; [c] Division of Gastroenterology, Massachusetts General Hospital, Harvard Medical School, MGH Crohn's and Colitis Center, 165 Cambridge Street, 9th Floor, Boston, MA 02114, USA
[1] Equal contribution co-first authors.
* Corresponding author.
E-mail address: aananthakrishnan@mgh.harvard.edu

Gastrointest Endoscopy Clin N Am 29 (2019) 447–470
https://doi.org/10.1016/j.giec.2019.02.006
1052-5157/19/© 2019 Elsevier Inc. All rights reserved.

INTRODUCTION

Crohn's disease (CD) and ulcerative colitis (UC) are immunologically mediated chronic inflammatory diseases that affect an estimated 1.6 million individuals in the United States and many more worldwide (**Table 1**). They progressively lead to irreversible bowel damage, strictures, and penetrating complications, causing hospitalization for medical or surgical treatment of disease in more than half the affected individuals.[1] Though disease activity can be quantified through patient-reported symptoms, it is recognized that such symptoms correlate poorly with objective evidence of inflammation, the latter being a more robust marker of disease severity and course.[2] Hence, treatment guidelines have incorporated objective markers of disease activity as a key component of both initial assessment and a therapeutic goal in the management of complex diseases.[3]

Traditionally, recognizing the near universal involvement of the ileum or colon in these diseases, ileocolonoscopy has been a gold standard test for determining the extent and severity of intestinal inflammation. However, there are many limitations to endoscopic evaluation, including poor patient acceptability, need for bowel preparation and sedation during procedures, and inability to visualize mucosa proximal to strictured segments. In addition, there is recognition that inflammation, particularly in CD, is not restricted to the lumen but is transmural and at times skipping the terminal ileum. Thus, for comprehensive assessment of disease status, evaluation of the entire thickness and length of the small bowel is necessary.[4] The past decade has witnessed a growth in the use of cross-sectional imaging through computed tomography (CT) or MRI scans for assessment of disease activity, extent, and complications.[5] Here, the authors review the role of such radiologic evaluation in assessing disease activity, prognostication, determination of therapeutic response, and detecting disease-related complications. Although there is also a select role for barium small bowel follow-through series, plain radiographic imaging, and in select cases, PET scans, the authors have focused this review on the commonly used CT and MRI modalities as well as the emerging modality of contrast-enhanced ultrasonography.

CROSS-SECTIONAL IMAGING MODALITIES

Computed tomography enterography (CTE) is a specialized protocol CT of the abdomen and pelvis designed to image the lumen and wall of the small bowel using a multidetector CT scanner with a minimum of 16 detector rows.[6] Patients ingest between 1500 and 2000 mL of a neutral enteric contrast administered in regularly divided doses 45 to 60 minutes before scanning, along with a timed injection of an iodinated intravenous contrast agent at 3 to 4 mL/s. Image acquisition from the enteric to the portal phase starts at 50 to 70 seconds after beginning of injection. The slice thickness of this protocol (axial, coronal, and sagittal) is usually around 2 to 3 mm. Recently, low-dose protocols have been developed that limit the radiation dose to less than 15 mGy for most patients weighing less than 220 pounds.

Magnetic resonance enterography (MRE) or enterocolonography is a noninvasive and radiation-free imaging technique primarily optimized to image the small bowel, although recent studies have also examined its use in assessing colonic inflammation. Standard MRE imaging protocols include rapidly acquired and motion-robust pulse sequences, including unenhanced T2-weighted sequences (with and without fat saturation), diffusion-weighted imaging (DWI), and gadolinium-enhanced T1-weighted sequences.[7] Similar to a CTE, an MRE requires ingestion of a large volume of neutral oral contrast, intravenous injection of an antiperistaltic agent (usually glucagon), and intravenous gadolinium contrast. Imaging acquisition generally occurs in the enteric phase

Table 1
Imaging modalities, indications, advantages, and disadvantages in ulcerative colitis and Crohn's disease

Imaging Modality	Ulcerative Colitis	When to Use Crohn's Disease	Advantages	Disadvantages
Plain film radiography	• Acute severe ulcerative colitis: to evaluate for colonic and small bowel air content and presence of complications of toxic megacolon or free perforation		• Universal availability • Short examination time • Low cost	• Lacks sensitivity for defining disease severity • Does not provide information about mural changes or extramural complications
Computed tomography CT abdomen/pelvis CTE	• Assessment of acute complications (perforation, toxic megacolon) • Assess disease activity • Evaluate for small bowel involvement (to rule out Crohn's disease) • Evaluate proximal colon for impassable stenosis or in those with severe comorbidities when colonoscopy may be contraindicated	• Assessment of severity and length of active CD in small bowel • Assessment of stricturing CD in small bowel and colon • Assessment of extraluminal complications, including internal penetrating disease, inflammatory collections and abscesses, and to guide abscess drainage • Evaluate response to medical therapy in comparison with pretreatment images	• Generally, universal availability • Short examination time • Assess luminal and extraluminal complications • Detailed cross-sectional images	• Radiation exposure is of concern particularly in children • Requires intravenous contrast (may not be appropriate in those with allergic reactions or renal insufficiency) • IV contrast limitation in renal disease
PET-CT	• May be used to assess disease activity. Similar in performance to non-PET-CT scan studies and not used clinically		• Assessment of inflammatory activity and extent	• Radiation exposure • Not widely available • Similar in performance to CT examinations

(continued on next page)

Table 1
(continued)

Imaging Modality	When to Use		Advantages	Disadvantages
	Ulcerative Colitis	Crohn's Disease		
MRI MRE DWI MRI pelvis fistula protocol	• Assess disease activity	• Assessment of severity and length of active CD in small bowel • Assessment of coexisting stricturing disease CD in small bowel and colon • Assessment of extraluminal complications, including internal penetrating disease, inflammatory collections and abscesses • Evaluate response to medical therapy in comparison with pretreatment images, preferred over CTE for serial monitoring of small bowel CD • Initial evaluation of perianal CD, guide management and follow-up after initial management	• No radiation exposure, preferred over CTE for serial monitoring of disease activity and response to therapy • Detailed imaging with qualitative and quantitative analysis	• Limited prospective data demonstrating usefulness in this indication • Not as sensitive as CT for extraluminal complications • Variable availability and insurance coverage in the community • IV contrast limitation in renal disease and pregnancy, may be overcome with DWI sequences with T2-weighted sequences • DWI sequences can be heterogenous between scanners and examinations, not recommended as sole sequence • Contraindicated with metal implants
Ultrasonography Elastography CEUS SICUS	• Assess disease activity, but limited information in ulcerative colitis	• Useful in centers with appropriate expertise in bowel ultrasonography • Primarily useful to evaluate disease activity in terminal ileum and colonic CD as point-of-care testing • Potential role for serial monitoring of response to therapy in select patients	• Low cost • Radiation free	• Degree of correlation with inflammation not well defined • Highly operator dependent • Limited by body habitus and bowel gas content

Abbreviations: CD, Crohn's disease; CEUS, contrast-enhanced ultrasonography; CT, computed tomography; CTE, computed tomography enterography; DWI, diffusion-weighted imaging; IVMRE, IV magnetic resonance enterography; PET-CT, positron emission tomography-computed tomography; SICUS, small intestine contrast ultrasonography.

of contrast enhancement with multiplanar images reconstructed in 3 planes, often with further acquisition of delayed postcontrast images. Diffusion-weighted imaging sequences provide additional qualitative and quantitative information complementing T1/T2-weighted images. A decrease in the apparent diffusion coefficient (ADC) indicates restricted diffusion and active disease. However, because of existing issues, including moderate sensitivity but low specificity to detect small bowel CD inflammation and interscanner reproducibility, recent consensus recommendations recommend the use of DWI as an adjunct but not the sole sequence to identify bowel inflammation in CD.[8]

Pelvic MRI is an additional, highly accurate noninvasive modality for the diagnosis and classification of perianal fistulas in CD.[9,10] This protocol consists of oblique axial and coronal T2-weighted fast spin echo sequences (with and without fat saturation), DWIs, and 2D or 3D T1-weighted images with fat saturation before and after administration of gadolinium-based contrast with additional optional fast spin echo T1-weighted sequences.[9]

Ultrasonography (USG) is a noninvasive, well-tolerated, low-cost, and radiation-free imaging technique that uses high-frequency sound waves to visualize tissues. It is particularly useful for visualizing terminal ileum and the colon; however, its performance is highly dependent on experienced sonographers and radiologists, and body habitus and the presence of bowel contents, including air, may both limit the quality of the examination.[11] Ultrasonography strain elastography measures the degree of tissue deformation with external compression, providing an estimation of stiffness.[12] Contrast-enhanced ultrasonography (CEUS) analyses tissue perfusion, using an intravenous contrast agent composed of innocuous microscopic gas bubbles that increase vascular contrast.[12–14] Small intestine contrast ultrasonography (SICUS) involves distending small bowel loops through ingestion of a hyperosmolar luminal contrast solution to enhance sonographic images.[15,16]

ULCERATIVE COLITIS
Plain Film Radiography

Historically, plain film radiography was used routinely in the care of patients with UC but has fallen out of favor since the emergence of cross-sectional imaging techniques. Plain film radiography may be useful in the setting of acute severe colitis to detect abdominal complications of toxic megacolon (defined as mid transverse colonic diameter >5.5 cm) or perforated bowel[17–20] (**Fig. 1**). Increased small bowel gas, persistent small bowel and gastric distension, mucosal islands, and colonic deep ulceration may predict severity and the need for urgent colectomy in patients with acute severe UC.[17–20]

Computed Tomography

Assessment of disease activity

Overall, CT imaging has moderate accuracy in defining disease activity in UC. Andersen and colleagues[21] examined the correlation between findings of multidetector CT colonography compared with colonoscopy in 21 patients with UC. Loss of haustration, a rigid bowel wall, and bowel thickness were moderately correlated with UC severity, as evaluated by endoscopy (r = 0.612). In a retrospective study of 35 patients with UC, CT had an overall sensitivity of 74% to detect colonic inflammation, with a sensitivity of 93% for detection of moderate and severe disease in well-distended colons.[22] Mild disease was defined as mucosal hyperenhancement only, moderate disease included wall thickening, and severe disease included

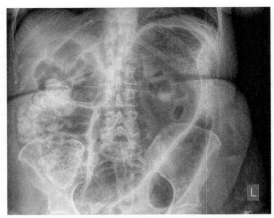

Fig. 1. Dilation of the transverse colon demonstrating toxic megacolon in a patient with acute severe ulcerative colitis.

pericolonic soft tissue stranding. The addition of PET to CT improves diagnostic performance. In small studies, 18-fluorodeoxyglucose (FDG) PET-CT demonstrated moderate correlation with extent of inflammation on colonoscopy (kappa 55%).[23] In a meta-analysis of 7 studies comprising 219 patients with inflammatory bowel disease, FDG PET-CT demonstrated a sensitivity of 85% and specificity of 87% in assessing UC on a per segment analysis.[24] In a recent study of 60 patients with UC, FDG PET-CT activity correlated with the total Mayo score (kappa = 0.465), endoscopic subscores (kappa = 0.526), histologic score (kappa = 0.496), and fecal calprotectin (kappa = 0.279).[25] However, the use of PET-CT remains limited by radiation exposure, particularly cumulative doses in young individuals over the course of their disease.

Prognostication
Few studies have examined whether radiographic findings can predict disease course in patients with UC. In a single-center retrospective study of 74 patients with acute, severe UC hospitalized for intravenous steroids who underwent a CT scan within 48 hours of hospitalization, the mean number of positive radiographic findings, including bowel wall thickening (BWT), stranding, hyperenhancement, mural stratification, mesenteric hyperemia, luminal narrowing, and proximal dilation, was modestly higher in those who required rescue therapy than those who did not (5.6 versus 5.0, $P = .03$).[26] Of these radiographic findings, mural stratification was significantly more common among those who required rescue therapy (57%) than those who did not (9%, $P<.001$).

Detection of complications
In addition to detecting complications of toxic megacolon and bowel perforation, CTE is useful for detecting the presence of small bowel inflammation in patients with UC with atypical symptoms, or endoscopic features raising suspicion for CD. Computed tomography imaging also has a role for evaluation of proximal colon in patients with impassable stricture in both CD and UC, staging of colorectal cancer, detecting intraabdominal complications such as mesenteric vein thrombosis,[27,28] and postoperative leak,[29] and in those with severe comorbidities in whom colonoscopy may be contraindicated.

MRI

Assessment of disease activity

MRI particularly when combined with DWI can be highly accurate in identifying colonic inflammation[30–35] (**Fig. 2**). A single-center observational study of 35 patients with UC and 61 patients with CD derived a segmental MRI score (MR-score-S) defined as the sum of 6 radiologic signs for each colonic segment.[30] These included DWI hyperintensity, rapid gadolinium enhancement after intravenous contrast medium administration, differentiation between the mucosa-submucosa complex and the muscularis propria, BWT, parietal edema, and the presence of ulceration(s). An MR-score-S greater than 1 detected endoscopic inflammation in UC with a sensitivity and specificity of 89% and 86%, respectively (area under the curve [AUC] = 0.92; $P<.001$). The total MR score correlated with the total modified Baron score (r = 0.813) and Walmsley index (r = 0.678). The presence of DWI hyperintensity predicted endoscopic inflammation in UC (odds ratio [OR] = 13.3; 95% CI: 3.6–48.9; AUC = 0.854; $P<.001$).[33] In a second prospective study of 50 patients with UC, MR colonography accurately assessed disease activity and severity using an index of MR parameters including colonic contrast uptake, mural edema, enlarged lymph nodes, and the presence of engorged perienteric vasculature with a sensitivity of 87% and specificity 88% (AUC = 0.95).[32]

Prognostication and monitoring

Studies have also examined whether MRI can be used to define mucosal healing in patients with UC. In a retrospective study of 29 patients with UC, a total Nancy score less than 7 had a sensitivity of 75% and a specificity 67% (AUC = 0.72; $P = .006$) for defining mucosal healing by sigmoidoscopy.[33] The mean Mayo endoscopic subscore and the mean Nancy score both decreased significantly in patients who achieved mucosal healing at reassessment, whereas there was no change in patients who did not achieve mucosal healing.[26] With these promising data, larger prospective studies are needed to robustly validate accuracy before more widespread use. In

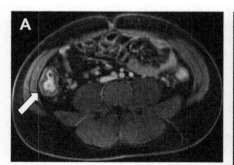
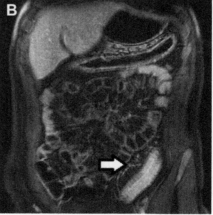

Fig. 2. Magnetic resonance enterography in a 24-year-old man with ulcerative colitis. (*A*) Colonic wall thickening (*white arrow*) and hyperenhancement of the right colon. (*B*) Engorgement of the pericolonic vasa recta (*white arrow*) with colonic wall thickening and hyperenhancement in the sigmoid colon. (*From* Deepak P, Bruining DH. Radiographical evaluation of ulcerative colitis. Gastroenterol Rep (Oxf) 2014;2(3):169–77; with permission.)

addition, the lack of availability of MR in many settings, associated cost, and radiologic expertise necessary for interpretation, limit its widespread use.

Ultrasonography

Assessment of disease activity

Ultrasonography may be useful in the evaluation of UC. Various sonographic features correlate with the presence of inflammation, including wall thickness and hypervascularity.[36–41] In a prospective, single-center study including 84 patients with UC or indeterminate colitis, the diagnostic accuracy of USG was superior for sigmoid/descending colonic disease (98% accuracy) compared with rectal disease (15%).[36] In a smaller study of 12 patients with UC, mean colonic wall thickness greater than 2.9 mm was predictive of moderate to severe disease on colonoscopy (positive predictive value 83%).[39] A composite ultrasound index, comprising the presence of colonic wall flow on Doppler and wall thickness, correlated with disease activity with a sensitivity of 0.71 and specificity of 1.00.[42]

Prognostication and monitoring

There are limited data on whether USG can be used to monitor disease response in UC. A prospective study evaluated 67 patients with UC, among whom 25 patients underwent repeat USG examination after 3 months.[41] Contrast-enhanced ultrasonography quantification of inflammatory hypervascularity of the bowel wall correlated well with both endoscopic and clinical improvement. In a study of 11 patients with UC, there was a significant correlation between histologic disease activity and the ratio of the time taken to reach peak activity to the value of the peak signal activity (r = −0.761, P<.01).[43]

CROHN'S DISEASE
Computed Tomography

Assessment of disease activity

Mural thickness and enhancement have been identified as the best CTE predictors of active disease, and in combination are superior to the routine clinical parameters (CD activity index, albumin, hematocrit, and C-reactive protein [CRP]) in identifying active disease.[44] However, there are no currently widely accepted scoring systems specific to CTE that combine these imaging features for quantitative assessment of disease activity. Faubion and colleagues[45] combined ileocolonoscopy with CTE assessment of disease severity in a manner similar to the simple endoscopic score for CD (SES-CD). This study demonstrated that such an approach correlated much better with biomarkers of inflammation than disease activity measured using ileocolonoscopy alone. Overall, CTE has a high sensitivity (>90%) and specificity (>90%) for the detection of small bowel CD, and has been validated against clinical, histologic, and endoscopic assessments.[46,47] The diagnostic accuracy in patients with suspected or established CD is comparable with that of MRE, with CTE reported to have higher and more consistent image quality less susceptible to motion artifacts.[48] A previous study evaluating ileocolonoscopy and CTE in 150 patients with CD identified active small bowel disease in more than half of the patients with endoscopically normal appearing ileum (36/67; 54%) termed "endoscopic skipping of the terminal ileum." This may be due to intramural inflammation in the terminal ileum that cannot be visualized at ileoscopy or due to more proximal small bowel disease than is evaluable by a colonoscope.[4] This highlights the complementary role of small bowel imaging in patients with CD in addition to ileocolonoscopy.

Prognostication and monitoring

Computed tomography enterography features consistently associated with active disease, including mural hyperenhancement and thickening and dilated vasa recta (comb sign), have been shown to improve after successful treatment, suggesting a potential role for CTE in monitoring of therapeutic efficacy.[49] Minordi and colleagues[50] performed CTE in 34 patients with suspected relapse following ileocolonic resection and developed a semiquantitative score system using the endoscopic Rutgeerts score. This was then validated second for its usefulness in predicting the rate of reoperation in a second study in a prospective cohort of 32 patients.[51]

Use for detection of complications

Computed tomography enterography has a sensitivity of 85% to 93% and specificity of 100% in detecting small bowel stenosis.[52] However, the accuracy for the number of strictures is only 83%, and there may be overestimation or underestimation of disease extent in 31% of patients with CD.[53] In addition, the absence of CTE findings of mesenteric hypervascularity, mural hyperenhancement, or stratification does not predict tissue fibrosis.[54] Computed tomography enterography has been shown to have a sensitivity and specificity of 70% and 97%, respectively, for the detection of internal penetrating disease, in a systematic review pooling data across 5 studies and using surgery and endoscopy as reference standards (**Fig. 3**).[55] Highlighting the importance

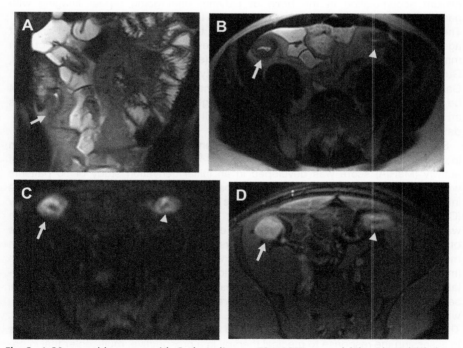

Fig. 3. A 30-year-old woman with Crohn's disease. T2-HASTE coronal (*A*) and axial (*B*) demonstrates a thickened and edematous terminal ileum. A skip lesion within the jejunum is incidentally noted (*arrowhead*). Diffusion-weighted images (*C*) and postcontrast T1-weighted axial images (*D*) demonstrate intense diffusion restriction and homogenous hyperenhancement of the terminal ileum (*arrow*). Similar findings are seen in the skip lesion involving the jejunum (*arrowhead*). The findings were interpreted as moderately active Crohn's disease.

of a cross-sectional assessment in CD, in a study of 357 consecutive patients with CD who had undergone a CTE, penetrating disease was detected in up to 20% of patients with CD, with this being a new finding compared with baseline evaluation in 50% of the cohort.[27] The detection of a concomitant stricture in the setting of an intraabdominal fistula is also associated with a 4- to 5-fold increase in the rate of surgery.[56] Finally, CT compared with surgery as a reference standard has demonstrated a sensitivity of ~85% for detection of intraabdominal abscesses, whereas specificity varied from 87.5% to 95%.[11]

MRI

Assessment of disease activity

Similar to CTE, conventional MRE has high sensitivity (>90%) and specificity (>90%) for the diagnosis of active small bowel inflammation in CD (**Fig. 4**).[46,47] As previously noted, DWI sequences are sensitive, but not specific for active disease. Seo and colleagues[57] performed a prospective, noninferiority study in 44 patients with known or suspected CD, with pairwise comparisons between conventional MRE features of inflammation with gadolinium contrast versus precontrast sequences alone with DWI. Precontrast sequences with DWI identified active inflammation in the terminal ileum with a sensitivity and specificity of 93% and 67%, respectively. There has been increasing interest in DWI because of recent studies showing evidence of gadolinium accumulation in the brain of patients undergoing repeat imaging with gadolinium-based contrast-enhanced MR, even in those with normal renal function.[58] The risk of accumulation seems to be limited to linear gadolinium-based contrast agents (eg, gadopentetate dimeglumine; Magnevist, Bayer Healthcare) and not with macrocyclic gadolinium-based contrast agents (eg, gadoterate meglumine; Dotarem, Guerbet).[59] Based on existing data, the Society of Abdominal Radiology-American Gastroenterological Association recommends that when intravenous contrast cannot be administered, noncontrast MRE with T2-weighted and DWI may be performed as an acceptable alternative for assessment of small bowel CD, but rated this recommendation as weak.[8]

Several MR-based scoring systems have been developed for potential application in clinical trials and clinical practice (**Table 2**).[47,60] The magnetic resonance index of activity (MaRIA) score was developed in an initial derivation study of 50 patients with established CD who underwent colonoscopy and whose MR features of active inflammation were correlated with Crohn's disease endoscopic index of severity (CDEIS).[61] In this study, the independent predictors for segmental CDEIS were wall thickness ($P = .007$), relative contrast enhancement (RCE) ($P = .01$), presence of edema ($P = .02$), and presence of ulcers at MR ($P = .003$). Using a regression model, the MaRIA score per segment was proposed as: 1.5*wall thickness (mm) + 0.02*RCE + 5*edema + 10*ulceration. The overall MaRIA score was calculated by adding individual segmental scores across 4 colonic segments and 1 ileal segment. In this study, overall MaRIA score was shown to have good correlation with total CDEIS ($r = 0.78$), CRP ($r = 0.53$), and Harvey-Bradshaw index ($r = 0.56$). This score has been subsequently validated and found to be reliable and responsive in assessing the response to medical therapy in a prospective, multicenter trial in patients with CD.[62,63] A Segmental MaRIA ≥ 11 predicted severe inflammatory lesions in a bowel segment with 96% accuracy, whereas a segmental MaRIA less than 7 detected segmental mucosal healing with 83% accuracy, 85% sensitivity, and 78% specificity.[62]

The Crohn's disease MRI index (CDMI) score was developed by correlating findings on MRE with transmural histopathology at the time of elective small bowel surgical

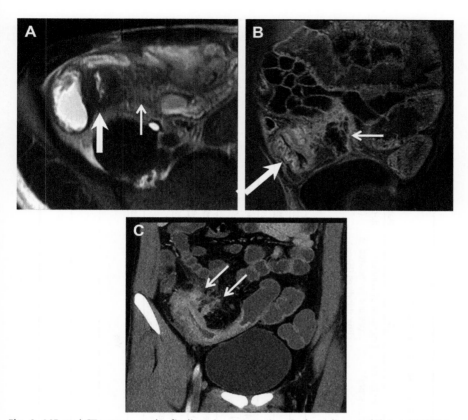

Fig. 4. MR and CT enterography findings in penetrating Crohn's disease. (*A*) Axial SSFSE image from MR enterography demonstrates marked wall thickening of the terminal ileum (*large arrow*) with prominence of the vasa recta (*small arrow*) in the adjacent mesenteric fat ("comb sign"). (*B*) Coronal postcontrast image from MR enterography demonstrates mural thickening with stratified mural hyperenhancement of the terminal ileum (*large arrow*), with inflammation and enhancement extending out into the perienteric fat. The small arrow points to a complex multiseptated perienteric abscess that was treated with percutaneous drainage. (*C*) Coronal postcontrast image from CT enterography demonstrates marked mural thickening and hyperenhancement of the terminal ileum over a length of 15 cm, with luminal narrowing and mild upstream small bowel dilatation. Arrows point to inflammatory sinus tracts that led to the abscess. (*From* Deepak P, Sheedy SP, Lightner AL, et al. Role of abdominal imaging in the diagnosis of IBD strictures, fistulas, and postoperative complications. In: Shen B, editors. Interventional inflammatory bowel disease: endoscopic management and treatment of complications. Elsevier: New York; 2018. p. 79–95; with permission.)

resection in patients with CD.[64] A simplified model (1.79 + 1.34 × mural thickness + 0.94 × mural T2 score) was developed to predict transmural inflammation. MR enterography global score (MEGS) is a further modification of the CDMI developed to include segmental disease length, evaluation of colonic haustral loss, and evaluation of extraenteric complications, such as enlarged mesenteric lymph nodes, abscesses, and fistulae.[65] MEGS is believed to better capture the full disease burden in patients with CD, and has been shown to be responsive to treatment in a

Table 2
Scoring systems using magnetic resonance imaging for assessment of disease activity in Crohn's disease

	MaRIA[61-63]	CDMI[64]	MEGS[65,66]	Nancy[30,70]	Clermont[67-69]
Reference standard	Ileocolonoscopy (CDEIS)	Surgical specimen (acute inflammation score)	Extension of London score and correlated to clinical indices (Harvey-Bradshaw index, fecal calprotectin, CRP, and CD activity score)	Ileocolonoscopy (SES-CD)	MaRIA
Validated	Yes	Yes	Yes	Yes	Yes
Responsive to treatment	Yes	No	Yes	Yes	Yes
Wall thickening	Yes	Yes	Yes	Yes	Yes
Enhancement	Yes (quantification of relative contrast enhancement)	Qualitative (4 different categories)	Qualitative (4 different categories)	Yes (qualitative evaluation)	Yes (qualitative evaluation)
High signal on T2	Yes (qualitative evaluation)	Yes (4 different categories)	Yes (4 different categories)	Yes (qualitative evaluation)	Yes (qualitative evaluation)
Ulcerations	Yes	–	–	Yes	Yes
T2 perimural signal	–	Yes (4 different categories)	Yes (4 different categories)	–	–
Mural stratification	–	–	–	Yes	–
Length of disease segment	–	–	Yes	–	–
Proximal small bowel disease assessed	–	–	–	–	Yes
Diffusion-weighted imaging hyperintensity	–	–	–	Yes	Yes

study of 36 patients with CD, in whom it demonstrated response to antitumor necrosis factor-alpha (TNF-α) therapy with good interobserver agreement, compared with clinical response assessment using the Physician's Global Assessment.[66]

Two current scoring systems, the Clermont and Nancy scores, use DWI as part of their scoring criteria. The Clermont score (1.646*bowel thickness − 1.321*ADC + 5.613*edema + 8.306*ulcers + 5.039) has shown high correlation (rho = 0.99) with high sensitivity (93.7%) and specificity (96.0%) for detecting active ileal and colonic CD compared with a reference standard of active disease defined as an Ma-RIA score ≥7, but without the need for an oral bowel preparation or enema.[67,68] A subsequent study correlating this score with endoscopic scoring systems (SES-CD and CDEIS), demonstrated the responsiveness of Clermont score and ADC to changes in ulcer size, especially in the ileum. A Clermont score greater than 18.9 detected ulcerations with sensitivity and specificity of 79% and 73%, respectively.[69] The Nancy score was developed in 40 patients with CD against a reference standard of SES-CD on colonoscopy and calculated as a score for 6 different radiological parameters (including DWI) across 5 colonic segments and ileum similar to UC, but with scores ranging from 0 to 36 in CD.[30] A segmental score greater than 2 detected endoscopic inflammation in the colon with a sensitivity and specificity of 58.3% and 84.5%, respectively (AUC = <0.78; P<.001). This score has been recently validated and found to be responsive to therapy.[70]

Recently, both GE and Siemens have incorporated MRI and PET scanning technologies into true hybrid machines with lower radiation exposure than for PET/CT, and with technical feasibility and good coregistration of bowel structures.[71,72] PET/MRE in a study across 35 patients with CD, compared with PET/CT, was more accurate in assessing extraluminal disease (P = .002), which was associated with higher need for stoma (P = .022) and allowed reduction in operative time (P = .022) as well as in detecting a fibrotic component compared with PET/CT-E (12/18 versus 5/18 patients, respectively, P = .04).[73] A second study highlighted the potential for a combined PET/MRE biomarker (ADC × SUV_{max}), with a cutoff of less than 3000 in differentiating between fibrosis and active inflammation, and with an accuracy, sensitivity, and specificity of 71%, 67%, and 73%, respectively.[74] The role of PET/MR in CD diagnostic and treatment algorithms requires further studies given the cost of scanning and also radiation exposure.

Prognostication and monitoring

The concept was using cross-sectional imaging to monitor transmural radiologic healing was explored in a retrospective study of 150 patients with small bowel CD undergoing serial CTE/MRE evaluation while on medical therapy across a median of 4 CTE/MRE and 4.6 years of follow-up.[75,76] Patients were classified as responders with second CTE/MRE and further serial scans if all individual lesions improved, nonresponders if any of the lesions worsened or a new lesion developed at second CTE/MRE, and partial responders if all lesions stayed the same or some but not all lesions improved. Responders at second CTE/MRE demonstrated a greater than 50% reduction in corticosteroid use (hazard ratio [HR] = 0.37; 95% CI: 0.21 to 0.64) along with a reduction by more than two-thirds in hospitalizations and surgery ([HR = 0.28; 95% CI: 0.15–0.50] and [HR = 0.34; 95% CI: 0.18–0.63], respectively).[75] MSE-based scoring systems, such as the MaRIA, MEGS, and Nancy scores have been validated to measure response to therapy in CD.[63,66,70]

Finally, recent efforts have also centered on the development of an index (Lémann index) that could reflect the cumulative permanent intestinal damage in CD.[77,78] The Lémann index was developed in 138 patients in a prospective, multicenter, cross-sectional study across 24 centers in 5 countries. The entire digestive tract was divided into 4 organs and subsequently into segments. This index accounts for previous operations, strictures, and penetrating lesions across the entire gastrointestinal tract by scoring each organ and segment based on historical, endoscopic, and MRE findings. A unit increase in disease burden was an independent prognostic factor for intestinal surgery and CD-related hospitalization.[79] It has also been shown to be responsive to anti-TNF therapy, with studies showing stabilization of bowel damage reflected by the Lémann index and improvement of the damage score in some.[80,81] This index is not structured currently for routine use in clinical practice and its use is restricted to research studies.

Use for detection of complications

The sensitivity for detection of strictures with an MRE ranges from 75% to 100%, whereas the specificity is 91% to 100%.[52,78] Magnetic resonance enterography findings of BWT have a positive association with small bowel fibrosis and a negative association with response to medical therapy.[52] Previous studies with preoperative MRE in a pediatric cohort of patients with CD with symptomatic strictures, who underwent surgery, demonstrated that prestenotic upstream small bowel dilatation greater than 3 cm was associated with confluent transmural fibrosis.[82] A recent study of 41 patients with an MRE within 4 months before surgery, correlated the percentage of gadolinium enhancement gain in the submucosa between 70 seconds and 7 minutes, and the pattern of enhancement at 7 minutes, with the degree of fibrosis ($P<.01$ for both).[83] Using the percentage of enhancement gain, MRE was able to discriminate between mild to moderate and severe fibrosis deposition with a sensitivity of 94% and a specificity of 89%. The CREOLE study analyzed the impact of MRE characteristics in 97 patients with CD with symptomatic small bowel strictures.[84] A prognostic score combining clinical and MRE-based imaging variables (stricture length <12 cm, prestenotic dilation <3 cm, lesion enhancement in delayed T1-weighted sequence and absence of associated small bowel fistula) indicated continued treatment with adalimumab at 24 weeks without change to other anti-TNFs, rescue corticosteroids, endoscopic dilation, or bowel resection. Magnetic resonance enterography also demonstrates a pooled sensitivity and specificity of 76% and 96%, respectively, for the diagnosis of small bowel fistulas against a reference standard of endoscopy or surgery.[55] Intraabdominal abscess using surgery as a reference standard was detected by MRE with a sensitivity of 86% and a specificity of 93%.[11]

Perianal Crohn's disease

Dedicated pelvic MRI has emerged as a cross-sectional imaging of choice in patients with established or suspected perianal CD (**Fig. 5**). This may provide additional information on luminal disease location, especially proctitis, disease severity, and fluid collections, and may prompt the need for an examination under anesthesia (EUA).[85] Actively inflamed fistulas are usually hyperintense on T2-weighted images and demonstrate avid contrast enhancement.[9] The Van Assche score is an MRI severity index of perianal disease that combines anatomic information based on the number and complexity of the tracts, the anatomy of the tract(s) relative to the anal sphincter, and the presence or absence of supralevator disease, with the degree of active inflammation within the fistula tracts on T2-weighted MR images, and the presence/absence of abscess and proctitis.[10] This score can also be used to assess response to medical therapy in perianal CD. Identification of abscess formation within the deep postanal space and supralevator compartment may prompt the need for an EUA.

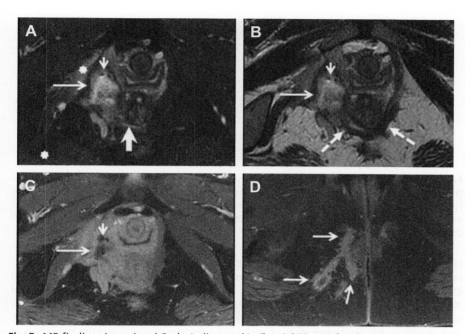

Fig. 5. MR findings in perianal Crohn's disease. (*A–C*) Axial T2-weighted image with fat saturation (*A*), T2-weighted image without fat saturation (*B*), and axial postcontrast images (*C*) demonstrate a right perianal/perivaginal fluid collection (*thin arrows*). The fluid collection abuts the right obturator internus muscle that demonstrates high signal from inflammation/edema (*A*) (*asterisk*). Note the small foci of gas anteriorly (*short arrows*) and the ring enhancement on the postgadolinium image (*C*), indicating the presence of pus. The T2-weighted images without fat saturation (*B*) allow for better delineation of the pelvic anatomy, and it is seen that the abscess involves the right side of the puborectalis muscle (*dashed arrow*). This abscess communicated with a fistula that initially tracked in the intersphincteric space (*A*) (*thick arrow*) from the posterior midline where the internal opening was identified (not shown). (*D*) Axial postcontrast image more caudally demonstrates multiple branching tracts in the ischioanal fossa (*arrows*), one of which extended out to the skin surface. (*From* Deepak P, Sheedy SP, Lightner AL, et al. Role of abdominal imaging in the diagnosis of IBD strictures, fistulas, and postoperative complications. In: Shen B, editors. Interventional inflammatory bowel disease: endoscopic management and treatment of complications. Elsevier: New York; 2018. p. 79–95; with permission.)

Ultrasonography

Assessment of disease activity

Ultrasonography imaging can be an accurate technique for diagnosis of CD, assessing location of involvement, quantifying disease activity, and for detection of complications.[86–89] Bowel wall thickening is the most important and frequently used sonographic parameter when diagnosing CD (**Fig. 6**), with sensitivities of 74% to 100% and specificities of 67% to 100%.[88–91] In a recent meta-analysis of 15 prospective studies, a cutoff value of 3 mm for BWT had a sensitivity and specificity of 89% and 96%, respectively, whereas 4 mm or more yielded a sensitivity of 87% and a specificity of 98% for detecting active CD.[92]

Contrast-enhanced ultrasonography may be helpful in estimating endoscopic activity and qualitatively distinguishing between fibrotic and inflammatory strictures.

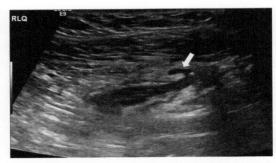

Fig. 6. Gray-scale bowel ultrasonographic image showing mural thickening and a penetrating ulcer in the terminal ileum (*arrow*) in a patient with Crohn's disease. (*From* Deepak P, Kolbe AB, Fidler JL, et al. Update on magnetic resonance imaging and ultrasound evaluation of Crohn's disease. Gastroenterol Hepatol (N Y) 2016;12(4):226–36; with permission.)

However, studies have demonstrated considerable heterogeneity with regard to technique and contrast parameters.[93–99] A recent meta-analysis examining the use of CEUS for the detection of CD activity in 332 patients found a pooled sensitivity of 94% and specificity of 79%.[100] Contrast-enhanced ultrasonography assessment of small bowel for quantifying disease activity correlated well with MRI (rho = 0.791), and, in particular, for parameters of wall thickness, comb sign, and the presence of lymph nodes.[101] In addition, good correlation was also found for layered wall appearance and fibro-adipose proliferation. Studies on the use of color Doppler to assess flow in the mesenteric and portal vein or mesenteric arteries are conflicting and their interpretation in CD is not well established. However, bowel wall vascularity seems to correlate well with inflammatory, endoscopic, clinical, and biochemical activity.[43,99,102–104]

Prognostication and monitoring

Several small studies have examined the use of USG strain elastography in assessing response to therapy and for detecting postoperative recurrence. This is a noninvasive method to differentiate inflammatory from fibrotic tissue based on strain under deformation and elastic modulus, with promising results in animal models and ex vivo human specimens. In a study of 30 patients that examined the response of ileal CD to anti-TNF therapy, an inverse correlation was observed between strain ratio values at baseline and BWT reduction following therapy ($P = .007$).[105] Moreover, patients achieving transmural healing (BWT ≤ 3 mm) at week 14 had significantly lower baseline strain ratio ($P<.05$). In another study of 24 patients with CD, anti-TNF therapy achieved a significant reduction in the BWT and Doppler flow.[106] However, sonographic normality was only achieved in 29% of patients with a clinical and biological response, and could not differentiate between those with and without clinical and biological response.[106]

Small intestine contrast ultrasonography has demonstrated high accuracy in assessing lesions (sensitivity 97.4%, specificity 100%), stenosis (sensitivity 92.3%, specificity 92.1%), penetrating complications such as abscesses (sensitivity 100%, specificity 91.5%), and postoperative recurrence (sensitivity 91.7%, specificity 94.0%).[15,16,107] Moreover, the SICUS-based sonographic lesion index for CD (SLIC) was higher in patients with CD activity index greater than 150 and CRP greater than 5 mg/L ($P<.003$).[108] Those with a higher SLIC were more likely to require surgery during a 1-year follow-up.[108] In a prospective study of 25 patients with CD over 3 years after ileo-colonic resection, SICUS demonstrated findings compatible with endoscopic recurrence using ileo-colonoscopy for CD.[15,109]

Use for detection of complications

Ultrasonography diagnostic criteria in detecting complications of penetrating disease include hypoechoic areas or tracts between ileal loops with or without internal gaseous artifacts, hypoechoic peri-intestinal tracts with or without gas, and hypoechoic peri-intestinal areas with a diameter less than 2 cm.[89–91] A systematic review of pooled results of 4 studies demonstrated a sensitivity of 74% and specificity of 95% for the diagnosis of fistula compared with surgery, barium studies, or colonoscopy.[55] In a larger study of 119 patients with internal fistula, USG showed a sensitivity of 71% and specificity of 96% in identifying fistula compared with surgery,[110] comparable with the previously reported accuracy of CT or MRI.

In abdominal abscesses, appearance by USG is characterized by hypoanechoic lesions containing fluid and gaseous artifacts, posterior enhancement, and irregular margins sometimes within hypertrophic mesentery.[88,91,110,111] A systematic review of 3 studies using surgery as a reference yielded a sensitivity of 84% and a specificity of 93%.[55] Contrast-enhanced ultrasonography may offer greater accuracy than standard ultrasonography, demonstrating diffuse enhancement in phlegmons compared with peripheral zone enhancement with an avascular central portion because of the fluid collection.[112] Several studies have also demonstrated high diagnostic accuracy for detection of small bowel and colonic stenoses with sensitivities of 75% and 100%, and specificities of 93% and 90%, respectively.[88,113,114] Ultrasonography elastography is useful in differentiating fibrotic from inflammatory strictures in CD.[12–14,114,115] In vivo strain measurements differed between normal and strictured segments, and correlated well with the severity of fibrosis.[14,116] Endo-anal US (EUS) is also an accurate and safe alternative to MRI or EUA for evaluation of perianal CD. A prospective, blinded study comparing EUA, MRI, and EUS demonstrated a diagnostic accuracy of 91%, 87%, and 91%, respectively, with 100% accuracy when any 2 of the tests were used together.[117] In a systematic review of 4 studies, there was a high degree of heterogeneity with a pooled sensitivity of 87% and specificity of 43% for the EUS diagnosis of a fistula.[118] Barriers to routine use of abdominal USG in the United States include need for operator training, challenges with regard to interobserver variability, and influence of body habitus, including obesity, on image acquisition and quality.

SUMMARY

Cross-sectional imaging is an important tool in diagnosing and monitoring patients with CD and UC. Although there is considerable literature supporting the sensitivity, specificity, and accuracy of CT and MRI for identifying inflammatory activity in the small bowel and colon, there is growing interest in using these modalities to longitudinally follow patients over time and assess response to treatment, disease activity, and cumulative irreversible damage attributable to the disease. Also, newer imaging modalities or modifications of existing modalities offer the ability to improve resolution in identifying inflammation and detecting fibrotic complications of the disease. In the future, such imaging modalities, in combination with other biomarkers, may allow for comprehensive evaluation of patients with these progressive diseases, which will facilitate more effective treatment and prevention of permanent damage and morbidity.

REFERENCES

1. Cosnes J, Gower-Rousseau C, Seksik P, et al. Epidemiology and natural history of inflammatory bowel diseases. Gastroenterology 2011;140:1785–94.
2. Gracie DJ, Williams CJ, Sood R, et al. Poor correlation between clinical disease activity and mucosal inflammation, and the role of psychological comorbidity, in inflammatory bowel disease. Am J Gastroenterol 2016;111:541–51.
3. Peyrin-Biroulet L, Sandborn W, Sands BE, et al. Selecting therapeutic targets in inflammatory bowel disease (STRIDE): determining therapeutic goals for treat-to-target. Am J Gastroenterol 2015;110:1324–38.
4. Samuel S, Bruining DH, Loftus EV Jr, et al. Endoscopic skipping of the distal terminal ileum in Crohn's disease can lead to negative results from ileocolonoscopy. Clin Gastroenterol Hepatol 2012;10:1253–9.
5. Deepak P, Bruining DH. Radiographical evaluation of ulcerative colitis. Gastroenterol Rep (Oxf) 2014;2:169–77.
6. Baker ME, Hara AK, Platt JF, et al. CT enterography for Crohn's disease: optimal technique and imaging issues. Abdom Imaging 2015;40:938–52.
7. Deepak P, Kolbe AB, Fidler JL, et al. Update on magnetic resonance imaging and ultrasound evaluation of Crohn's disease. Gastroenterol Hepatol (N Y) 2016;12:226–36.
8. Bruining DH, Zimmermann EM, Loftus EV Jr, et al. Consensus recommendations for evaluation, interpretation, and utilization of computed tomography and magnetic resonance enterography in patients with small bowel Crohn's disease. Gastroenterology 2018;154:1172–94.
9. Sheedy SP, Bruining DH, Dozois EJ, et al. MR imaging of perianal Crohn disease. Radiology 2017;282:628–45.
10. Gecse KB, Bemelman W, Kamm MA, et al. A global consensus on the classification, diagnosis and multidisciplinary treatment of perianal fistulising Crohn's disease. Gut 2014;63:1381–92.
11. Panes J, Bouhnik Y, Reinisch W, et al. Imaging techniques for assessment of inflammatory bowel disease: joint ECCO and ESGAR evidence-based consensus guidelines. J Crohns Colitis 2013;7:556–85.
12. Pescatori LC, Mauri G, Savarino E, et al. Bowel sonoelastography in patients with crohn's disease: a systematic review. Ultrasound Med Biol 2018;44:297–302.
13. Lu C, Gui X, Chen W, et al. Ultrasound shear wave elastography and contrast enhancement: effective biomarkers in Crohn's disease strictures. Inflamm Bowel Dis 2017;23:421–30.
14. Sconfienza LM, Cavallaro F, Colombi V, et al. In-vivo axial-strain sonoelastography helps distinguish acutely-inflamed from fibrotic terminal ileum strictures in patients with Crohn's disease: preliminary results. Ultrasound Med Biol 2016;42:855–63.
15. Biancone L, Onali S, Calabrese E, et al. Non-invasive techniques for assessing postoperative recurrence in Crohn's disease. Dig Liver Dis 2008;40(Suppl 2):S265–70.
16. Zhu C, Ma X, Xue L, et al. Small intestine contrast ultrasonography for the detection and assessment of Crohn disease: a meta-analysis. Medicine 2016;95:e4235.
17. Latella G, Vernia P, Viscido A, et al. GI distension in severe ulcerative colitis. Am J Gastroenterol 2002;97:1169–75.
18. Chew CN, Nolan DJ, Jewell DP. Small bowel gas in severe ulcerative colitis. Gut 1991;32:1535–7.

19. Kumar S, Ghoshal UC, Aggarwal R, et al. Severe ulcerative colitis: prospective study of parameters determining outcome. J Gastroenterol Hepatol 2004;19: 1247–52.
20. Autenrieth DM, Baumgart DC. Toxic megacolon. Inflamm Bowel Dis 2012;18: 584–91.
21. Andersen K, Vogt C, Blondin D, et al. Multi-detector CT-colonography in inflammatory bowel disease: prospective analysis of CT-findings to high-resolution video colonoscopy. Eur J Radiol 2006;58:140–6.
22. Johnson KT, Hara AK, Johnson CD. Evaluation of colitis: usefulness of CT enterography technique. Emerg Radiol 2009;16:277–82.
23. Das CJ, Makharia GK, Kumar R, et al. PET/CT colonography: a novel non-invasive technique for assessment of extent and activity of ulcerative colitis. Eur J Nucl Med Mol Imaging 2010;37:714–21.
24. Treglia G, Quartuccio N, Sadeghi R, et al. Diagnostic performance of fluorine-18-fluorodeoxyglucose positron emission tomography in patients with chronic inflammatory bowel disease: a systematic review and a meta-analysis. J Crohns Colitis 2013;7:345–54.
25. Berry N, Sinha SK, Bhattacharya A, et al. Role of positron emission tomography in assessing disease activity in ulcerative colitis: comparison with biomarkers. Dig Dis Sci 2018;63:1541–50.
26. Cushing KC, Gee M, Kordbacheh H, et al. Su1808 - mural stratification on CT scan independently predicts need for medical or surgical rescue therapy in acute severe ulerative colitis. Gastroenterology 2018;154:S-592.
27. Bruining DH, Siddiki HA, Fletcher JG, et al. Prevalence of penetrating disease and extraintestinal manifestations of Crohn's disease detected with CT enterography. Inflamm Bowel Dis 2008;14:1701–6.
28. Navaneethan U, Shen B. Hepatopancreatobiliary manifestations and complications associated with inflammatory bowel disease. Inflamm Bowel Dis 2010;16: 1598–619.
29. Khoury W, Ben-Yehuda A, Ben-Haim M, et al. Abdominal computed tomography for diagnosing postoperative lower gastrointestinal tract leaks. J Gastrointest Surg 2009;13:1454–8.
30. Oussalah A, Laurent V, Bruot O, et al. Diffusion-weighted magnetic resonance without bowel preparation for detecting colonic inflammation in inflammatory bowel disease. Gut 2010;59:1056–65.
31. Yu L-L, Yang H-S, Zhang B-T, et al. Diffusion-weighted magnetic resonance imaging without bowel preparation for detection of ulcerative colitis. World J Gastroenterol 2015;21:9785–92.
32. Ordás I, Rimola J, García-Bosch O, et al. Diagnostic accuracy of magnetic resonance colonography for the evaluation of disease activity and severity in ulcerative colitis: a prospective study. Gut 2013;62:1566–72.
33. Laurent V, Naudé S, Vuitton L, et al. Accuracy of diffusion-weighted magnetic resonance colonography in assessing mucosal healing and the treatment response in patients with ulcerative Colitis. J Crohns Colitis 2017;11:716–23.
34. Nozue T, Kobayashi A, Takagi Y, et al. Assessment of disease activity and extent by magnetic resonance imaging in ulcerative colitis. Pediatr Int 2000;42:285–8.
35. Maccioni F, Colaiacomo MC, Parlanti S. Ulcerative colitis: value of MR imaging. Abdom Imaging 2005;30:584–92.
36. Parente F, Greco S, Molteni M, et al. Role of early ultrasound in detecting inflammatory intestinal disorders and identifying their anatomical location within the bowel. Aliment Pharmacol Ther 2003;18:1009–16.

37. Parente F, Molteni M, Marino B, et al. Are colonoscopy and bowel ultrasound useful for assessing response to short-term therapy and predicting disease outcome of moderate-to-severe forms of ulcerative colitis? A prospective study. Am J Gastroenterol 2010;105:1150–7.

38. Parente F, Molteni M, Marino B, et al. Bowel ultrasound and mucosal healing in ulcerative colitis. Dig Dis 2009;27:285–90.

39. Bremner AR, Griffiths M, Argent JD, et al. Sonographic evaluation of inflammatory bowel disease: a prospective, blinded, comparative study. Pediatr Radiol 2006;36:947–53.

40. Civitelli F, Di Nardo G, Oliva S, et al. Ultrasonography of the colon in pediatric ulcerative colitis: a prospective, blind, comparative study with colonoscopy. J Pediatr 2014;165:78–84.e2.

41. Socaciu M, Ciobanu L, Diaconu B, et al. Non-invasive assessment of inflammation and treatment response in patients with Crohn's disease and ulcerative colitis using contrast-enhanced ultrasonography quantification. J Gastrointest Liver Dis 2015;24:457–65.

42. Allocca M, Fiorino G, Bonovas S, et al. Accuracy of Humanitas Ultrasound Criteria in assessing disease activity and severity in ulcerative colitis: a prospective study. J Crohns Colitis 2018;12(12):1385–91.

43. Girlich C, Jung EM, Huber E, et al. Comparison between preoperative quantitative assessment of bowel wall vascularization by contrast-enhanced ultrasound and operative macroscopic findings and results of histopathological scoring in Crohn's disease. Ultraschall Med 2011;32:154–9.

44. Bruining DH, Loftus EV Jr. Technology insight: new techniques for imaging the gut in patients with IBD. Nat Clin Pract Gastroenterol Hepatol 2008;5:154–61.

45. Faubion WA Jr, Fletcher JG, O'Byrne S, et al. EMerging BiomARKers in Inflammatory Bowel Disease (EMBARK) study identifies fecal calprotectin, serum MMP9, and serum IL-22 as a novel combination of biomarkers for Crohn's disease activity: role of cross-sectional imaging. Am J Gastroenterol 2013;108: 1891–900.

46. Fletcher JG, Fidler JL, Bruining DH, et al. New concepts in intestinal imaging for inflammatory bowel diseases. Gastroenterology 2011;140:1795–806.

47. Deepak P, Fletcher JG, Fidler JL, et al. Computed tomography and magnetic resonance enterography in Crohn's disease: assessment of radiologic criteria and endpoints for clinical practice and trials. Inflamm Bowel Dis 2016;22: 2280–8.

48. Siddiki HA, Fidler JL, Fletcher JG, et al. Prospective comparison of state-of-the-art MR enterography and CT enterography in small-bowel Crohn's disease. AJR Am J Roentgenol 2009;193:113–21.

49. Bruining DH, Loftus EV Jr, Ehman EC, et al. Computed tomography enterography detects intestinal wall changes and effects of treatment in patients with Crohn's disease. Clin Gastroenterol Hepatol 2011;9:679–83.e1.

50. Minordi LM, Vecchioli A, Poloni G, et al. Enteroclysis CT and PEG-CT in patients with previous small-bowel surgical resection for Crohn's disease: CT findings and correlation with endoscopy. Eur Radiol 2009;19:2432–40.

51. Mao R, Gao X, Zhu ZH, et al. CT enterography in evaluating postoperative recurrence of Crohn's disease after ileocolic resection: complementary role to endoscopy. Inflamm Bowel Dis 2013;19:977–82.

52. Rieder F, Zimmermann EM, Remzi FH, et al. Crohn's disease complicated by strictures: a systematic review. Gut 2013;62:1072–84.

53. Vogel J, da Luz Moreira A, Baker M, et al. CT enterography for Crohn's disease: accurate preoperative diagnostic imaging. Dis Colon Rectum 2007;50:1761–9.
54. Adler J, Punglia DR, Dillman JR, et al. Computed tomography enterography findings correlate with tissue inflammation, not fibrosis in resected small bowel Crohn's disease. Inflamm Bowel Dis 2012;18:849–56.
55. Pénes J, Bouzas R, Chaparro M, et al. Systematic review: the use of ultrasonography, computed tomography and magnetic resonance imaging for the diagnosis, assessment of activity and abdominal complications of Crohn's disease. Aliment Pharmacol Ther 2011;34:125–45.
56. Yaari S, Benson A, Aviran E, et al. Factors associated with surgery in patients with intra-abdominal fistulizing Crohn's disease. World J Gastroenterol 2016; 22:10380–7.
57. Seo N, Park SH, Kim KJ, et al. MR enterography for the evaluation of small-bowel inflammation in Crohn disease by using diffusion-weighted imaging without intravenous contrast material: a prospective noninferiority study. Radiology 2016;278:762–72.
58. Kanda T, Fukusato T, Matsuda M, et al. Gadolinium-based contrast agent accumulates in the brain even in subjects without severe renal dysfunction: evaluation of autopsy brain specimens with inductively coupled plasma mass spectroscopy. Radiology 2015;276:228–32.
59. Radbruch A, Weberling LD, Kieslich PJ, et al. Gadolinium retention in the dentate nucleus and globus pallidus is dependent on the class of contrast agent. Radiology 2015;275:783–91.
60. Deepak P, Fowler KJ, Fletcher JG, et al. Novel imaging approaches in inflammatory bowel diseases. Inflamm Bowel Dis 2019;25(2):248–60.
61. Rimola J, Rodriguez S, Garcia-Bosch O, et al. Magnetic resonance for assessment of disease activity and severity in ileocolonic Crohn's disease. Gut 2009; 58:1113–20.
62. Rimola J, Ordas I, Rodriguez S, et al. Magnetic resonance imaging for evaluation of Crohn's disease: validation of parameters of severity and quantitative index of activity. Inflamm Bowel Dis 2011;17:1759–68.
63. Ordas I, Rimola J, Rodriguez S, et al. Accuracy of magnetic resonance enterography in assessing response to therapy and mucosal healing in patients with Crohn's disease. Gastroenterology 2014;146:374–82.e1.
64. Steward MJ, Punwani S, Proctor I, et al. Non-perforating small bowel Crohn's disease assessed by MRI enterography: derivation and histopathological validation of an MR-based activity index. Eur J Radiol 2012;81:2080–8.
65. Makanyanga JC, Pendse D, Dikaios N, et al. Evaluation of Crohn's disease activity: initial validation of a magnetic resonance enterography global score (MEGS) against faecal calprotectin. Eur Radiol 2014;24:277–87.
66. Prezzi D, Bhatnagar G, Vega R, et al. Monitoring Crohn's disease during anti-TNF-alpha therapy: validation of the magnetic resonance enterography global score (MEGS) against a combined clinical reference standard. Eur Radiol 2016;26(7):2107–17.
67. Buisson A, Joubert A, Montoriol PF, et al. Diffusion-weighted magnetic resonance imaging for detecting and assessing ileal inflammation in Crohn's disease. Aliment Pharmacol Ther 2013;37:537–45.
68. Hordonneau C, Buisson A, Scanzi J, et al. Diffusion-weighted magnetic resonance imaging in ileocolonic Crohn's disease: validation of quantitative index of activity. Am J Gastroenterol 2014;109:89–98.

69. Buisson A, Hordonneau C, Goutte M, et al. Diffusion-weighted magnetic resonance imaging is effective to detect ileocolonic ulcerations in Crohn's disease. Aliment Pharmacol Ther 2015;42:452–60.

70. Thierry ML, Rousseau H, Pouillon L, et al. Accuracy of diffusion-weighted magnetic resonance imaging in detecting mucosal healing and treatment response, and in predicting surgery, in Crohn's disease. J Crohns Colitis 2018;12(10): 1180–90.

71. Mansi L, Ciarmiello A. Perspectives on PET/MR imaging: are we ready for clinical use? J Nucl Med 2014;55:529–30.

72. Beiderwellen K, Kinner S, Gomez B, et al. Hybrid imaging of the bowel using PET/MR enterography: Feasibility and first results. Eur J Radiol 2016;85:414–21.

73. Pellino G, Nicolai E, Catalano OA, et al. PET/MR versus PET/CT imaging: impact on the clinical management of small-bowel Crohn's disease. J Crohns Colitis 2016;10:277–85.

74. Catalano OA, Gee MS, Nicolai E, et al. Evaluation of quantitative PET/MR enterography biomarkers for discrimination of inflammatory strictures from fibrotic strictures in Crohn disease. Radiology 2016;278:792–800.

75. Deepak P, Fletcher JG, Fidler JL, et al. Radiological response is associated with better long-term outcomes and is a potential treatment target in patients with small bowel Crohn's disease. Am J Gastroenterol 2016;111:997–1006.

76. Deepak P, Fletcher JG, Fidler JL, et al. Predictors of durability of radiological response in patients with small bowel Crohn's disease. Inflamm Bowel Dis 2018;24(8):1815–25.

77. Pariente B, Cosnes J, Danese S, et al. Development of the Crohn's disease digestive damage score, the Lemann score. Inflamm Bowel Dis 2011;17: 1415–22.

78. Pariente B, Mary JY, Danese S, et al. Development of the Lemann index to assess digestive tract damage in patients with Crohn's disease. Gastroenterology 2015;148:52–63.e3.

79. Fiorino G, Morin M, Bonovas S, et al. Prevalence of bowel damage assessed by cross-sectional imaging in early Crohn's disease and its impact on disease outcome. J Crohns Colitis 2017;11:274–80.

80. Bodini G, Giannini EG, De Maria C, et al. Anti-TNF therapy is able to stabilize bowel damage progression in patients with Crohn's disease. A study performed using the Lemann Index. Dig Liver Dis 2017;49:175–80.

81. Fiorino G, Bonifacio C, Allocca M, et al. Bowel damage as assessed by the Lemann index is reversible on anti-TNF therapy for Crohn's disease. J Crohns Colitis 2015;9:633–9.

82. Barkmeier DT, Dillman JR, Al-Hawary M, et al. MR enterography-histology comparison in resected pediatric small bowel Crohn disease strictures: can imaging predict fibrosis? Pediatr Radiol 2016;46:498–507.

83. Rimola J, Planell N, Rodriguez S, et al. Characterization of inflammation and fibrosis in Crohn's disease lesions by magnetic resonance imaging. Am J Gastroenterol 2015;110:432–40.

84. Bouhnik Y, Carbonnel F, Laharie D, et al, GETAID CREOLE Study Group. Efficacy of adalimumab in patients with Crohn's disease and symptomatic small bowel stricture: a multicentre, prospective, observational cohort (CREOLE) study. Gut 2018;67(1):53–60.

85. Deepak P, Park SH, Ehman EC, et al. Crohn's disease diagnosis, treatment approach, and management paradigm: what the radiologist needs to know. Abdom Radiol (N Y) 2017;42:1068–86.

86. Calabrese E, Maaser C, Zorzi F, et al. Bowel ultrasonography in the management of Crohn's disease. A review with Recommendations of an International Panel of Experts. Inflamm Bowel Dis 2016;22:1168–83.

87. Di Mizio R, Maconi G, Romano S, et al. Small bowel Crohn disease: sonographic features. Abdom Imaging 2004;29:23–35.

88. Maconi G, Bollani S, Bianchi Porro G. Ultrasonographic detection of intestinal complications in Crohn's disease. Dig Dis Sci 1996;41:1643–8.

89. Maconi G, Nylund K, Ripolles T, et al. EFSUMB recommendations and clinical guidelines for intestinal ultrasound (GIUS) in inflammatory bowel diseases. Ultraschall Med 2018;39:304–17.

90. Maconi G, Parente F, Bollani S, et al. Abdominal ultrasound in the assessment of extent and activity of Crohn's disease: clinical significance and implication of bowel wall thickening. Am J Gastroenterol 1996;91:1604–9.

91. Maconi G, Radice E, Greco S, et al. Bowel ultrasound in Crohn's disease. Best practice and research. Clin Gastroenterol 2006;20:93–112.

92. Dong J, Wang H, Zhao J, et al. Ultrasound as a diagnostic tool in detecting active Crohn's disease: a meta-analysis of prospective studies. Eur Radiol 2014;24:26–33.

93. Cheng W, Gao X, Wang W, et al. Preliminary analysis of clinical situations involved in quantification of contrast-enhanced ultrasound in Crohn's disease. Ultrasound Med Biol 2016;42:1784–91.

94. Quaia E, Migaleddu V, Baratella E, et al. The diagnostic value of small bowel wall vascularity after sulfur hexafluoride-filled microbubble injection in patients with Crohn's disease. Correlation with the therapeutic effectiveness of specific anti-inflammatory treatment. Eur J Radiol 2009;69:438–44.

95. Quaia E, Sozzi M, Angileri R, et al. Time-intensity curves obtained after microbubble injection can be used to differentiate responders from nonresponders among patients with clinically active Crohn disease after 6 weeks of pharmacologic treatment. Radiology 2016;281:606–16.

96. Migaleddu V, Scanu AM, Quaia E, et al. Contrast-enhanced ultrasonographic evaluation of inflammatory activity in Crohn's disease. Gastroenterology 2009;137:43–52.

97. Castiglione F, Bucci L, Pesce G, et al. Oral contrast-enhanced sonography for the diagnosis and grading of postsurgical recurrence of Crohn's disease. Inflamm Bowel Dis 2008;14:1240–5.

98. Gatta G, Di Grezia G, Di Mizio V, et al. Crohn's disease imaging: a review. Gastroenterol Res Pract 2012;2012:816920.

99. Kratzer W, von Tirpitz C, Mason R, et al. Contrast-enhanced power Doppler sonography of the intestinal wall in the differentiation of hypervascularized and hypovascularized intestinal obstructions in patients with Crohn's disease. J Ultrasound Med 2002;21:149–57 [quiz: 158].

100. Serafin Z, Białecki M, Białecka A, et al. Contrast-enhanced ultrasound for detection of Crohn's disease activity: systematic review and meta-analysis. J Crohns Colitis 2016;10:354–62.

101. Martínez MJ, Ripollés T, Paredes JM, et al. Assessment of the extension and the inflammatory activity in Crohn's disease: comparison of ultrasound and MRI. Abdom Imaging 2009;34:141–8.

102. Drews BH, Barth TFE, Hänle MM, et al. Comparison of sonographically measured bowel wall vascularity, histology, and disease activity in Crohn's disease. Eur Radiol 2009;19:1379–86.

103. Malagò R, D'Onofrio M, Mantovani W, et al. Contrast-enhanced ultrasonography (CEUS) vs. MRI of the small bowel in the evaluation of Crohn's disease activity. Radiol Med 2012;117:268–81.
104. Neye H, Voderholzer W, Rickes S, et al. Evaluation of criteria for the activity of Crohn's disease by power Doppler sonography. Dig Dis 2004;22:67–72.
105. Orlando S, Fraquelli M, Coletta M, et al. Ultrasound elasticity imaging predicts therapeutic outcomes of patients with Crohn's disease treated with anti-tumour necrosis factor antibodies. J Crohns Colitis 2018;12:63–70.
106. Paredes JM, Ripollés T, Cortés X, et al. Abdominal sonographic changes after antibody to tumor necrosis factor (anti-TNF) alpha therapy in Crohn's disease. Dig Dis Sci 2010;55:404–10.
107. Calabrese E, Petruzziello C, Onali S, et al. Severity of postoperative recurrence in Crohn's disease: correlation between endoscopic and sonographic findings. Inflamm Bowel Dis 2009;15:1635–42.
108. Calabrese E, Zorzi F, Zuzzi S, et al. Development of a numerical index quantitating small bowel damage as detected by ultrasonography in Crohn's disease. J Crohns Colitis 2012;6:852–60.
109. Parente F, Sampietro GM, Molteni M, et al. Behaviour of the bowel wall during the first year after surgery is a strong predictor of symptomatic recurrence of Crohn's disease: a prospective study. Aliment Pharmacol Ther 2004;20:959–68.
110. Maconi G, Sampietro GM, Parente F, et al. Contrast radiology, computed tomography and ultrasonography in detecting internal fistulas and intra-abdominal abscesses in Crohn's disease: a prospective comparative study. Am J Gastroenterol 2003;98:1545–55.
111. Carnevale Maffè G, Brunetti L, Formagnana P, et al. Ultrasonographic findings in Crohn's disease. J Ultrasound 2015;18:37–49.
112. Ripollés T, Martínez-Pérez MJ, Paredes JM, et al. Contrast-enhanced ultrasound in the differentiation between phlegmon and abscess in Crohn's disease and other abdominal conditions. Eur J Radiol 2013;82:e525–31.
113. Gasche C, Moser G, Turetschek K, et al. Transabdominal bowel sonography for the detection of intestinal complications in Crohn's disease. Gut 1999;44:112–7.
114. Coelho R, Ribeiro H, Maconi G. Bowel thickening in crohn's disease: fibrosis or inflammation? diagnostic ultrasound imaging tools. Inflamm Bowel Dis 2017;23:23–34.
115. Sousa HTD, Brito J, Magro F. New cross-sectional imaging in IBD. Curr Opin Gastroenterol 2018;34:194–207.
116. Stidham RW, Xu J, Johnson LA, et al. Ultrasound elasticity imaging for detecting intestinal fibrosis and inflammation in rats and humans with Crohn's disease. Gastroenterology 2011;141:819–26.e1.
117. Schwartz DA, Wiersema MJ, Dudiak KM, et al. A comparison of endoscopic ultrasound, magnetic resonance imaging, and exam under anesthesia for evaluation of Crohn's perianal fistulas. Gastroenterology 2001;121:1064–72.
118. Siddiqui MRS, Ashrafian H, Tozer P, et al. A diagnostic accuracy meta-analysis of endoanal ultrasound and MRI for perianal fistula assessment. Dis Colon Rectum 2012;55:576–85.

Capsule Endoscopy and Small Bowel Enteroscopy
Have They Rendered the Radiologist Obsolete?

George Ou, MD, Robert Enns, MD*

KEYWORDS

- Capsule endoscopy • Double balloon enteroscopy • Single balloon enteroscopy
- Magnetic resonance enterography • Crohn's disease • Small bowel ulcers

KEY POINTS

- Capsule endoscopy (CE) provides a noninvasive means of visualizing the small bowel, which can aid in diagnosis of small bowel Crohn's disease and monitor therapeutic response with validated scoring systems.
- CE and magnetic resonance enterography (MRE) provide complementary details on Crohn's disease phenotype. CE can detect subtle mucosal lesions, whereas MRE can detect extraluminal disease.
- Patency capsule and cross-sectional imaging should be used to exclude significant stricture before administering CE if there is clinical suspicion of stenotic disease.
- Device-assisted enteroscopy has limited role in the diagnosis and management of small bowel Crohn's disease.

BACKGROUND

The diagnosis of Crohn's disease (CD) requires consideration of a combination of clinical history, symptoms, and evidence of intestinal inflammation based on imaging, endoscopy, histology, and biochemical parameters.[1,2] Given that most patients with CD have ileocolonic involvement, endoscopic and histologic confirmation can usually be achieved through ileocolonoscopy, which is recommended as the first step in the diagnostic algorithm.[1–4] However, approximately 30% of patients have isolated small bowel (SB) disease,[5,6] which can be difficult to access through standard endoscopies including esophagogastroduodenoscopy and ileocolonoscopy. The diagnosis can therefore be missed on the basis of ileocolonoscopy alone.

Noninvasive evaluation of the SB for CD in the past was, however, limited due to technological constraints. Conventional radiologic imaging, such as SB follow-

Disclosure Statement: The authors have no disclosure to report.
Division of Gastroenterology, Department of Medicine, St Paul's Hospital, University of British Columbia, 770-1190 Hornby Street, Vancouver, British Columbia V6Z 2K5, Canada
* Corresponding author.
E-mail address: rob.enns@ubc.ca

through and conventional enteroclysis, lacked sensitivity. The introduction of cross-sectional imaging techniques such as computed tomography (CT) enterography/enteroclysis and magnetic resonance (MR) enterography/enteroclysis enhanced overall bowel wall evaluation with greater accuracy, but subtle mucosal changes can still be missed.

The development of capsule endoscopy (CE) and device-assisted enteroscopy revolutionized the approach to SB diseases. Before their development, intraoperative enteroscopy was the only means of visualizing mid-SB mucosa; deep enteroscopy was achieved by pleating the SB along an endoscope inserted through a surgical enterostomy or mouth/anus. Its invasiveness prevented routine incorporation of enteroscopy into the diagnostic algorithm for SB CD. However, this changed when much less-invasive techniques became available and were adapted into routine clinical practice.

CAPSULE ENDOSCOPY

Small bowel CE was first introduced in 2000 as a noninvasive means of assessing the SB.[7] CE is a capsule-shaped camera that takes several images per second as it passively traverses the gastrointestinal (GI) tract through a combination of bowel peristalsis and gravity. Currently, multiple similar CE systems are available worldwide, most of which wirelessly transmit and store images in an external recorder that patients carry during the recording. The images are then downloaded to a workstation at the end of the procedure to be reviewed in rapid sequence like a motion picture. There are several notable differences in the design of various CE systems, including battery life (8–15 h), image retrieval method (wireless vs stored in camera), frames-per-second recording (2–6 fps), and viewing angle (150°–360°) (**Table 1**).

Patient preparation for CE is straightforward and usually involves taking bowel preparation the day before the procedure. On ingesting the capsule, patients are free to resume normal activity, and resume oral intake several hours into the recording. The procedure ends when the capsule is evacuated from the GI tract, or when the battery life is exhausted. Most CE systems have disposable cameras, so patients do not have to retrieve the camera endoscope unless otherwise specified.

Commonly cited contraindications for CE include implantable cardiac devices, pregnancy, swallowing disorders, and known/suspected strictures. At present, cohort studies and case series/reports have not demonstrated adverse effects among patients with implantable cardiac devices, so the use of CE in this patient population is currently accepted in the most recent guideline.[8] Swallowing difficulty, in absence of structural causes, can also be overcome by deploying the CE directly into the SB with the aid of standard endoscopy. There is no formal guideline recommendation for the use of CE in pregnant women, because of exclusion of this population from previous studies; however, CE seems to be safe during pregnancy based on an isolated case report[9] and anecdotal evidence in clinical practice.

Scoring Systems

In the first few years of experience with CE in CD, there was no standardized scoring system. Thus, studies used various criteria to define positive findings in keeping with CD. This ranged from subjective global evaluation of inflammatory findings[10] to arbitrary assignment of greater than 3 ulcers[11] as diagnostic. Without a standardized language to report the findings on CE, objective quantification of inflammatory burden and precise communication of disease severity were lacking.

Table 1
Examples of small bowel capsule endoscopy systems

	PillCam SB3	EndoCapsule EC-S10	MiroCam MC1600/MC2000	CapsoCam Plus	OMOM Capsule
Dimensions, mm × mm	26.2 × 11.4	26 × 11	24.5 × 10.8/30.1 × 10.8	31 × 11	25.4 × 11
Battery life, h	>8	12	12	15	12
Camera orientation	End view	End view	End view/2× end views	Side view camera ×4	End view
Field of view, °	156	160	170/170 per camera	360	150
Data storage/communication	Radiofrequency	Radiofrequency	Human body communication	Stored in capsule	Radiofrequency
Frame per second	2–6	2	6/3 per camera	3–5 per camera	2
Retrieval postprocedure	Not necessary	Not necessary	Not necessary	Yes for image retrieval	Not necessary

There are currently 2 validated scoring systems for reporting severity of SB CD: the Lewis score (LS)[12–14] and CE Crohn's disease activity index (CECDAI).[15,16] LS, also known as the CE severity index, divides the SB into 3 tertiles based on the time it takes the CE to traverse the SB (ie, SB transit time). Each tertile is then assigned a score based on the 3 parameters (villous edema, ulcers, and stenosis) and their respective extent of involvement. The tertile with the highest score constitutes the final LS. A score <135 is considered normal; 135 to 789 is considered mild; and ≥790 is considered moderate-severe.[12] LS ≥135 has a sensitivity of 89.5% and specificity of 78.9% for the diagnosis of CD among patients who present with suspicious clinical features[14] (**Table 2**).

CECDAI, also known as Niv score, divides the SB into proximal and distal segments, and scores each segment based on 3 parameters (severity of inflammation, extent of disease, and presence of stricture); the segmental scores are then added for a total score.[15] Good correlation has been demonstrated between the 2 scores[17–20] (**Table 3**).

DEVICE-ASSISTED ENTEROSCOPY

Yamamoto and colleagues[21] described the first device-assisted enteroscopy using a double balloon enteroscope (DBE) around the time when CE was introduced. DBE is a 200-cm flexible enteroscope with a latex-based balloon at the end of the enteroscope, and a second balloon on an overtube that slides over the enteroscope. A push-and-pull technique using the 2 balloons for traction allows the enteroscope to advance deep into the SB by pleating the bowel on the overtube like a "curtain on a rod," thereby reducing loop formation. DBE can proceed in antegrade and/or retrograde direction depending on the location of the target lesion, and can examine the entire length of the SB between 18% and 66% of the time.[22]

DBE is considered the reference standard for endoscopic evaluation of SB mucosa, providing the benchmark for comparison of other modalities' performance (eg, MRE

Table 2
Lewis score

Tertile-Specific Parameters	Number	Longitudinal Extent[a]	Descriptor
Villous appearance score per tertile	Normal (0) Edematous (1)	Short segment (8) Long segment (12) Whole tertile (20)	Single (1) Patchy (14) Diffuse (17)
Ulcer score per tertile	None (0) Single (3) Few (5) Multiple (10)	Short segment (5) Long segment (10) Whole tertile (15)	<1/4 (9) 1/4–1/2 (12) >1/2 (18)

Whole-Length Stenosis	Number	Ulceration	Obstruction
Stenosis score for whole length	None (0) Single (14) Multiple (20)	Ulcerated (24) Nonulcerated (2)	Traversed (7) Not traversed (10)

Lewis score = score from worst tertile (villous number × extent × descriptor + ulcer number × extent × descriptor) + whole-length stenosis score (stenosis number × ulceration × obstruction).
[a] Short segment defined as ≤10% of a tertile; long segment defined as 11% to 50% of a tertile; whole tertile defined as >50% of tertile.
From Gralnek IM, Defranchis R, Seidman E, et al. Development of a capsule endoscopy scoring index for small bowel mucosal inflammatory change. Aliment Pharmacol Ther 2008;27(2):150; with permission.

Table 3	
Capsule endoscopy Crohn's disease activity index	
Inflammation score per segment[a]	None (0)
	Mild to moderate edema/hyperemia/denudation (1)
	Severe edema/hyperemia/denudation (2)
	Bleeding, exudate, aphthae, erosion, small ulcer (<0.5 cm) (3)
	Moderate ulcer (0.5–2 cm), pseudopolyp (4)
	Large ulcer (>2 cm) (5)
Extent of disease score per segment[a]	None (0)
	Focal disease (single segment) (1)
	Patchy disease (multiple segment) (2)
	Diffuse disease (3)
Narrowing (stricture) per segment[a]	None (0)
	Single-passed (1)
	Multiple-passed (2)
	Obstruction (3)

Total score = (A1 × B1 × C1) + (A2 + B2 + C2).

[a] Small bowel divided into proximal and distal segments. Segmental score = A × B × C.

From Gal E, Geller A, Fraser G, et al. Assessment and validation of the new capsule endoscopy Crohn's disease activity index (CECDAI). Dig Dis Sci 2008;53(7):1934; with permission.

and CE).[23] However, given its relative invasiveness with an overall major complication rate of approximately 1% (eg, perforation, pancreatitis, bleeding, ileus),[24] its clinical usefulness in the management of CD is limited. Application of DBE in this patient population includes therapeutic dilation of SB stricture,[25,26] retrieval of retained CE,[27,28] and targeted tissue sampling guided by either cross-sectional imaging or CE when histologic diagnosis is required.[1]

Single balloon enteroscopy (SBE) was introduced in 2008, with a similar operating concept as DBE but with 1 significant difference: there is only 1 silicone-based balloon on the overtube and none at the end of the enteroscope.[29] A "hooking maneuver" with the tip of the enteroscope is used to provide the traction in place of the distal balloon. Aside from the design difference and lower rate of complete enteroscopy, SBE has been shown to be equivalent to DBE in many aspects, including diagnostic yield, therapeutic yield, and complication rate.[22]

Spiral enteroscopy (SE) refers to the use of an overtube lined with spiral ridges over either an enteroscope or a pediatric colonoscope. The overtube rotates independently of the endoscope within the SB. The rotational energy is converted into a linear force moving the whole unit (overtube + endoscope) forward together.[30] A significant advantage of SE over both SBE and DBE is the relative ease of use and shorter procedural time; otherwise they all have similar diagnostic yield, therapeutic yield, and depth of endoscope insertion.[31] A motorized SE has also been developed.[32]

Last but not least, an on-demand enteroscopy is available in the form of a catheter-based latex-free balloon that can be introduced through the accessory channel >3.7 mm.[33] Although this system has the advantage of being compatible with standard endoscopes, a potential drawback is the risk of accidental blind dilation of a stricture during balloon inflation because balloon obstructs the view.

CAPSULE ENDOSCOPY IN SUSPECTED/NEWLY DIAGNOSED CROHN'S DISEASE
Small Bowel Ulcerating Disease

CE is becoming increasingly used in the evaluation and management of SB CD, which is the second most common indication for CE.[34] Endoscopic features of CD include mucosal erythema, villous edema, mucosal denudation, erosion, aphthous ulceration, deep ulceration, bleeding, pseudopolyp, and strictures[12,15] (**Fig. 1**). However, many of these features are nonspecific and can be seen in other conditions affecting the SB. Differential diagnoses of SB ulcers/stenoses include nonsteroidal anti-inflammatory drug-induced injury, celiac disease/ulcerative jejunoileitis, chronic mesenteric ischemia, enteric infection, malignancy, hypersecretory disorders, and traumatic injury.[35] Moreover, Goldstein and colleagues[36] elegantly demonstrated that incidental SB lesions of no clinical significance can be seen in 13.8% of healthy volunteers. Among the remaining healthy volunteers in this study, 55% developed small bowel mucosal breaks after receiving 2 weeks of naproxen and omeprazole, while 7% developed new mucosal breaks after receiving 2 weeks of placebo. Thus, CE should be conducted after stopping nonsteroidal anti-inflammatory drugs for at least a month.[1,4] It is also imperative to consider clinical history and other investigations collectively before committing to the diagnosis of CD. Suspicious clinical features of CD include chronic diarrhea, abdominal pain, weight loss, anorexia, anemia, malaise, fever, leukocytosis, increased C-reactive protein/erythrocyte sedimentation rate, and increased fecal calprotectin.[2,37]

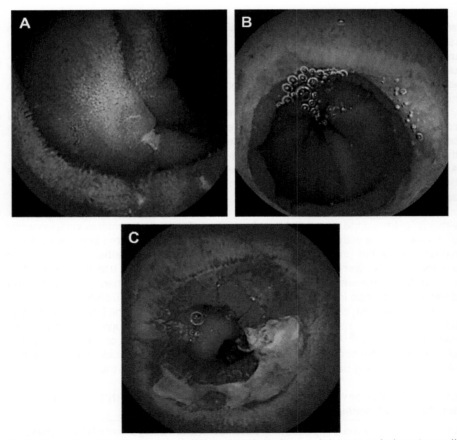

Fig. 1. Examples of CE images of small bowel Crohn's disease. (*A*) Scattered ulcers in small bowel; (*B, C*) ulcerated strictures in small bowel.

Diagnosis of Small Bowel Crohn's Disease

SB evaluation plays an integral part in the work-up of suspected, as well as newly diagnosed CD. For example, it is recommended to assess for isolated SB CD in the setting of suspicious clinical features (ie, symptoms and/or inflammatory markers) after negative standard endoscopic evaluation.[1,3,4] Ileocolonoscopy can miss the diagnosis of CD when lesions "skip" the ileocolonic region and only manifest in the SB, as was demonstrated in 54% of the patients with negative ileocolonoscopy in 1 study.[38]

Further SB evaluation is also recommended once ileal and/or colonic CD is confirmed.[1,4] Up to 66% of these patients can have concomitant proximal SB disease.[39–42] Establishing the extent of CD involvement accurately in each patient has important prognostication and management implications.

Diagnostic Performance

Currently, accepted diagnostic tools for SB evaluation include cross-sectional imaging (MR enterography/enteroclysis or CT enterography/enteroclysis) and SB endoscopy (CE and device-assisted enteroscopy). Enteroclysis differs from enterography in the use of a nasoenteric tube to deliver contrast directly into the proximal SB instead of taking oral contrast. Although enteroclysis has the advantage of achieving better distension of proximal SB loops, CT enterography (CTE) and MR enterography (MRE) provide similar diagnostic characteristics as their respective counterparts while offering patients generally more favorable experience.[43,44]

Since CE was brought into clinical use, many studies have attempted to compare CE with other diagnostic modalities. In absence of a single reference standard for the diagnosis of SB CD, many studies relied on incremental change in diagnostic yield as a surrogate measure of performance. In a meta-analysis by Dionisio and colleagues,[45] CE provides higher diagnostic yield compared with SB barium study (52% vs 16%; incremental yield [IY] = 32%; 95% CI, 16%–48%) and CT enterography/enteroclysis (68% vs 21%; IY = 47%; 95% CI, 31%–63%) in patients with suspected SB CD, but not in comparison with MR enterography/enteroclysis (55% vs 45%; IY = 10%; 95% CI, −14%–34%). In a more recent meta-analysis, CE was shown to have comparable diagnostic yield as MR enterography/enteroclysis (odds ratio [OR] = 1.17; 95% CI, 0.83–1.67) and small intestine contrast ultrasound (OR = 0.88; 95% CI, 0.51–1.53).[46]

Choosing the Test

Despite the similarity in overall diagnostic yields between CE and MRE, there are features of each that provide complementary information. The choice of initial test for SB evaluation therefore should be individualized based on patient factors, associated symptoms, and clinical question to be addressed.

By virtue of high-resolution visualization, CE is able to detect more cases of mild CD activity with subtle mucosal abnormalities than MRE.[23] CE has a high negative predictive value in patients with suspected CD, making it an excellent "rule-out" test.[47,48] CE is also able to detect more cases of proximal SB CD than MRE.[46,49] This is a potential advantage of CE for prognostication purposes because proximal CD is associated with higher risk of stricture formation and need for surgical intervention.[50] Early identification of this high-risk group may allow for earlier aggressive therapy to reduce risk of CD complications. CE may also still have a place in the diagnostic algorithm when there is persistent clinical suspicion despite negative ileocolonoscpoy and cross-sectional imaging. In a prospective study of patients with persistent perianal disease but negative standard work-up, CE had an incremental diagnostic yield of 24% following negative ileocolonoscopy and radiology imaging.[51]

In contrast to CE, which can only detect mucosal changes, cross-sectional imaging can also identify transmural abnormalities and extraintestinal pathologies of CD, such as fistula formation and intra-abdominal abscess. MRE can also detect luminal stricture that would otherwise preclude safe administration of CE.[23] Thus, patients with features of sepsis including tachycardia, fever, and leukocytosis, and patients with obstructive symptoms should undergo MRE or CTE to look for these complicated pathologies, which may lead to a shift from medical management to a more surgical approach.[1,2]

Without a history of obstructive symptoms or known strictures, CE can be administered in patients with suspected CD without significantly increased risk of capsule retention, defined as the presence of CE in the GI tract after 2 weeks. The rate of capsule retention in patients with suspected CD was reported to be approximately 3.6% (95% CI, 1.7%–8.6%) compared with 2.1% (95% CI, 1.5%–2.8%) in patients with suspected SB bleeding.[52] If there are concerns of stricturing disease due to history of obstructive symptoms or suspicious finding on other investigations, then functional patency of the bowel should be demonstrated first using a dissolvable patency capsule that mimics the actual diagnostic CE. Alternatively, cross-sectional imaging can be used to assess for SB disease while avoiding the risk of capsule retention, as discussed earlier.

In summary, CE and cross-sectional imaging are complementary diagnostic tools for the work-up of suspected SB CD; CE is able to detect subtle mucosal lesions as well as those located in the proximal SB; cross-sectional imaging can detect more severe disease activity and better characterize the CD phenotype in terms of extraluminal involvement (**Table 4**). Availability of local expertise/resources, specific clinical question (eg, rule out concomitant SB disease or assess for extraluminal manifestations), and patient factors (eg, pacemaker or claustrophobia precluding MRE) need to be considered in choosing the appropriate diagnostic tool.

CAPSULE ENDOSCOPY IN MONITORING ESTABLISHED CROHN'S DISEASE
Mucosal Healing

Mucosal healing, as determined by endoscopic evaluation with ileocolonoscopy, has become the therapeutic target in the management of CD.[2] It is associated with improved outcomes in terms of long-term clinical remission, steroid-free clinical remission, endoscopic remission, and reduced surgical intervention.[53–55] A similar concept is extrapolated to SB CD; limited evidence has shown that normal CE at baseline predicts fewer clinical relapses at 1 year (0% vs 23%)[56] and lower CE score

Table 4			
Advantages and disadvantages of capsule endoscopy versus MR enterography versus CT enterography			
	Capsule Endoscopy	**MR Enterography**	**CT Enterography**
Advantage	• Endoscopic view may detect subtle lesion • Superior proximal SB lesion detection	• Extraluminal finding	• Extraluminal finding • Widespread availability
Disadvantage	• Risk of capsule retention and bowel obstruction • Distal small bowel view may be obscured by debris	• Long scan time in tight space (claustrophobia) • Intravenous contrast • Metal foreign object contraindicated • Underdistention of bowel loops can compromise view	• Ionizing radiation • Intravenous contrast

at baseline predicts mucosal healing at follow-up between 12 weeks and 24 months (OR = 11.06; 95% CI, 3.74–32.73).[57]

Although the accuracy of CE in monitoring proximal SB CD over time has not been formally compared with device-assisted enteroscopy because of the latter procedure's invasiveness, distal SB mucosal changes seen on CE seem to correlate with those seen on ileocolonoscopy, which is the reference standard in terminal ileal CD.[58] The diagnostic superiority, or at least equivalency, of CE to radiologic imaging has also been repeatedly demonstrated in patients with established CD. In an early meta-analysis, CE had superior diagnostic yield compared with SB barium study (71% vs 36%; IY = 38%; 95% CI, 22%–54%) and CT enterography/enteroclysis (71% vs 39%; IY = 32%; 95% CI, 16%–47%), but not when compared with MR enteroclysis/enterography (70% vs 79%; IY = −6%; 95% CI, −30%–19%).[45] In a more recent analysis of studies comparing CE's diagnostic yield to that of radiology techniques, Kopylov and colleagues[46] found the diagnostic yield of CE to be similar to that of MR enterography/enteroclysis (OR = 0.88; 95% CI, 0.53–1.48) and small intestine contrast ultrasound (OR = 0.57; 95% CI, 0.27–1.20).

Considering the similar testing characteristics of CE and MRE in established CD, the choice of test may again be influenced by additional factors (see **Table 4**). For example, MRE may be more appropriate for patients with a history of fibrostenotic and/or penetrating CD; CE may assess proximal SB lesions more accurately; and CE may be preferred over other cross-sectional imaging modalities in patients with contraindications for MRE. Another important factor to consider is patient preference in order to improve adherence to therapy/follow-up. In a prospective study of patients with CD experiencing mild/no clinical symptoms, CE was better tolerated and preferred because of less side effects.[59]

Postoperative Recurrence Surveillance

CE has also shown some promise in postoperative recurrence surveillance, with excellent sensitivity but relatively poor specificity compared with the other modalities including intestinal ultrasound and MRE.[60] Considering the risk of capsule retention and the inability to obtain tissue samples, CE is unlikely to overtake ileocolonoscopy as the standard of practice for patients who have undergone ileocolonic resection. However, there may still be a role in patients who have undergone SB resection with entero-enteral anastomosis that is beyond the reach of a standard endoscope.

Reclassification of Inflammatory Bowel Disease

CE can potentially clarify SB status in patients with unclassified inflammatory bowel disease (IBD),[61] which accounts for approximately 10% of patients with IBD at diagnosis.[62] In a multicenter retrospective study, 25% (9/36) of patients with unclassified IBD were found to have features on CE (ie, LS ≥135) consistent with CD.[63] All these patients were subsequently reclassified to CD based on overall clinical presentation and investigations, and the immunosuppressive therapy of many patients was adjusted as a result. In 2 other smaller studies, 50% of patients with colonic inflammation were also reclassified to having SB CD after CE.[64,65] Although a positive CE can lead to immediate clinical impact through reclassification of IBD, a negative result does not exclude the diagnosis of CD in unclassified IBD, which may become evident in the future.[63]

Clinical Impact Based on Capsule Endoscopy Findings

New information from CE often leads to a significant clinical impact in patients with CD by directing their medical therapy. Retrospective studies showed CE conferring an impact on medical management in 40% to 64% of patients,[40,65–69] with associated positive outcome at 1-year reported in 1 study due to the therapeutic changes.[65] In a prospective study of 50 adult patients with CD who underwent CE after ileocolonoscopy and MRE/CTE, additional findings on CE led care-providers to change treatment plan in 34% of the patients.[49] In another small prospective study with 18 pediatric patients with suspected or established CD, CE led to change in medical management in 14 (78%) patients.[64] Given these observations, patients with persistent clinical/biochemical features suspicious for CD but negative findings on standard evaluations should undergo CE to assess for SB CD activity.[3,70]

Assessing Bowel Patency

In patients with established CD, the prevalence of strictures has been shown to be approximately 25%.[23,69,71] Capsule retention rate has been reported to be as high as 13%,[72] but a meta-analysis found a pooled rate of 8.2% (95% CI, 6%–11%).[52] Predictors of capsule retention in patients with SB CD seem to be the presence of stricturing and penetrating phenotypes (OR ~ 10 in both).[73,74]

Risk of capsule retention can be stratified using cross-sectional imaging such as MRE/CTE or patency capsule, both of which have high negative predictive value,[75] and can lower the overall risk of retention to 2.7% (95% CI, 1.1%–6.4%).[1–4,52,70]

Nonselective use of patency capsule in all patients with established CD did not reduce the rate of capsule retention compared with a selective approach based on history of obstructive symptoms, previous obstruction, or previous abdominal surgery.[76] Patency capsule was shown to have a high false-positive rate (because of bowel motility) in the same study, with only 11.1% retention rate after the actual diagnostic CE. This false positivity may preclude patients from undergoing an otherwise useful diagnostic test. Patency capsule also only matches the dimensions of PillCam SB3 (Medtronic, Minneapolis, MN, USA), limiting its applicability to other CE systems.

Another consideration is that capsule retention, which is arbitrarily defined as nonexcretion of CE after a 14-day period, does not always lead to clinical symptoms. In a large multicenter retrospective study of CE-related adverse events, 61.5% of patients remained asymptomatic despite retention, 37.5% of the events resolved spontaneously after a mean of 42 days, and 19.2% resolved with medical therapy after a mean of 24 days.[77] Initial conservative management with medical therapy for capsule retention is therefore recommended, before attempting endoscopic retrieval with device-assisted enteroscopy.[4]

With the above considerations in mind, a more selective approach of assessing risk of retention in patients with CD will likely suffice. This includes patients with obstructive symptoms,[2,70] known strictures,[70] and/or history of bowel resection.[1,70]

REFERENCES

1. Maaser C, Sturm A, Vavricka SR, et al. ECCO-ESGAR guideline for diagnostic assessment in IBD Part 1: initial diagnosis, monitoring of known IBD, detection of complications. J Crohns Colitis 2019;13:144–64.
2. Lichtenstein GR, Loftus EV, Isaacs KL, et al. ACG clinical guideline: management of Crohn's disease in adults. Am J Gastroenterol 2018;113(4):481–517.
3. American Society for Gastrointestinal Endoscopy Standards of Practice Committee, Shergill AK, Lightdale JR, et al. The role of endoscopy in inflammatory bowel disease. Gastrointest Endosc 2015;81(5):1101–21.e1-13.
4. Pennazio M, Spada C, Eliakim R, et al. Small-bowel capsule endoscopy and device-assisted enteroscopy for diagnosis and treatment of small-bowel

disorders: European Society of Gastrointestinal Endoscopy (ESGE) clinical guideline. Endoscopy 2015;47(4):352–76.

5. Steinhardt HJ, Loeschke K, Kasper H, et al. European Cooperative Crohn's Disease Study (ECCDS): clinical features and natural history. Digestion 1985; 31(2–3):97–108.

6. Cheifetz AS. Management of active Crohn disease. JAMA 2013;309(20):2150–8.

7. Iddan G, Meron G, Glukhovsky A, et al. Wireless capsule endoscopy. Nature 2000;405(6785):417.

8. Rondonotti E, Spada C, Adler S, et al. Small-bowel capsule endoscopy and device-assisted enteroscopy for diagnosis and treatment of small-bowel disorders: European Society of Gastrointestinal Endoscopy (ESGE) technical review. Endoscopy 2018;50(4):423–46.

9. Hogan RB, Ahmad N, Hogan RB 3rd, et al. Video capsule endoscopy detection of jejunal carcinoid in life-threatening hemorrhage, first trimester pregnancy. Gastrointest Endosc 2007;66(1):205–7.

10. Solem CA, Loftus EV Jr, Fletcher JG, et al. Small-bowel imaging in Crohn's disease: a prospective, blinded, 4-way comparison trial. Gastrointest Endosc 2008;68(2):255–66.

11. Mow WS, Lo SK, Targan SR, et al. Initial experience with wireless capsule enteroscopy in the diagnosis and management of inflammatory bowel disease. Clin Gastroenterol Hepatol 2004;2(1):31–40.

12. Gralnek IM, Defranchis R, Seidman E, et al. Development of a capsule endoscopy scoring index for small bowel mucosal inflammatory change. Aliment Pharmacol Ther 2008;27(2):146–54.

13. Rosa B, Moreira MJ, Rebelo A, et al. Lewis score: a useful clinical tool for patients with suspected Crohn's disease submitted to capsule endoscopy. J Crohns Colitis 2012;6(6):692–7.

14. Monteiro S, Boal Carvalho P, Dias de Castro F, et al. Capsule endoscopy: diagnostic accuracy of Lewis score in patients with suspected Crohn's disease. Inflamm Bowel Dis 2015;21(10):2241–6.

15. Gal E, Geller A, Fraser G, et al. Assessment and validation of the new capsule endoscopy Crohn's disease activity index (CECDAI). Dig Dis Sci 2008;53(7):1933–7.

16. Niv Y, Ilani S, Levi Z, et al. Validation of the capsule endoscopy Crohn's disease activity index (CECDAI or Niv score): a multicenter prospective study. Endoscopy 2012;44(1):21–6.

17. Yablecovitch D, Lahat A, Neuman S, et al. The Lewis score or the capsule endoscopy Crohn's disease activity index: which one is better for the assessment of small bowel inflammation in established Crohn's disease? Therap Adv Gastroenterol 2018;11. 1756283X17747780.

18. Arieira C, Dias de Castro F, Rosa B, et al. Can we rely on inflammatory biomarkers for the diagnosis and monitoring Crohn's disease activity? Rev Esp Enferm Dig 2017;109(12):828–33.

19. Ponte A, Pinho R, Rodrigues A, et al. Evaluation and comparison of capsule endoscopy scores for assessment of inflammatory activity of small-bowel in Crohn's disease. Gastroenterol Hepatol 2018;41(4):245–50.

20. Koulaouzidis A, Douglas S, Plevris JN. Lewis score correlates more closely with fecal calprotectin than capsule endoscopy Crohn's disease activity index. Dig Dis Sci 2012;57(4):987–93.

21. Yamamoto H, Sekine Y, Sato Y, et al. Total enteroscopy with a nonsurgical steerable double-balloon method. Gastrointest Endosc 2001;53(2):216–20.

22. Wadhwa V, Sethi S, Tewani S, et al. A meta-analysis on efficacy and safety: single-balloon vs. double-balloon enteroscopy. Gastroenterol Rep (Oxf) 2015;3(2): 148–55.

23. Wiarda BM, Mensink PB, Heine DG, et al. Small bowel Crohn's disease: MR enteroclysis and capsule endoscopy compared to balloon-assisted enteroscopy. Abdom Imaging 2012;37(3):397–403.

24. Xin L, Liao Z, Jiang YP, et al. Indications, detectability, positive findings, total enteroscopy, and complications of diagnostic double-balloon endoscopy: a systematic review of data over the first decade of use. Gastrointest Endosc 2011; 74(3):563–70.

25. Hirai F, Andoh A, Ueno F, et al. Efficacy of endoscopic balloon dilation for small bowel strictures in patients with Crohn's disease: a nationwide, multi-centre, open-label, prospective cohort study. J Crohns Colitis 2018;12(4):394–401.

26. Bettenworth D, Gustavsson A, Atreja A, et al. A pooled analysis of efficacy, safety, and long-term outcome of endoscopic balloon dilation therapy for patients with stricturing Crohn's disease. Inflamm Bowel Dis 2017;23(1):133–42.

27. Mitsui K, Fujimori S, Tanaka S, et al. Retrieval of retained capsule endoscopy at small bowel stricture by double-balloon endoscopy significantly decreases surgical treatment. J Clin Gastroenterol 2016;50(2):141–6.

28. Makipour K, Modiri AN, Ehrlich A, et al. Double balloon enteroscopy: effective and minimally invasive method for removal of retained video capsules. Dig Endosc 2014;26(5):646–9.

29. Tsujikawa T, Saitoh Y, Andoh A, et al. Novel single-balloon enteroscopy for diagnosis and treatment of the small intestine: preliminary experiences. Endoscopy 2008;40(1):11–5.

30. Akerman PA, Agrawal D, Chen W, et al. Spiral enteroscopy: a novel method of enteroscopy by using the endo-ease discovery SB overtube and a pediatric colonoscope. Gastrointest Endosc 2009;69(2):327–32.

31. Baniya R, Upadhaya S, Subedi SC, et al. Balloon enteroscopy versus spiral enteroscopy for small-bowel disorders: a systematic review and meta-analysis. Gastrointest Endosc 2017;86(6):997–1005.

32. Neuhaus H, Beyna T, Schneider M, et al. Novel motorized spiral enteroscopy: first clinical case. VideoGIE 2016;1(2):32–3.

33. Tontini GE, Grauer M, Akin H, et al. Extensive small-bowel diverticulosis identified with the newly introduced on demand enteroscopy system. Endoscopy 2013; 45(Suppl 2 UCTN):E350–1.

34. Liao Z, Gao R, Xu C, et al. Indications and detection, completion, and retention rates of small-bowel capsule endoscopy: a systematic review. Gastrointest Endosc 2010;71(2):280–6.

35. Freeman HJ. Multifocal stenosing ulceration of the small intestine. World J Gastroenterol 2009;15(39):4883–5.

36. Goldstein JL, Eisen GM, Lewis B, et al. Video capsule endoscopy to prospectively assess small bowel injury with celecoxib, naproxen plus omeprazole, and placebo. Clin Gastroenterol Hepatol 2005;3(2):133–41.

37. Gomollon F, Dignass A, Annese V, et al. European evidence-based consensus on the diagnosis and management of Crohn's disease 2016: part 1: diagnosis and medical management. J Crohns Colitis 2017;11(1):3–25.

38. Samuel S, Bruining DH, Loftus EV Jr, et al. Endoscopic skipping of the distal terminal ileum in Crohn's disease can lead to negative results from ileocolonoscopy. Clin Gastroenterol Hepatol 2012;10(11):1253–9.

39. Cotter J, Dias de Castro F, Moreira MJ, et al. Tailoring Crohn's disease treatment: the impact of small bowel capsule endoscopy. J Crohns Colitis 2014;8(12): 1610–5.
40. Kopylov U, Nemeth A, Koulaouzidis A, et al. Small bowel capsule endoscopy in the management of established Crohn's disease: clinical impact, safety, and correlation with inflammatory biomarkers. Inflamm Bowel Dis 2015;21(1):93–100.
41. Flamant M, Trang C, Maillard O, et al. The prevalence and outcome of jejunal lesions visualized by small bowel capsule endoscopy in Crohn's disease. Inflamm Bowel Dis 2013;19(7):1390–6.
42. Petruzziello C, Onali S, Calabrese E, et al. Wireless capsule endoscopy and proximal small bowel lesions in Crohn's disease. World J Gastroenterol 2010;16(26): 3299–304.
43. Arrive L, El Mouhadi S. MR enterography versus MR enteroclysis. Radiology 2013;266(2):688.
44. Minordi LM, Vecchioli A, Mirk P, et al. CT enterography with polyethylene glycol solution vs CT enteroclysis in small bowel disease. Br J Radiol 2011;84(998): 112–9.
45. Dionisio PM, Gurudu SR, Leighton JA, et al. Capsule endoscopy has a significantly higher diagnostic yield in patients with suspected and established small-bowel Crohn's disease: a meta-analysis. Am J Gastroenterol 2010;105(6): 1240–8 [quiz: 1249].
46. Kopylov U, Yung DE, Engel T, et al. Diagnostic yield of capsule endoscopy versus magnetic resonance enterography and small bowel contrast ultrasound in the evaluation of small bowel Crohn's disease: systematic review and meta-analysis. Dig Liver Dis 2017;49(8):854–63.
47. Hall B, Holleran G, Costigan D, et al. Capsule endoscopy: high negative predictive value in the long term despite a low diagnostic yield in patients with suspected Crohn's disease. United European Gastroenterol J 2013;1(6):461–6.
48. Tukey M, Pleskow D, Legnani P, et al. The utility of capsule endoscopy in patients with suspected Crohn's disease. Am J Gastroenterol 2009;104(11):2734–9.
49. Hansel SL, McCurdy JD, Barlow JM, et al. Clinical benefit of capsule endoscopy in Crohn's disease: impact on patient management and prevalence of proximal small bowel involvement. Inflamm Bowel Dis 2018;24(7):1582–8.
50. Lazarev M, Huang C, Bitton A, et al. Relationship between proximal Crohn's disease location and disease behavior and surgery: a cross-sectional study of the IBD Genetics Consortium. Am J Gastroenterol 2013;108(1):106–12.
51. Adler SN, Yoav M, Eitan S, et al. Does capsule endoscopy have an added value in patients with perianal disease and a negative work up for Crohn's disease? World J Gastrointest Endosc 2012;4(5):185–8.
52. Rezapour M, Amadi C, Gerson LB. Retention associated with video capsule endoscopy: systematic review and meta-analysis. Gastrointest Endosc 2017; 85(6):1157–68.e2.
53. Schnitzler F, Fidder H, Ferrante M, et al. Mucosal healing predicts long-term outcome of maintenance therapy with infliximab in Crohn's disease. Inflamm Bowel Dis 2009;15(9):1295–301.
54. Froslie KF, Jahnsen J, Moum BA, et al. Mucosal healing in inflammatory bowel disease: results from a Norwegian population-based cohort. Gastroenterology 2007;133(2):412–22.
55. Baert F, Moortgat L, Van Assche G, et al. Mucosal healing predicts sustained clinical remission in patients with early-stage Crohn's disease. Gastroenterology 2010;138(2):463–8 [quiz: e10–1].

56. Aggarwal V, Day AS, Connor S, et al. Role of capsule endoscopy and fecal bio-markers in small-bowel Crohn's disease to assess remission and predict relapse. Gastrointest Endosc 2017;86(6):1070–8.

57. Niv Y. Small-bowel mucosal healing assessment by capsule endoscopy as a predictor of long-term clinical remission in patients with Crohn's disease: a systematic review and meta-analysis. Eur J Gastroenterol Hepatol 2017;29(7):844–8.

58. Melmed GY, Dubinsky MC, Rubin DT, et al. Utility of video capsule endoscopy for longitudinal monitoring of Crohn's disease activity in the small bowel: a prospective study. Gastrointest Endosc 2018;88(6):947–55.e2.

59. Lahat A, Kopylov U, Amitai MM, et al. Magnetic resonance enterography or video capsule endoscopy - what do Crohn's disease patients prefer? Patient Prefer Adherence 2016;10:1043–50.

60. Yung DE, Har-Noy O, Tham YS, et al. Capsule endoscopy, magnetic resonance enterography, and small bowel ultrasound for evaluation of postoperative recurrence in Crohn's disease: systematic review and meta-analysis. Inflamm Bowel Dis 2017;24(1):93–100.

61. Silverberg MS, Satsangi J, Ahmad T, et al. Toward an integrated clinical, molecular and serological classification of inflammatory bowel disease: report of a Working Party of the 2005 Montreal World Congress of Gastroenterology. Can J Gastroenterol 2005;19(Suppl A):5A–36A.

62. Prenzel F, Uhlig HH. Frequency of indeterminate colitis in children and adults with IBD - a metaanalysis. J Crohns Colitis 2009;3(4):277–81.

63. Monteiro S, Dias de Castro F, Boal Carvalho P, et al. Essential role of small bowel capsule endoscopy in reclassification of colonic inflammatory bowel disease type unclassified. World J Gastrointest Endosc 2017;9(1):34–40.

64. Gralnek IM, Cohen SA, Ephrath H, et al. Small bowel capsule endoscopy impacts diagnosis and management of pediatric inflammatory bowel disease: a prospective study. Dig Dis Sci 2012;57(2):465–71.

65. Min SB, Le-Carlson M, Singh N, et al. Video capsule endoscopy impacts decision making in pediatric IBD: a single tertiary care center experience. Inflamm Bowel Dis 2013;19(10):2139–45.

66. Dussault C, Gower-Rousseau C, Salleron J, et al. Small bowel capsule endoscopy for management of Crohn's disease: a retrospective tertiary care centre experience. Dig Liver Dis 2013;45(7):558–61.

67. Long MD, Barnes E, Isaacs K, et al. Impact of capsule endoscopy on management of inflammatory bowel disease: a single tertiary care center experience. Inflamm Bowel Dis 2011;17(9):1855–62.

68. Lorenzo-Zuniga V, de Vega VM, Domenech E, et al. Impact of capsule endoscopy findings in the management of Crohn's disease. Dig Dis Sci 2010;55(2):411–4.

69. Santos-Antunes J, Cardoso H, Lopes S, et al. Capsule enteroscopy is useful for the therapeutic management of Crohn's disease. World J Gastroenterol 2015; 21(44):12660–6.

70. Enns RA, Hookey L, Armstrong D, et al. Clinical practice guidelines for the use of video capsule endoscopy. Gastroenterology 2017;152(3):497–514.

71. Voderholzer WA, Beinhoelzl J, Rogalla P, et al. Small bowel involvement in Crohn's disease: a prospective comparison of wireless capsule endoscopy and computed tomography enteroclysis. Gut 2005;54(3):369–73.

72. Cheifetz AS, Kornbluth AA, Legnani P, et al. The risk of retention of the capsule endoscope in patients with known or suspected Crohn's disease. Am J Gastroenterol 2006;101(10):2218–22.

73. Rozendorn N, Klang E, Lahat A, et al. Prediction of patency capsule retention in known Crohn's disease patients by using magnetic resonance imaging. Gastrointest Endosc 2016;83(1):182–7.

74. Albuquerque A, Cardoso H, Marques M, et al. Predictive factors of small bowel patency in Crohn's disease patients. Rev Esp Enferm Dig 2016;108(2):65–70.

75. Yadav A, Heigh RI, Hara AK, et al. Performance of the patency capsule compared with nonenteroclysis radiologic examinations in patients with known or suspected intestinal strictures. Gastrointest Endosc 2011;74(4):834–9.

76. Nemeth A, Kopylov U, Koulaouzidis A, et al. Use of patency capsule in patients with established Crohn's disease. Endoscopy 2016;48(4):373–9.

77. Fernandez-Urien I, Carretero C, Gonzalez B, et al. Incidence, clinical outcomes, and therapeutic approaches of capsule endoscopy-related adverse events in a large study population. Rev Esp Enferm Dig 2015;107(12):745–52.

Endoscopy in Postoperative Patients with Crohn's Disease or Ulcerative Colitis. Does It Translate to Better Outcomes?

Abhik Bhattacharya, MD, Bo Shen, MD, Miguel Regueiro, MD*

KEYWORDS

- Postoperative Crohn's disease • Postoperative recurrence
- Postoperative ulcerative colitis • J pouch • Pouchitis • Needle knife • Stricturotomy
- Fistulotomy

KEY POINTS

- Postoperative recurrence occurs in nearly 60% of patients undergoing resection for Crohn's disease.
- It is important for gastroenterologists to know the findings and appropriate language associated with postoperative recurrence (ie, Rutgeert score).
- It is important for endoscopists to understand different postoperative anatomies of Crohn's disease, in order to identify the landmarks that help in determining postoperative recurrence of disease.
- Because 30% of patients with ulcerative colitis require colectomy over their lifetimes, it is important for endoscopists to understand the ileal pouch anal anastomosis (IPAA) anatomy and its variations.
- IPAA can develop a variety of complications, including pouchitis, recurrence of Crohn's disease in the neoterminal ileum, irritable pouch syndrome, strictures, and fistulas. It is important for gastroenterologists to recognize the endoscopic appearance of these complications in order to better manage these patients.

Disclosures: A. Bhattacharya has nothing to disclose. B. Shen is a consultant for Janssen, AbbVie, and Takeda. M. Regueiro has received research support from AbbVie, Janssen, and Takeda; unrestricted educational grants from AbbVie, Janssen, UCB, Pfizer, Takeda, Salix, and Shire; and is on the Advisory Boards and is a consultant for AbbVie, Janssen, UCB, Takeda, Pfizer, Miraca Labs, Amgen, Celgene, Seres, and Allergan.
Department of Gastroenterology, Hepatology, and Nutrition, Cleveland Clinic Foundation, 9500 Euclid Avenue, A30, Cleveland, OH 44195, USA
* Corresponding author.
E-mail address: regueim@ccf.org

Gastrointest Endoscopy Clin N Am 29 (2019) 487–514
https://doi.org/10.1016/j.giec.2019.02.013
1052-5157/19/© 2019 Elsevier Inc. All rights reserved.

INTRODUCTION

Both Crohn's disease (CD) and ulcerative colitis (UC) are chronic inflammatory disorders of the gastrointestinal system. Although CD can involve the mouth to the anus, UC is limited only to the colon. Approximately 54% of patients with CD develop an intestinal complication, such as stricture, fistula, or abscess.[1] This complication leads to surgery, with the cumulative risk for resection as high as 70% in 15 years, most commonly an ileocecal resection.[2] Intestinal surgery is not curative and most patients have recurrence after surgery. In patients with UC, the 5-year, 10-year, and 20-year actuarial risk of requiring colectomy has been reported as around 7.5%, 10.4%, and 14.8%, respectively.[3] In UC, surgery is thought to be curative; however, complications are common; for example, the risk of pouchitis in patients who undergo colectomy with ileal pouch anal anastomosis (IPAA). This article discusses the management of postoperative inflammatory bowel diseases (IBDs), focusing on the medical and endoscopic aspects of management.

CROHN'S DISEASE
Natural History of Postoperative Crohn's Disease

In the pre–biologic therapy era, the risk of postoperative surgical recurrence (POR) in CD was as high as 60% (**Fig. 1**).[4] Recent reports indicate that the clinical recurrence (CR) is approximately 40% and endoscopic recurrence as high as 90% by 5 years.[5] POR is often clinically silent with histologic recurrence (HR) occurring as early as 1 week after surgery.[6] In a study published by Rutgeerts and colleagues,[7,8] it was observed that 72% of patients had endoscopic recurrence within 1 year of an ileocolonic resection and primary anastomosis. The endoscopic recurrence is seen in the preanastomotic region and graded based on severity.[7] Often the endoscopic recurrence is clinically silent with most patients asymptomatic; only 35% to 50% of patients developed clinical symptoms of recurrence by 5 years.[7–10] There is very poor correlation between endoscopic disease activity and clinical activity.[9,11] Approximately 35% of patients require another surgical resection by 10 years.[12] In the biologic era the POR seems to be lower, but, despite this, patients still develop endoscopic recurrence and subsequent need for surgery.[13]

Definition of Recurrence

There are several definitions of postoperative CD recurrence: histologic, endoscopic, clinical, and surgical.

Histologic recurrence

This is defined as the presence of disease activity histologically from ileocolonoscopy mucosal "pinch" biopsies or resected intestine from surgery. HR may be present in the absence of endoscopic recurrence; that is, macroscopically normal-appearing neo-terminal ileum on endoscopy, but active CD on histopathology. A scoring system has been developed for quantifying histologic disease activity.[6,14] The significance

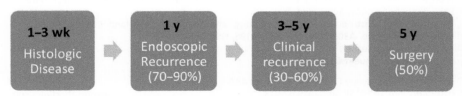

Fig. 1. Natural history of postoperative CD. (*Data from* Refs.[6–8])

of histologic POR in endoscopically normal neoterminal ileum from patients who are asymptomatic is not known. However, it is the authors' practice to use histologic activity to decide on who to continue on postoperative medications rather than deescalate or stop therapy. Patients in an endoscopic remission for at least 3 years without histologic inflammation are those with whom we have a discussion about stopping therapy. If treatment is stopped, we routinely perform the next colonoscopy 1 year later. Those patients with histologic activity in the neoterminal ileum but normal-appearing mucosa present a dilemma. For those patients who have had more than 2 resections, we continue therapy indefinitely because of the high risk of future recurrence.

Endoscopic recurrence

Endoscopic findings represent the primary end point of most postoperative CD studies and is a clinically practical target for gastroenterologists managing such patients. The endoscopic activity determines when medical therapy needs to be initiated, escalated, or potentially deescalated. The scoring system developed by Rutgeerts and colleagues[7] is the most widely applied to postoperative CD. This endoscopic score was derived from a prospective cohort study of 89 patients who underwent ileocolonic resections to assess predictors of recurrent disease. The strongest predictor of clinical POR was endoscopically active CD within 10 cm of ileum above the anastomosis (neoterminal ileum) 1 year after surgery (**Fig. 2** and **Table 1**). Patients with normal mucosa or mild inflammation of less than 5 aphthous ulcers (i0, i1) had less than 10% risk of clinical symptom recurrence at 5 to 10 years, whereas those with very severe diseases (i3, i4) had greater than 90% risk of recurrence at 5 to 10 years. There is good intraobserver reliability for the Rutgeerts scoring system with kappa coefficients of 0.43 and 0.67[15,16]. However, the score has not been validated to define recurrence or remission, but prognosticates future clinical and surgical recurrence. Despite the lack of validation, most studies have defined endoscopic remission as a score of i0 or i1 with recurrence as i2, 3, and 4. Limiting the validity of the score is the fact that a patient with a score of i2 is deemed as recurrence, whereas another patient with i1 is remission. This scoring means that remission and recurrence may be separated by 2 aphthous ulcers; for example, i1 = 4 aphthae and i2 = 6 aphthae. In this context a more robust separation would be to separate any inflammation from complete absence of inflammation or no Crohn recurrence (i0) from those with severe recurrence (i3 or i4).

Clinical recurrence

CR has been measured by the CD Activity Index (CDAI),[17] Harvey Bradshaw Index,[18] and patient-reported outcome measures.[19] Measurement of CR is imperfect in postoperative CD because patients may have symptoms related to the surgical resection; for example, bile salt diarrhea or altered motility, or they may be asymptomatic despite endoscopic activity (eg, clinically silent). In the study by Regueiro and colleagues,[11] there was very low agreement (kappa coefficient, 0.12) between patient endoscopic score and CDAI. Therefore, endoscopic outcomes should be the measure by which postoperative remission or recurrence is defined.

Other markers of postoperative Crohn's disease recurrence

Other less invasive modalities of determining postoperative recurrence have been studied. These modalities include the use of fecal calprotectin, small bowel ultrasonography, video capsule endoscopy (VCE), magnetic resonance enterography (MRE) and computed tomography enterography (CTE). Fecal calprotectin level less than 100 µg/g had good negative predictive value and correlated with remission.[20–23]

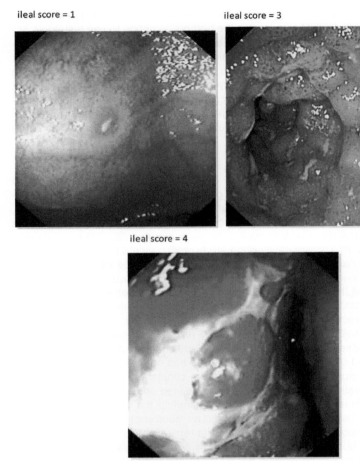

Fig. 2. Endoscopic views of postoperative CD recurrence in the ileum.

Table 1	
Postoperative ileal endoscopic recurrence score	
Endoscopic Score[a]	**Definition**
i0	No lesions
i1	≤5 aphthous lesions
i2	>5 aphthous lesions with normal mucosa between the lesions or skip areas of larger lesions or lesions confined to the ileocolonic anastomosis
i3	Diffuse aphthous ileitis with diffusely inflamed mucosa
i4	Diffuse inflammation with already larger ulcers, nodules, and/or narrowing

[a] Remission, endoscopic score of i0 or i1; recurrence, endoscopic score of i2, i3, or i4.

(*From* Rutgeerts P, Geboes K, Vantrappen G, et al. Natural history of recurrent Crohn's disease at the ileocolonic anastomosis after curative surgery. Gut 1984;25(6):665–72; with permission.)

Similarly bowel wall thickness of greater than 3 mm on small bowel ultrasonography predicts POR with greater than 6-mm bowel thickness having a 40% risk of surgical recurrence.[24–26] Both CTE and MRE have shown variable correlation with endoscopic and clinical activity scores, but lack sensitivity and specificity for accurately assessing POR.[27,28] VCE may be used for assessment of CD in the postoperative situation but is limited by the inability to biopsy, the risk of retention within an area of stricture (5%–13%) requiring subsequent endoscopic extraction or surgery,[29] and decreased/limited visualization of terminal ileum.[30,31]

Risk Factors for Recurrence

There are risk factors that portend a higher risk of POR. A summary of pertinent risk factors is given in **Table 2**.

Patient-related factors

High risk:
1. Smoking, especially in women and those who smoke more than 15 cigarettes per day[32–35]
2. Younger age at onset and younger age at time of primary surgery[10,36,37]
3. Shorter disease duration before surgery[38]

Equivocal to no effect:
1. Gender[39,40]
2. Family history of IBD[41,42]

Table 2
Factors associated with risk of postoperative recurrence in Crohn's disease

Patient	
Smoking	+++
Gender	~
Age at onset	~
Disease Duration before surgery	~
Family history	~
Visceral adiposity	+
Disease	
Penetrating/perforating	+++
Prior CD surgery (>2)	+++
Small bowel involvement	++
Perianal disease	++
Histopathology	
Myenteric plexitis	+
Granulomas present	+
Surgery	
Anastomosis type	~
Open vs laparoscopic	~
Length of resected segment	+

Symbols: ~, equivocal or unknown; +, weak; ++, moderate; +++, strong.

Adapted from Click BH, Regueiro M. Use of biologics in the postoperative management of Crohn's disease. In: Cheifetz AS, Feuerstein JD, editors. Treatment of inflammatory bowel disease with biologics. Cham (Switzerland): Springer International Publishing; 2018. p. 59–79; with permission.

Disease-related factors

High risk
1. History of multiple prior surgeries[43,44]
2. Disease location, especially extensive small bowel involvement[45–47]
3. Penetrating/perforating disease[48,49]
4. Perianal disease[50,51]

Histopathology-related factors

1. Granulomas (not crypt rupture)[49,52,53]
2. Myenteric plexitis[54,55]

Surgery-related factors

High risk
1. Length of bowel resected or extent of diseased segment[51,56]
Equivocal to no effect
1. Type of anastomosis (side to side vs end to end)[44,57,58]

General Principles of Management

The basic guiding principle in the management of postoperative CD is preventing recurrence and future surgery (**Fig. 3**). Endoscopic monitoring remains the gold

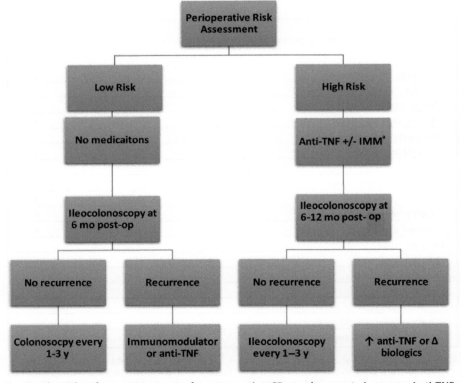

Fig. 3. Algorithm for management of postoperative CD. Δ, change; ↑, increase; Anti-TNF, anti–tumor necrosis factor alpha; Postop, postoperative. [a] Monotherapy with therapeutic drug monitoring or combination with immunomodulators (IMM).

standard assessment for recurrence. Prevention with postoperative initiation of anti-tumor necrosis factor (TNF) therapy and 6-month ileocolonoscopy for high-risk patients is prudent, whereas low-risk patients (first surgery) may be monitored with fecal calprotectin and ileocolonoscopy 3 to 6 months after surgery.

When to start treatment?
There are 2 approaches for the monitoring and management of postoperative CD:

1. Early postoperative prophylactic anti-TNF within 2 to 4 weeks of surgery for high-risk patients followed by a 6 to 12 month ileocolonoscopy[13,59]
2. No postoperative therapy for low-risk patients but ileocolonoscopy at 6 months with initiation of treatment of recurrence[60]

Endoscopic Surveillance

Ileocolonoscopy is the best modality for evaluating disease activity in postoperative CD. One of the landmark postoperative endoscopy studies was the multicenter, double-blind, randomized controlled trial across 17 centers in Australia and New Zealand (POCER trial).[60] Patients were randomized into 2 endoscopy surveillance arms, active versus standard care, and stratified by risk of POR. The primary end point was endoscopic recurrence 18 months after surgery. The active care arm patients had an ileocolonoscopy at 6 months with escalation of medical therapy if there was endoscopic recurrence ($\geq$ i2). The standard care arm did not have a 6-month interval ileocolonoscopy. Patients were stratified to postoperative treatment based on risk factors. All patients, independent of risk strata, received 3 months of metronidazole. High-risk patients had 1 of 3 risk factors (active smoking, penetrating disease, and/or previous surgery) and received azathioprine within 1 month of surgery, and low-risk patients had none of these factors and received no additional therapy. If high-risk patients had previously received azathioprine and had failed, or were intolerant, they received adalimumab within 1 month of surgery. There was a lower endoscopic recurrence rate at 18 months in the patients randomized to the active care arm compared with the standard care arm (49% vs 67%; P = .03)[60]. The results from the POCER and prior studies led to the American Gastroenterological Association guidelines recommending an ileocolonoscopy at 6 months in all postoperative patients with CD.[61]

Technical aspects: endoscopy of the anastomosis
The 3 most commonly encountered anastomoses in the postoperative setting are side-to-side anastomosis, end-to-end anastomosis, and end-to-side anastomosis. It is important to understand the anatomy of each when performing endoscopy. For purposes of this description, the authors refer to the most common ileocolonic resection with primary anastomosis between the ileum and colon.

1. End-to-end anastomosis: in this type of anastomosis, the intestine is connected in continuity as a straight anastomosis and often hand sewn rather than stapled. Consequently, the endoscope is passed directly from the colon through the anastomosis into the neoterminal ileum without the need for special manipulation (**Fig. 4**A, B).
2. Side-to-side anastomosis: in this type of anastomosis, a stapling device is often used to connect the ileum to colon in a parallel fashion. This type results in a wider luminal diameter with a blind end of the colon and blind end of the ileum. It often requires a partial or full retroflexion of the colonoscope to pass from the colon through the anastomosis into the ileum. At times, this can be technically

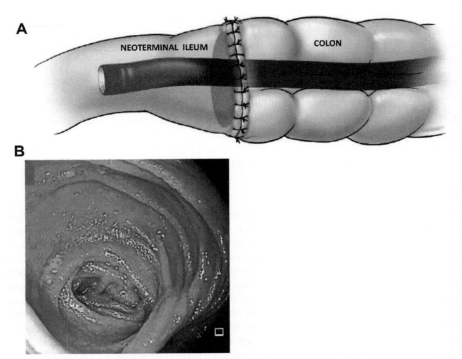

Fig. 4. (*A*) End-to-end anastomosis showing direction of endoscopic passage. Reprinted with permission, Cleveland Clinic Center for Medical Art & Photography © 1997-2018. All Rights Reserved. (*B*) Forward endoscopic view of an end-to-end anastomosis.

challenging and, unless the clinician is aware of the type of anastomosis, the blind end of the ileum may be mistaken for the neoterminal ileum and further evaluation of the ileum for CD not performed (**Fig. 5**).
3. End-to-side anastomosis: this is the least common type. The neoterminal ileum is attached perpendicularly to the colonic lumen resulting in a colonic blind end. Depending on the configuration, the anastomosis and ileum may not be readily identified and require special colonoscopic manipulation (**Fig. 6**).

Special scenarios of postoperative Crohn's disease ileocolonoscopy
Anastomotic ulcers Anastomotic ulcers refers to ulceration present at the anastomosis without involving the preanastomotic area. There is much debate as to the significance of anastomotic ulceration and differentiation between ischemic changes and recurrent CD. The anastomotic changes were not described in the original study by Rutgeerts and colleagues,[7] and were considered i0 to i1 in the absence of any disease in the preanastomotic region. However, recent data suggest that multiple (>5) ulcerations along the anastomosis represent an i2 recurrence. To further delineate the finding of anastomotic ulcers, the ileal score has been subclassified as i2a when there are ulcerations only along the anastomoses without ileal inflammation, or i2b when there are ulcerations along the anastomosis and extending into the neoterminal ileum[62,63](**Fig. 7**). Although anastomotic-only ulcerations (i2a) were once thought to carry a low risk for recurrence, there are emerging data that there may be progression to significant CD recurrence. In one such retrospective cohort study it was reported that anastomotic ulcerations on the first

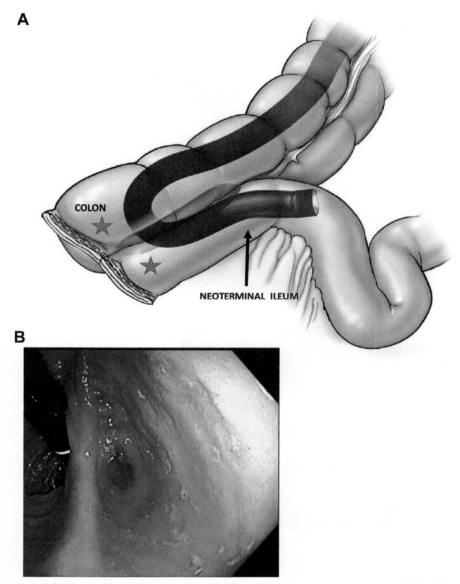

Fig. 5. (*A*) Side-to-side anastomosis showing direction of endoscopic passage and blind ends (*red stars*). Reprinted with permission, Cleveland Clinic Center for Medical Art & Photography © 1997-2018. All Rights Reserved. (*B*) Retroflexed endoscopic view of a side-to-side anastomosis.

ileocolonoscopy after surgery correlated with higher risk of endoscopic recurrence and repeat surgical resection.[64] The study concluded that anastomotic ulceration should be treated as a true endoscopic recurrence and treatment escalated accordingly. It is the authors' opinion that i2a is ischemiclike CD recurrence at the anastomosis. We do not initiate CD medications for i2a in isolation but do suggest another colonoscopy 1 year after finding the i2a recurrence. If there is progression of

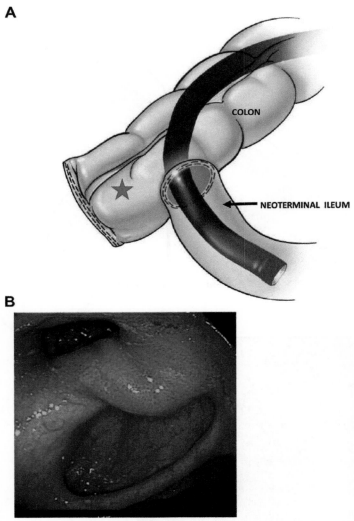

Fig. 6. (*A*) End-to-side anastomosis showing direction of endoscopic passage and blind ends (*red star*). Reprinted with permission, Cleveland Clinic Center for Medical Art & Photography © 1997-2018. All Rights Reserved. (*B*) Forward endoscopic view of an end-to-side anastomosis.

inflammation beyond the anastomosis greater than i2b, we initiate anti-TNF at that time. Often these i2a recurrence develop a ringlike stricture at the anastomosis that may be safely balloon dilated. We consider i2b an immune-mediated CD recurrence and treat this as any POR with medical therapy.

Ulcerations in the blind end of the ileum The management of isolated ulcerations in the blind end of a side-to-side anastomosis is not known. It is our opinion that, as with the anastomotic ulcerations, the blind-end inflammation represents CD recurrence. We think that the blind-end inflammation likely occurs at a stapled end or dog-ear closure and may be a nidus for future abscess/fistula. In patients with blind-end

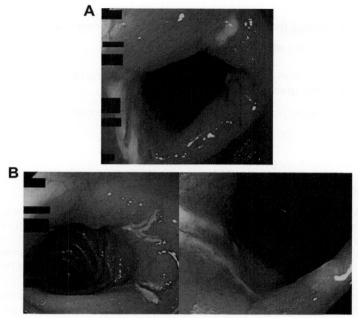

Fig. 7. Endoscopic view of anastomotic ulcers. (*A*) Ulcer at the anastomosis without any neo-terminal ileal involvement of i2a. (*B*) Ulcer at the anastomosis extending into the neotermi-nal ileum i2b.

inflammation and subsequent abscess, surgical resection of the anastomosis is often required. The authors currently suggest that the blind end be counted in our reporting of recurrence and an i1 could be monitored with a 6-month to 12-month repeat ileoco-lonoscopy and a greater than or equal to i2 initiation or escalation of therapy (**Fig. 8**).

Summary

Based on available data, the authors recommend risk stratifying patients as low risk versus high risk based on following factors[61]:

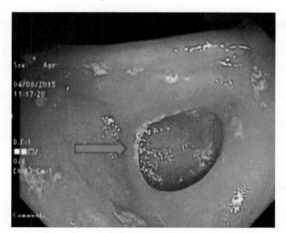

Fig. 8. Endoscopic view of ulceration (*arrow*) in the blind ileal region of a side-to-side anastomosis.

Low risk (hypothetical risk at 18 months: CR 20% and endoscopic recurrence 30%)

1. Older patient (>50 years)
2. Nonsmoker
3. First surgery for short-segment fibrostenotic, nonpenetrating disease (<10–20 cm)
4. Disease duration greater than 20 years

High risk (hypothetical risk at 18 months: CR 50% and endoscopic recurrence 80%)

1. Younger patient (<30 years)
2. Smoker
3. More than 2 prior surgeries
4. Penetrating disease in the absence of a stricture
5. Perianal disease

After risk stratification, the authors recommend immediate postoperative prophylaxis with an anti-TNF agent in combination with an immune-modulator within 4 weeks of surgery for high-risk patients. Low-risk patients do not need treatment prophylactically. We recommend that all patients, regardless of their risk factors, undergo regular endoscopic surveillance at 6 months to assess the anastomosis and POR in the neoterminal ileum.

Ileocolonoscopy still remains the most accurate measure of POR. The timing may vary between 6 and 12 months depending on risk assessment. In case there is worsening of disease on surveillance, we recommend escalating treatment. Fecal calprotectin can be used as a useful noninvasive tool to determine whether patients are in remission.

The best modality of treatment of postoperative recurrence based on studies are biologics, namely anti–TNF alpha agents (infliximab and adalimumab).[13,59,65,66] Vedolizumab in a recent study by Yamada and colleagues[67] showed that, compared with anti–TNF alpha agents, patients had higher rates of postoperative recurrence. However, these data were retrospective, had small sample sizes, and had considerable heterogeneity in patient population and disease behavior. Data are awaited from randomized controlled trials to determine the effectiveness of vedolizumab in treatment and prevention of POR. Most data on ustekinumab are on the effect of preoperative ustekinumab on postoperative outcomes. So far the data suggest this is a safe medication preoperatively, without any increase in postoperative complications; however, data on treatment of postoperative recurrence are lacking.[68–70]

Endoscopic evaluation of postoperative CD continues to evolve. A more nuanced and validated endoscopic scoring system is needed for postoperative recurrence. For example, the subtle differences of only 1 ulceration between an i1 remission and i2 recurrence, the uncertain significance of anastomotic ulcers (i2a vs i2b), and blind limb ulcerations require further exploration. Better optics, improved endoscopes, and enhanced understanding of the correlation between endoscopic findings and disease progression have led to ongoing postoperative endoscopic study.

ULCERATIVE COLITIS

Around 31% of patients with UC over their lifetimes require colectomy.[71] As mentioned before, colectomy is curative for UC, but postoperatively patients can develop various complications. It is important for gastroenterologists to recognize these complications and their medical/endoscopic managements. Restorative proctocolectomy with IPAA was first described in 1978 and since then has become the surgery of choice in patients with UC.[72] The various complications and management of conditions of the pouch are discussed here.

Types of Pouch

J pouch

J pouch is the most commonly performed pouch surgery (**Fig. 9**). It is constructed from a double loop of ileum, each measuring around 15 to 20 cm. On pouchoscopy it is identified by the presence of a blind limb and afferent limb. It has a characteristic double-lumen appearance on endoscopy. The landmarks to know are the following:

1. Afferent limb: the part of the small intestine that leads to remaining small bowel proximally
2. Blind limb: the area of the ileum that ends blindly
3. Pouch body: the area of the pouch from the limbs to the rectal cuff, which stores the stool
4. Rectal cuff/anal transition zone: the final 2 to 2.5 cm up from the body to the anus (this is a remnant of the rectum)

S pouch

Less commonly seen is the S pouch, which consists of 3 loops of small intestine each measuring 15 cm in length (**Fig. 10**). It appears like a large single lumen during endoscopy with a pouch inlet leading to the terminal ileum.

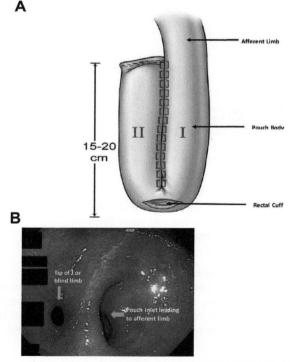

Fig. 9. (*A*) Anatomy of J pouch. Reprinted with permission, Cleveland Clinic Center for Medical Art & Photography © 1997-2018. All Rights Reserved. (*B*) Endoscopic view of J pouch showing characteristic owl's eye appearance.

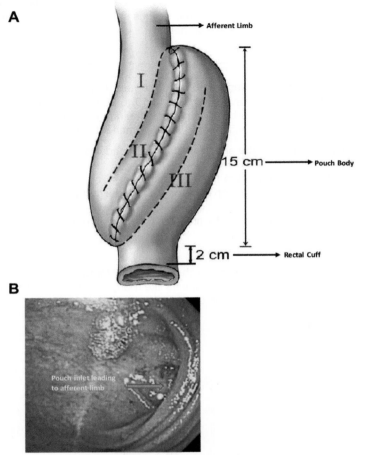

Fig. 10. (A) Anatomy of S pouch. Reprinted with permission, Cleveland Clinic Center for Medical Art & Photography © 1997-2018. All Rights Reserved. (B) Endoscopic view of S pouch.

1. Pouch inlet: the opening into the small intestine proximally
2. Pouch body: the large reservoir leading up to the inlet
3. Rectal cuff/anal transition zone (refer to J pouch)

Kock pouch or continent ileostomy

The Kock pouch is a continent ileostomy created from the terminal ileum (**Fig. 11**). On pouchoscopy it appears like a single lumen after entering through a tight ileostomy. On entry, the scope can be retroflexed to see the valve that is created near the entry site. There is a large lumen that leads into a pouch inlet. Landmarks to remember are:

1. Pouch inlet: opening into the remaining proximal small bowel
2. Pouch body: the large reservoir leading up to the inlet
3. Valve or nipple: seen on retroflexion

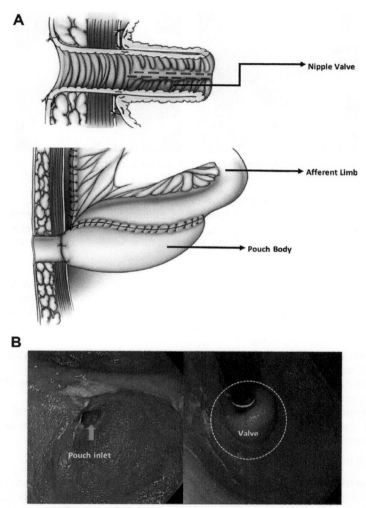

Fig. 11. (*A*) Anatomy of K pouch. Reprinted with permission, Cleveland Clinic Center for Medical Art & Photography © 1997-2018. All Rights Reserved. (*B*) Endoscopic view of K pouch showing pouch inlet on the left and retroflexed view of valve on the right.

Inflammatory Complications

Pouchitis

Exclusively occurs in patients with underlying UC, and rarely in those with familial adenomatous polyposis,[73,74] and is defined as the inflammation of the ileal pouch reservoir of an IPAA (**Fig. 12**). Around 50% patients with IPAA develop pouchitis.[75] The condition presents with increased stool frequency, rectal bleeding, urgency, fevers, and appearance of extraintestinal manifestations.[76]

Pouchitis is classified into:

1. Acute (<4 weeks) or chronic (>4 weeks)
2. Antibiotic responsive versus antibiotic dependent versus antibiotic refractory
3. Infrequent (<3 flares/y) versus relapsing pouchitis (>3 episodes/y)

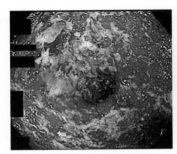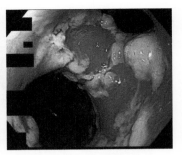

Fig. 12. Endoscopic views showing pouchitis of the body of the pouch.

4. Pouchitis only versus pouchitis with concurrent prepouch ileitis
5. Idiopathic versus secondary (cytomegalovirus, nonsteroidal antiinflammatory drugs [NSAIDs], ischemia, fecal diversion, immunoglobulin [Ig] G4 related, primary sclerosing cholangitis [PSC] associated, Crohn, cuffitis, fistula, prolapse, twisted pouch)

Risk factors for pouchitis:

- History of UC: pouchitis rarely occurs in patients who have IPAA for familial adenomatous polyposis syndrome. Patients with extensive colitis have as much as 3-fold risk of pouchitis compared with those with more limited disease.[77]
- PSC: patients who have concomitant UC with PSC have higher risk of pouchitis compared with UC alone.[73]
- Smoking: increased risk of acute, but decreased risk of chronic, pouchitis has been seen with smoking.[78,79]
- NSAID: increased risk of pouchitis with use of NSAIDs has been seen.[80]
- Gender: men have higher risk for chronic pouchitis.[81]
- Autoimmune serologies: high serum IgG4, autoantibodies to bacterial antigens, and positive antineutrophil cytoplasmic antibody serology are associated with higher risk of pouchitis.[75,77,79,82]

Medical management:

- Most robust data are present on the use of antibiotics such as metronidazole, tinidazole, and ciprofloxacin.[83–85] These data can be used for acute pouchitis, as well as a long-term course for chronic/antibiotic-dependent pouchitis.[86–88]
- For refractory or chronic pouchitis and CD of the pouch refractory to antibiotic therapy, the authors use biologics. There are data on infliximab,[89–94] adalimumab,[95] vedolizumab,[96–99] as well as ustekinumab for treatment.[100]
- If there is underlying IgG4 pouchitis, oral budesonide, 6-mercaptopurine, or methotrexate can be used.[101,102]

Irritable pouch syndrome

This syndrome is a functional disorder of the pouch especially seen in patients who are on antidepressants or antianxiety medications, suggesting a strong psychological component to this disorder. It presents as perianal or pelvic pain, urgency, and increased frequency of stools. Histology may show enterochromaffin cells on pouch biopsy[103]

Medical management: once this is confirmed after ruling out other causes of symptoms, patients can be treated empirically with antidiarrheals, antispasmodics, or tricyclic antidepressants.

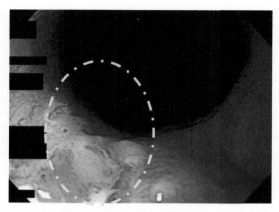

Fig. 13. Endoscopic view of showing cuffitis (*dashed circle*) at the anal transition zone or the rectal cuff.

Cuffitis

Cuffitis is the presence of inflammation in the remaining rectal cuff presenting with hematochezia and urgency (**Fig. 13**). This condition is basically recurrence of UC in the remaining rectum. It may be steroid/mesalamine responsive, steroid/mesalamine dependent, or steroid/mesalamine refractory.[104]

Medical management: typical cuffitis can be treated with 5-aminosalicylate agents or topical corticosteroids.[105] Patients refractory to treatment need to be evaluated for other disorders.

Diversion pouchitis

This condition is inflammation seen when IPAA is associated with diverting ileostomy. The pathogenesis is speculated to be related to deficiency in short-chain fatty acids caused by fecal diversion. This condition can lead to bloody or mucous discharge from the anus and urgency.

Crohn's disease of pouch

This condition is often the cause of refractory or recurrent pouchitis, and can occur either because of a missed diagnosis (especially in patients with family history of CD) or as a de novo phenomenon.[106,107] It endoscopically appear like ulcers and strictures in the afferent limb or prepouch ileum, in the absence of the use of NSAIDs. Patients may develop fistulas and abscesses, requiring pouch revisions.

Medical management: limited data are present on the medical management of pouch CD, including biologics as mentioned earlier (refer to the management of refractory/chronic pouchitis in medical management of pouchitis).

Endoscopic management of inflammatory conditions The most important goal is to distinguish between inflammatory disorders and functional disorder. Symptoms of pouchitis have poor correlation with disease.[108,109] Furthermore, clinicians also need to be able to differentiate different inflammatory conditions of the pouch (ie, pouchitis/cuffitis or CD of pouch). The diagnosis needs to be confirmed by typical endoscopic and histologic features.[108] The endoscopic evaluation of pouch should include the following:

- Evaluation of distensibility of pouch body, and severity, extent, and distribution of mucosal inflammation

- Assessment of prepouch ileum for possible CD or backwash enteritis
- Inspection of rectal cuff to rule out cuffitis
- Biopsies should be obtained from a normal looking pouch also, because there may be histologic inflammation seen with endoscopic evidence of disease

Key features on endoscopy:

- Diffuse erythema, friability, granularity, exudates, erosions, and/or ulcerations
- Chronic pouchitis may have mucosal bridging, inflammatory polyps, poor distensibility of the pouch body, or the loss of owls'-eye configuration of a J pouch
- Features suggesting CD of pouch include afferent limb ulcer and/or stricture, ulcers or strictures in other parts of small bowel in the absence of NSAID use[110,111]
- Morphology of ulcers cannot reliably differentiate between pouchitis or CD
- Biopsy taken from suture lines can show foreign body granulomas and should be avoided
- It is important to distinguish backwash ileitis from CD ileitis
    1. CD ileitis shows discrete ulcers in neoterminal ileum (>10 cm from pouch inlet), with stricture of inlet
    2. Backwash is contiguous inflammation from the pouch to distal neoterminal ileum (within 10 cm of pouch inlet) with patent inlet
- Surgery-related strictures can be difficult to distinguish from CD-related stricture

Mechanical and Surgical Complications

Anastomotic leak
Anastomotic separation leading to exodus of pouch contents. Common location is pouch anal anastomosis, tip of the J, and body of pouch along staple line.[112] Surgical intervention is often required.

Pouch sinus
This is a blind tract that can lead to an abscess, typically occurring as a consequence of anastomotic leaks (**Fig. 14**). The most common site is the pouch anal anastomotic site. Careful examination on pouchoscopy can detect these openings, but contrasted radiographic examination via MRI is often required to differentiate it from a fistula. A flexible jag wire can be used to access this opening, but careful examination needs to be performed because these sinuses can perforate and turn into a fistula. These fistulas require periodic incision and drainage and may take 9 to 12 months to heal.

Pouch fistulas
In patients with IPAA, fistulas can occur anywhere in the pouch and can extend into surrounding organs or skin (**Figs. 15** and **16**).[76,113] Fistulas can occur either at the level of anastomosis or below the level of anastomosis.[114,115] Fistulas can be difficult to manage either medically or surgically.[115,116] Endoscopic fistulotomy (see **Fig. 16**) has recently been shown to be an effective treatment strategy for fistulas, with 89% of patients in the study by Kochhar and Shen[117] showing complete resolution of fistula.

Strictures
Around 11% of patients with IPAA for UC develop strictures (**Fig. 17**).[118] They can occur at multiple locations, including anastomotic/pouch outlet, midpouch, pouch inlet, and afferent limb.[113] They can be inflammatory or fibrotic and can be caused by NSAIDs, CD, ischemia, or inappropriate surgical techniques. These strictures

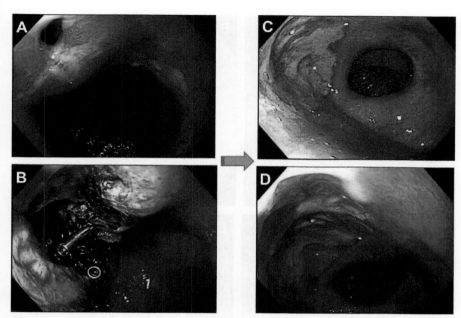

Fig. 14. Endoscopic sinusotomy. (*A*) The opening of the deep presacral sinus. (*B*) Needle knife electroincision of the wall between the sinus and pouch body with endoclips deployed along the incised edges of the sinus. (*C*) and (*D*) Follow-up endoscopies showed complete healing of the sinus. (*Adapted from* Lan N, Hull TL, Shen B. Endoscopic sinusotomy versus redo surgery for the treatment of chronic pouch anastomotic sinus in ulcerative colitis patients. Gastrointestinal Endoscopy 2019;89(1):144–56; with permission; and *Data from* Heriot AG, Tekkis PP, Smith JJ, et al. Management and outcome of pouch-vaginal fistulas following restorative proctocolectomy. Dis Colon Rectum 2005;48(3):451–58.)

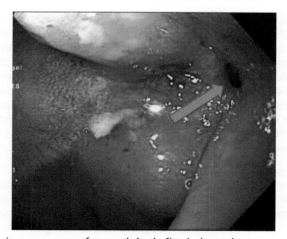

Fig. 15. Endoscopic appearance of a pouch body fistula (*arrow*).

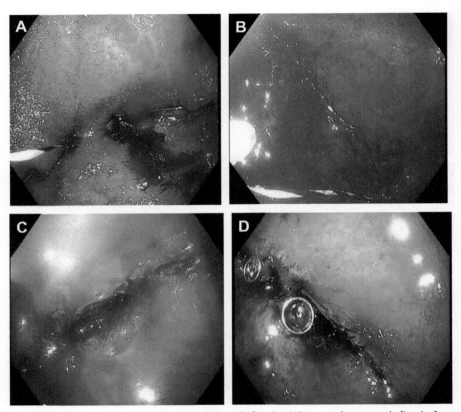

Fig. 16. Endoscopic fistulotomy for pouch-pouch fistula. (*A*) A pouch-to-pouch fistula from staple line leak was detected with a guidewire. (*B*) Needle knife in action. (*C*) Completed fistulotomy. (*D*) Deployment of endoclips (*circle*). (*Adapted from* Kochhar G, Shen B. Endoscopic fistulotomy in inflammatory bowel disease (with video). Gastrointest Endosc 2018;88(1):87–94; with permission; and *Data from* Shen B, Fazio VW, Remzi FH, et al. Endoscopic balloon dilation of ileal pouch strictures. Am J Gastroenterol 2004;99(12):2340–47.)

can lead to symptoms of bowel obstruction. These strictures can be dilated endoscopically with balloon dilation[119] or bougie dilations.[113] Surgical stricturoplasty and pouch diversion or excision are other options.[113] In a study by Shen and colleagues[119] it was shown that endoscopic balloon dilations improved quality of life and had very low complication rates. These patients often require multiple sessions of dilation to achieve optimal effect. Endoscopic stricturotomy with needle knife or insulated-tip knife can also be performed for fibrotic strictures. A study of 85 patients showed that needle knife stricturotomy was an effective and safe treatment strategy for IBD-related fibrotic strictures.[120] These treatments should not be done for inflammatory strictures because of high risk of perforation.

Afferent limb syndrome
This syndrome refers to acute angulation, prolapse, or intussusception of the afferent limb at the junction to the pouch. It can lead to symptoms of bowel obstruction. In a study of 567 patients with IPAA, 122 patients had symptoms of bowel obstruction, of which 6 were caused by afferent limb syndrome.[121] During endoscopy such angulations can make intubating the afferent limb very difficult.

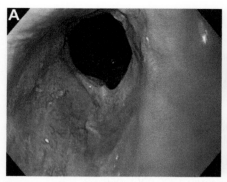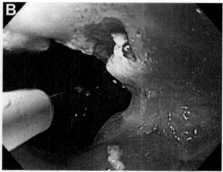

Fig. 17. Endoscopic views of pouch anastomosis stricture. (*A*) Before needle knife stricturotomy. (*B*) After needle knife stricturotomy. (*Adapted from* Bharadwaj S, Shen B. Medical, endoscopic, and surgical management of ileal pouch strictures (with video). Gastrointest Endosc 2017;86(1):59–73; with permission; and *Data from* Lan N, Shen B. Endoscopic stricturotomy with needle knife in the treatment of strictures from inflammatory bowel disease. Inflamm Bowel Dis 2017;23(4):502–13).

Efferent limb syndrome

Efferent limb syndrome typically occurs in patients with S pouches with long redundant efferent limbs. It can occur in J pouches with long rectal stumps. Surgical correction is needed for both afferent and efferent limb syndromes.[122]

Adenocarcinoma

The incidence of colorectal cancer in pouch patients is very low. There are no recommendations for surveillance. It is almost exclusively limited to the anal transition zone or cuff. Some risk factors include prior history of colorectal cancer, PSC, chronic pouchitis/cuffitis, and family history of colorectal cancer.[123,124] In a surveillance program of 106 high-risk patients, only 1 had multifocal low-grade dysplasia but no adenocarcinoma.[125] During endoscopy of the pouch it is important to take biopsies from the rectal cuff.

SUMMARY

Restorative proctocolectomy with IPAA can cure patients with UC, but adverse sequelae are common. It is important for endoscopists to be well versed in the anatomy of different pouches and understand the endoscopic landmarks. It is also important to understand the different endoscopic treatments that can be provided and the contexts in which to use them; for example, stricturotomy only for fibrotic strictures.

REFERENCES

1. Thia KT, Sandborn WJ, Harmsen WS. Risk factors associated with progression to intestinal complications of Crohn's disease in a population-based cohort. Gastroenterology 2010;139(4):1147–55.
2. Munkholm P, Langholz E, Davidsen M. Intestinal cancer risk and mortality in patients with Crohn's disease. Gastroenterology 1993;105(6):1716–23.
3. Targownik LE, Singh H, Nugent Z, et al. The epidemiology of colectomy in ulcerative colitis: results from a population-based cohort. Am J Gastroenterol 2012; 107(8):1228–35.

4. Lennard-Jones JE, Stalder GA. Prognosis after resection of chronic regional ileitis. Gut 1967;8(4):332–6.
5. Buisson A, Chevaux J-B, Allen PB, et al. Review article: the natural history of postoperative Crohn's disease recurrence. Aliment Pharmacol Ther 2012; 35(6):625–33.
6. D'Haens GR, Geboes K, Peeters M, et al. Early lesions of recurrent Crohn's disease caused by infusion of intestinal contents in excluded ileum. Gastroenterology 1998;114(2):262–7.
7. Rutgeerts P, Geboes K, Vantrappen G, et al. Natural history of recurrent Crohn's disease at the ileocolonic anastomosis after curative surgery. Gut 1984;25(6): 665–72.
8. Rutgeerts P, Geboes K, Vantrappen G, et al. Predictability of the postoperative course of Crohn's disease. Gastroenterology 1990;99(4):956–63.
9. Olaison G, Smedh K, Sjödahl R. Natural course of Crohn's disease after ileocolic resection: endoscopically visualised ileal ulcers preceding symptoms. Gut 1992;33(3):331–5.
10. Greenstein AJ, Sachar DB, Pasternack BS, et al. Reoperation and recurrence in Crohn's colitis and ileocolitis — Crude and cumulative rates. N Engl J Med 1975; 293(14):685–90.
11. Regueiro M, Kip KE, Schraut W, et al. Crohn's disease activity index does not correlate with endoscopic recurrence one year after ileocolonic resection. Inflamm Bowel Dis 2011;17(1):118–26.
12. Frolkis AD, Lipton DS, Fiest KM, et al. Cumulative incidence of second intestinal resection in Crohn's disease: a systematic review and meta-analysis of population-based studies. Am J Gastroenterol 2014;109(11):1739–48.
13. Regueiro M, Feagan BG, Zou B, et al. infliximab reduces endoscopic, but not clinical, recurrence of Crohn's disease after ileocolonic resection. Gastroenterology 2016;150(7):1568–78.
14. Geboes K, Dalle I. Influence of treatment on morphological features of mucosal inflammation. Gut 2002;50(Suppl 3):III37–42.
15. Daperno M, Comberlato M, Bossa F, et al. Inter-observer agreement in endoscopic scoring systems: preliminary report of an ongoing study from the Italian Group for Inflammatory Bowel Disease (IG-IBD). Dig Liver Dis 2014;46(11): 969–73.
16. Marteau P, Laharie D, Colombel J-F, et al. Interobserver variation study of the Rutgeerts score to assess endoscopic recurrence after surgery for Crohn's disease. J Crohns Colitis 2016;10(9):1001–5.
17. Best WR, Becktel JM, Singleton JW, et al. Development of a Crohn's disease activity index. National Cooperative Crohn's Disease Study. Gastroenterology 1976;70(3):439–44.
18. Harvey RF, Bradshaw JM. A simple index of Crohn's-disease activity. Lancet 1980;1(8167):514.
19. Higgins PDR, Harding G, Leidy NK, et al. Development and validation of the Crohn's disease patient-reported outcomes signs and symptoms (CD-PRO/SS) diary. J Patient Rep Outcomes 2017;2(1):24.
20. Boschetti G, Laidet M, Moussata D, et al. Levels of fecal calprotectin are associated with the severity of postoperative endoscopic recurrence in asymptomatic patients with Crohn's disease. Am J Gastroenterol 2015;110(6):865–72.
21. Qiu Y, Mao R, Chen B, et al. Fecal calprotectin for evaluating postoperative recurrence of Crohn's disease: a meta-analysis of prospective studies. Inflamm Bowel Dis 2015;21(2):315–22.

22. Garcia-Planella E, Mañosa M, Cabré E, et al. Fecal calprotectin levels are closely correlated with the absence of relevant mucosal lesions in postoperative Crohn's disease. Inflamm Bowel Dis 2016;22(12):2879–85.
23. Wright EK, Kamm MA, De Cruz P, et al. Measurement of fecal calprotectin improves monitoring and detection of recurrence of Crohn's disease after surgery. Gastroenterology 2015;148(5):938–47.e1.
24. Cammarota T, Ribaldone DG, Resegotti A, et al. Role of bowel ultrasound as a predictor of surgical recurrence of Crohn's disease. Scand J Gastroenterol 2013;48(5):552–5.
25. Paredes JM, Ripollés T, Cortés X, et al. Contrast-enhanced ultrasonography: usefulness in the assessment of postoperative recurrence of Crohn's disease. J Crohns Colitis 2013;7(3):192–201.
26. Andreoli A, Cerro P, Falasco G, et al. Role of ultrasonography in the diagnosis of postsurgical recurrence of Crohn's disease. Am J Gastroenterol 1998;93(7): 1117–21.
27. Choi IY, Park SH, Park SH, et al. CT enterography for surveillance of anastomotic recurrence within 12 months of bowel resection in patients with Crohn's disease: an observational study using an 8-year registry. Korean J Radiol 2017;18(6): 906–14.
28. Baillet P, Cadiot G, Goutte M, et al. Faecal calprotectin and magnetic resonance imaging in detecting Crohn's disease endoscopic postoperative recurrence. World J Gastroenterol 2018;24(5):641–50.
29. Annese V, Manetti N. Capsule endoscopy in Crohn's disease: is there enough light in the tunnel? J Crohns Colitis 2014;8(12):1598–600.
30. Cotter J, Dias de Castro F, Moreira MJ, et al. Tailoring Crohn's disease treatment: the impact of small bowel capsule endoscopy. J Crohns Colitis 2014;8(12): 1610–5.
31. Niv E, Fishman S, Kachman H, et al. Sequential capsule endoscopy of the small bowel for follow-up of patients with known Crohn's disease. J Crohns Colitis 2014;8(12):1616–23.
32. Sutherland LR, Ramcharan S, Bryant H, et al. Effect of cigarette smoking on recurrence of Crohn's disease. Gastroenterology 1990;98(5 Pt 1):1123–8.
33. Cottone M, Rosselli M, Orlando A, et al. Smoking habits and recurrence in Crohn's disease. Gastroenterology 1994;106(3):643–8.
34. Cosnes J, Beaugerie L, Carbonnel F, et al. Smoking cessation and the course of Crohn's disease: an intervention study. Gastroenterology 2001;120(5):1093–9.
35. Reese GE, Nanidis T, Borysiewicz C, et al. The effect of smoking after surgery for Crohn's disease: a meta-analysis of observational studies. Int J Colorectal Dis 2008;23(12):1213–21.
36. De Dombal FT, Burton I, Goligher JC. Recurrence of Crohn's disease after primary excisional surgery. Gut 1971;12(7):519–27.
37. Lautenbach E, Berlin JA, Lichtenstein GR. Risk factors for early postoperative recurrence of Crohn's disease. Gastroenterology 1998;115(2):259–67.
38. Poggioli G, Laureti S, Selleri S, et al. Factors affecting recurrence in Crohn's disease. Results of a prospective audit. Int J Colorectal Dis 1996;11(6):294–8.
39. Wettergren A, Christiansen J. Risk of recurrence and reoperation after resection for ileocolic Crohn's disease. Scand J Gastroenterol 1991;26(12):1319–22.
40. Sachar DB, Wolfson DM, Greenstein AJ, et al. Risk factors for postoperative recurrence of Crohn's disease. Gastroenterology 1983;85(4):917–21.
41. Unkart JT, Anderson L, Li E, et al. Risk factors for surgical recurrence after ileocolic resection of Crohn's disease. Dis Colon Rectum 2008;51(8):1211–6.

42. Kurer MA, Stamou KM, Wilson TR, et al. Early symptomatic recurrence after intestinal resection in Crohn's disease is unpredictable. Colorectal Dis 2007;9(6): 567–71.

43. Ng SC, Lied GA, Arebi N, et al. Clinical and surgical recurrence of Crohn's disease after ileocolonic resection in a specialist unit. Eur J Gastroenterol Hepatol 2009;21(5):551–7.

44. McLeod RS, Wolff BG, Ross S, et al. Investigators of the CAST Trial. Recurrence of Crohn's disease after ileocolic resection is not affected by anastomotic type: results of a multicenter, randomized, controlled trial. Dis Colon Rectum 2009; 52(5):919–27.

45. Lock MR, Farmer RG, Fazio VW, et al. Recurrence and reoperation for Crohn's disease: the role of disease location in prognosis. N Engl J Med 1981; 304(26):1586–8.

46. Keh C, Shatari T, Yamamoto T, et al. Jejunal Crohn's disease is associated with a higher postoperative recurrence rate than ileocaecal Crohn's disease. Colorectal Dis 2005;7(4):366–8.

47. Borley NR, Mortensen NJM, Chaudry MA, et al. Recurrence after abdominal surgery for Crohn's disease: relationship to disease site and surgical procedure. Dis Colon Rectum 2002;45(3):377–83.

48. Aeberhard P, Berchtold W, Riedtmann HJ, et al. Surgical recurrence of perforating and nonperforating Crohn's disease. A study of 101 surgically treated Patients. Dis Colon Rectum 1996;39(1):80–7.

49. Simillis C, Yamamoto T, Reese GE, et al. A meta-analysis comparing incidence of recurrence and indication for reoperation after surgery for perforating versus nonperforating Crohn's disease. Am J Gastroenterol 2008;103(1):196–205.

50. Parente F, Sampietro GM, Molteni M, et al. Behaviour of the bowel wall during the first year after surgery is a strong predictor of symptomatic recurrence of Crohn's disease: a prospective study. Aliment Pharmacol Ther 2004;20(9): 959–68.

51. Bernell O, Lapidus A, Hellers G. Risk factors for surgery and recurrence in 907 patients with primary ileocaecal Crohn's disease. Br J Surg 2000;87(12): 1697–701.

52. Johnson CM, Hartman DJ, Ramos-Rivers C, et al. Epithelioid granulomas associate with increased severity and progression of Crohn's disease, based on 6-year follow-up. Clin Gastroenterol Hepatol 2018;16(6):900–7.e1.

53. Cullen G, O'Toole A, Keegan D, et al. Long-term clinical results of ileocecal resection for Crohn's disease. Inflamm Bowel Dis 2007;13(11):1369–73.

54. Ferrante M, de Hertogh G, Hlavaty T, et al. The value of myenteric plexitis to predict early postoperative Crohn's disease recurrence. Gastroenterology 2006; 130(6):1595–606.

55. Sokol H, Polin V, Lavergne-Slove A, et al. Plexitis as a predictive factor of early postoperative clinical recurrence in Crohn's disease. Gut 2009;58(9):1218–25.

56. D'Haens GR, Gasparaitis AE, Hanauer SB. Duration of recurrent ileitis after ileocolonic resection correlates with presurgical extent of Crohn's disease. Gut 1995;36(5):715–7.

57. Gajendran M, Bauer AJ, Buchholz BM, et al. Ileocecal anastomosis type significantly influences long-term functional status, quality of life, and healthcare utilization in postoperative Crohn's disease patients independent of inflammation recurrence. Am J Gastroenterol 2018;113(4):576–83.

58. Muñoz-Juárez M, Yamamoto T, Wolff BG, et al. Wide-lumen stapled anastomosis vs. conventional end-to-end anastomosis in the treatment of Crohn's disease. Dis Colon Rectum 2001;44(1):20–5 [discussion: 25–6].
59. Regueiro M, Schraut W, Baidoo L, et al. Infliximab prevents Crohn's disease recurrence after ileal resection. Gastroenterology 2009;136(2):441–50.e1 [quiz: 716].
60. De Cruz P, Kamm MA, Hamilton AL, et al. Crohn's disease management after intestinal resection: a randomised trial. Lancet 2015;385(9976):1406–17.
61. Regueiro M, Velayos F, Greer JB, et al. American Gastroenterological Association Institute technical review on the management of Crohn's disease after surgical resection. Gastroenterology 2017;152(1):277–95.e3.
62. Bayart P, Duveau N, Nachury M, et al. Ileal or anastomotic location of lesions does not impact rate of postoperative recurrence in Crohn's disease patients classified i2 on the Rutgeerts score. Dig Dis Sci 2016;61(10):2986–92.
63. Domènech E, Mañosa M, Bernal I, et al. Impact of azathioprine on the prevention of postoperative Crohn's disease recurrence: results of a prospective, observational, long-term follow-up study. Inflamm Bowel Dis 2008;14(4):508–13.
64. Lopatin S, Mayorga DC, Cohen B, et al. Anastamotic ulcers after ileocolic resection predict Crohn's disease recurrence: 572. American Journal of Gastroenterology 2018;113:S329–30.
65. Asada T, Nakayama G, Tanaka C, et al. Postoperative adalimumab maintenance therapy for Japanese patients with Crohn's disease: a single-center, single-arm phase II trial (CCOG-1107 study). Surg Today 2018;48(6):609–17.
66. Papamichael K, Archavlis E, Lariou C, et al. Adalimumab for the prevention and/ or treatment of post-operative recurrence of Crohn's disease: a prospective, two-year, single center, pilot study. J Crohns Colitis 2012;6(9):924–31.
67. Yamada A, Komaki Y, Patel N, et al. The use of vedolizumab in preventing postoperative recurrence of Crohn's disease. Inflamm Bowel Dis 2018;24(3):502–9.
68. Novello M, Stocchi L, Holubar S, et al. Surgical outcomes of patients treated with ustekinumab vs. vedolizumab in inflammatory bowel disease: a matched case analysis. Int J Colorectal Dis 2018. https://doi.org/10.1007/s00384-018-3212-6.
69. Shim HH, Ma C, Kotze PG, et al. preoperative ustekinumab treatment is not associated with increased postoperative complications in Crohn's Disease: a Canadian multi-centre observational cohort study. J Can Assoc Gastroenterol 2018;1(3):115–23.
70. Shim H, Ma C, Al-Farhan H, et al. A107 Postoperative outcomes among ustekinumab treated Crohn's disease patients: a multicentre Canadian provincial experience. J Can Assoc Gastroenterol 2018;1(suppl_1):185–7.
71. Hendriksen C, Kreiner S, Binder V. Long term prognosis in ulcerative colitis—based on results from a regional patient group from the county of Copenhagen. Gut 1985;26(2):158–63.
72. Parks AG, Nicholls RJ. Proctocolectomy without ileostomy for ulcerative colitis. Br Med J 1978;2(6130):85–8.
73. Penna C, Dozois R, Tremaine W, et al. Pouchitis after ileal pouch-anal anastomosis for ulcerative colitis occurs with increased frequency in patients with associated primary sclerosing cholangitis. Gut 1996;38(2):234–9.
74. Tjandra JJ, Fazio VW, Church JM, et al. Similar functional results after restorative proctocolectomy in patients with familial adenomatous polyposis and mucosal ulcerative colitis. Am J Surg 1993;165(3):322–5.
75. Fleshner PR, Vasiliauskas EA, Kam LY, et al. High level perinuclear antineutrophil cytoplasmic antibody (pANCA) in ulcerative colitis patients before colectomy

predicts the development of chronic pouchitis after ileal pouch-anal anastomosis. Gut 2001;49(5):671–7.

76. Fazio VW, Tekkis PP, Remzi F, et al. Quantification of risk for pouch failure after ileal pouch anal anastomosis surgery. Ann Surg 2003;238(4):605–14 [discussion: 614–7].

77. Hashavia E, Dotan I, Rabau M, et al. Risk factors for chronic pouchitis after ileal pouch-anal anastomosis: a prospective cohort study. Colorectal Dis 2012; 14(11):1365–71.

78. Merrett MN, Mortensen N, Kettlewell M, et al. Smoking may prevent pouchitis in patients with restorative proctocolectomy for ulcerative colitis. Gut 1996;38(3): 362–4.

79. Fleshner P, Ippoliti A, Dubinsky M, et al. A prospective multivariate analysis of clinical factors associated with pouchitis after ileal pouch-anal anastomosis. Clin Gastroenterol Hepatol 2007;5(8):952–8 [quiz: 887].

80. Achkar J-P, Al-Haddad M, Lashner B, et al. Differentiating risk factors for acute and chronic pouchitis. Clin Gastroenterol Hepatol 2005;3(1):60–6.

81. Wu X-R, Ashburn J, Remzi FH, et al. Male gender is associated with a high risk for chronic antibiotic-refractory pouchitis and ileal pouch anastomotic sinus. J Gastrointest Surg 2016;20(3):631–9.

82. Shen B, Remzi FH, Nutter B, et al. Association between immune-associated disorders and adverse outcomes of ileal pouch-anal anastomosis. Am J Gastroenterol 2009;104(3):655–64.

83. Holubar SD, Cima RR, Sandborn WJ, et al. Treatment and prevention of pouchitis after ileal pouch-anal anastomosis for chronic ulcerative colitis. Cochrane Database Syst Rev 2010;(6):CD001176.

84. Shen B, Achkar JP, Lashner BA, et al. A randomized clinical trial of ciprofloxacin and metronidazole to treat acute pouchitis. Inflamm Bowel Dis 2001;7(4):301–5.

85. Pardi DS, D'Haens G, Shen B, et al. Clinical guidelines for the management of pouchitis. Inflamm Bowel Dis 2009;15(9):1424–31.

86. Gionchetti P, Rizzello F, Venturi A, et al. Antibiotic combination therapy in patients with chronic, treatment-resistant pouchitis. Aliment Pharmacol Ther 1999;13(6):713–8.

87. Abdelrazeq AS, Kelly SM, Lund JN, et al. Rifaximin-ciprofloxacin combination therapy is effective in chronic active refractory pouchitis. Colorectal Dis 2005; 7(2):182–6.

88. Mimura T, Rizzello F, Helwig U, et al. Four-week open-label trial of metronidazole and ciprofloxacin for the treatment of recurrent or refractory pouchitis. Aliment Pharmacol Ther 2002;16(5):909–17.

89. Segal JP, Penez L, Mohsen Elkady S, et al. Long term outcomes of initial infliximab therapy for inflammatory pouch pathology: a multi-Centre retrospective study. Scand J Gastroenterol 2018;53(9):1051–8.

90. Huguet M, Pereira B, Goutte M, et al. Systematic review with meta-analysis: anti-TNF therapy in refractory pouchitis and Crohn's disease-like complications of the pouch after ileal pouch-anal anastomosis following colectomy for ulcerative colitis. Inflamm Bowel Dis 2018;24(2):261–8.

91. Kelly OB, Rosenberg M, Tyler AD, et al. Infliximab to treat refractory inflammation after pelvic pouch surgery for ulcerative colitis. J Crohns Colitis 2016; 10(4):410–7.

92. Viazis N, Giakoumis M, Koukouratos T, et al. Long term benefit of one year infliximab administration for the treatment of chronic refractory pouchitis. J Crohns Colitis 2013;7(10):e457–60.

93. Barreiro-de Acosta M, García-Bosch O, Souto R, et al. Efficacy of infliximab rescue therapy in patients with chronic refractory pouchitis: a multicenter study. Inflamm Bowel Dis 2012;18(5):812–7.

94. Ferrante M, D'Haens G, Dewit O, et al. Efficacy of infliximab in refractory pouchitis and Crohn's disease-related complications of the pouch: a Belgian case series. Inflamm Bowel Dis 2010;16(2):243–9.

95. Barreiro-de Acosta M, García-Bosch O, Gordillo J, et al. Efficacy of adalimumab rescue therapy in patients with chronic refractory pouchitis previously treated with infliximab: a case series. Eur J Gastroenterol Hepatol 2012;24(7):756–8.

96. Khan F, Gao X-H, Singh A, et al. Vedolizumab in the treatment of Crohn's disease of the pouch. Gastroenterol Rep (Oxf) 2018;6(3):184–8.

97. Bär F, Kühbacher T, Dietrich NA, et al. Vedolizumab in the treatment of chronic, antibiotic-dependent or refractory pouchitis. Aliment Pharmacol Ther 2018; 47(5):581–7.

98. Coletta M, Paroni M, Caprioli F. Successful treatment with vedolizumab in a patient with chronic refractory pouchitis and primary sclerosing cholangitis. J Crohns Colitis 2017;11(12):1507–8.

99. Philpott J, Ashburn J, Shen B. Efficacy of vedolizumab in patients with antibiotic and anti-tumor necrosis alpha refractory pouchitis. Inflamm Bowel Dis 2017; 23(1):E5–6.

100. Weaver KN, Gregory M, Syal G, et al. Ustekinumab is effective for the treatment of Crohn's disease of the pouch in a multicenter cohort. Inflamm Bowel Dis 2018. https://doi.org/10.1093/ibd/izy302.

101. Sambuelli A, Boerr L, Negreira S, et al. Budesonide enema in pouchitis–a double-blind, double-dummy, controlled trial. Aliment Pharmacol Ther 2002; 16(1):27–34.

102. Navaneethan U, Venkatesh PGK, Bennett AE, et al. Impact of budesonide on liver function tests and gut inflammation in patients with primary sclerosing cholangitis and ileal pouch anal anastomosis. J Crohns Colitis 2012;6(5):536–42.

103. Shen B, Liu W, Remzi FH, et al. Enterochromaffin cell hyperplasia in irritable pouch syndrome. Am J Gastroenterol 2008;103(9):2293–300.

104. Wu B, Lian L, Li Y, et al. Clinical course of cuffitis in ulcerative colitis patients with restorative proctocolectomy and ileal pouch-anal anastomoses. Inflamm Bowel Dis 2013;19(2):404–10.

105. Shen B, Lashner BA, Bennett AE, et al. Treatment of rectal cuff inflammation (cuffitis) in patients with ulcerative colitis following restorative proctocolectomy and ileal pouch-anal anastomosis. Am J Gastroenterol 2004;99(8):1527–31.

106. Subramani K, Harpaz N, Bilotta J, et al. Refractory pouchitis: does it reflect underlying Crohn's disease? Gut 1993;34(11):1539–42.

107. Melmed GY, Fleshner PR, Bardakcioglu O, et al. Family history and serology predict Crohn's disease after ileal pouch-anal anastomosis for ulcerative colitis. Dis Colon Rectum 2008;51(1):100–8.

108. Moskowitz RL, Shepherd NA, Nicholls RJ. An assessment of inflammation in the reservoir after restorative proctocolectomy with ileoanal ileal reservoir. Int J Colorectal Dis 1986;1(3):167–74.

109. Shen B, Achkar JP, Lashner BA, et al. Endoscopic and histologic evaluation together with symptom assessment are required to diagnose pouchitis. Gastroenterology 2001;121(2):261–7.

110. Wolf JM, Achkar J-P, Lashner BA, et al. Afferent limb ulcers predict Crohn's disease in patients with ileal pouch-anal anastomosis. Gastroenterology 2004; 126(7):1686–91.

111. Shen B, Fazio VW, Remzi FH, et al. Risk factors for clinical phenotypes of Crohn's disease of the ileal pouch. Am J Gastroenterol 2006;101(12):2760–8.

112. Paye F, Penna C, Chiche L, et al. Pouch-related fistula following restorative proctocolectomy. Br J Surg 1996;83(11):1574–7.

113. Lolohea S, Lynch AC, Robertson GB, et al. Ileal pouch-anal anastomosis-vaginal fistula: a review. Dis Colon Rectum 2005;48(9):1802–10.

114. Heriot AG, Tekkis PP, Smith JJ, et al. Management and outcome of pouch-vaginal fistulas following restorative proctocolectomy. Dis Colon Rectum 2005; 48(3):451–8.

115. O'Kelly TJ, Merrett M, Mortensen NJ, et al. Pouch-vaginal fistula after restorative proctocolectomy: aetiology and management. Br J Surg 1994;81(9):1374–5.

116. Burke D, van Laarhoven CJ, Herbst F, et al. Transvaginal repair of pouch-vaginal fistula. Br J Surg 2001;88(2):241–5.

117. Kochhar G, Shen B. Endoscopic fistulotomy in inflammatory bowel disease (with video). Gastrointest Endosc 2018;88(1):87–94.

118. Prudhomme M, Dozois RR, Godlewski G, et al. Anal canal strictures after ileal pouch-anal anastomosis. Dis Colon Rectum 2003;46(1):20–3.

119. Shen B, Fazio VW, Remzi FH, et al. Endoscopic balloon dilation of ileal pouch strictures. Am J Gastroenterol 2004;99(12):2340–7.

120. Lan N, Shen B. Endoscopic stricturotomy with needle knife in the treatment of strictures from inflammatory bowel disease. Inflamm Bowel Dis 2017;23(4): 502–13.

121. Read TE, Schoetz DJ, Marcello PW, et al. Afferent limb obstruction complicating ileal pouch-anal anastomosis. Dis Colon Rectum 1997;40(5):566–9.

122. Baixauli J, Delaney CP, Wu JS, et al. Functional outcome and quality of life after repeat ileal pouch-anal anastomosis for complications of ileoanal surgery. Dis Colon Rectum 2004;47(1):2–11.

123. Kariv R, Remzi FH, Lian L, et al. Preoperative colorectal neoplasia increases risk for pouch neoplasia in patients with restorative proctocolectomy. Gastroenterology 2010;139(3):806–12, 812.e1-2.

124. Liu Z-X, Kiran RP, Bennett AE, et al. Diagnosis and management of dysplasia and cancer of the ileal pouch in patients with underlying inflammatory bowel disease. Cancer 2011;117(14):3081–92.

125. Thompson-Fawcett MW, Marcus V, Redston M, et al. Risk of dysplasia in long-term ileal pouches and pouches with chronic pouchitis. Gastroenterology 2001;121(2):275–81.

Advances in Perianal Disease Associated with Crohn's Disease-Evolving Approaches

Xinying Wang, MD, PhD[a], Bo Shen, MD[b],*

KEYWORDS

- Crohn's disease • Endoscopic therapy • Fistula • Perianal disease • Stem cells

KEY POINTS

- Perianal diseases, among the most common complications of Crohn's disease, are difficult to diagnose and manage.
- Patients with perianal Crohn's disease suffer from persistent pain and drainage, recurrent perianal sepsis, impaired quality of life, and financial burden.
- Conventional medical and surgical therapies for the condition carry risk for infection, myelosuppression, incontinence, and disease recurrence.
- Although the treatment of the phenotype of Crohn's disease has been extensively studied, the reported outcomes are inconsistent.
- In addition to conventional CT and MRI, endoanal ultrasonography is becoming popular thanks to its low cost and its ability to acquire images in real time.
- Emerging management strategies for treatment including laser therapy, local injection of agents, use of hyperbaric oxygen, and stem cell therapy, have demonstrated efficacy.

INTRODUCTION

Crohn's disease (CD) is a chronic inflammatory, refractory, and disabling disease associated with an abnormal immune response to altered gut microbiome in a genetically susceptible host. Perianal disease is one of the most common complications of CD, which can present as fistulae-in-ano, abscesses, fissures, and perineal sepsis. First described by Penner and Crohn in 1938, perianal fistulizing Crohn's disease (PFCD), is associated with severe medical, psychological, and social consequences, significantly impairing the patient's quality of life (QOL).[1] Perianal fistulizing Crohn's disease presents in up to 43% of patients with CD and it

Disclosure: The authors declared no financial conflict of interest.
[a] Department of Gastroenterology, Zhujiang Hospital, Southern Medical University, Guangzhou, China; [b] The Center for Inflammatory Bowel Diseases-A31, Digestive Disease and Surgery Institute, Cleveland Clinic, 9500 Euclid Avenue, Cleveland, OH 44195, USA
* Corresponding author.
E-mail address: shenb@ccf.org

Gastrointest Endoscopy Clin N Am 29 (2019) 515–530
https://doi.org/10.1016/j.giec.2019.02.011
1052-5157/19/© 2019 Elsevier Inc. All rights reserved.

may be the sole representation of CD in proximately 5% of patients.[2] The rate of occurrence for PFCD is time-dependent; the longer a patient has CD, the more likely he is to have perianal manifestations.[3–5] The cumulative incidence of PFCD 1 year after diagnosis is estimated to be 12%; and this rate doubles 20 years after diagnosis.[6] The proposed Perianal Disease Activity Index has been used to measure severity of perianal involvement with CD, especially in clinical trials.[7] Patients with perianal CD often have persistent pain, drainage, recurrent perianal sepsis, significant financial burden, and impaired QOL. The ultimate outcome of treatment is complete closure, without infection, abscess, or recurrence. Reported success rates of conventional medical and surgical treatments range from 30% to 80%. Intensive medical treatment, such as the use of immunomodulators or biological agents, albeit given their modest efficacy, have significant adverse effects, whereas surgical therapy carries an increased risk for postoperative complications, such as incontinence, as well as postoperative disease recurrence.[8] In this article, the authors review recent developments in PFCD management.

CLASSIFICATION OF PERIANAL FISTULAE

Although there is no consensus for classifying perianal fistulas in CD, 3 major anatomic classifications have been used: the Parks classification, the St. James's University Hospital classification, and the American Gastroenterological Association (AGA) classification[1,9,10] (**Table 1**). The Parks' classification describes 5 types of fistulas, which are distinguished according to surgical anatomy (superficial, intersphincteric, transsphincteric, suprasphincteric, and extrasphincteric).[10] According to the AGA classification, perianal fistulas are divided into 2 categories: simple fistulas or complex fistulas.[1] A simple fistula is a superficial, intersphincteric, or transsphincteric fistula, with a single external orifice and without complicating features (abscess, rectovaginal fistula, and rectal or anal stricture), located below the dentate line. A complex fistula is an intersphincteric, transsphincteric, suprasphincteric, or extrasphincteric fistula, above the dentate line, which may have multiple external orifices or complicating features. Complex fistulas are encountered more commonly than simple fistulas in patients with CD. Classification and identification of fistulas are essential for determining therapeutic approaches.

DIAGNOSIS

The methods recommended for characterization of perianal fistulizing disease and preoperative evaluation for appropriate surgical interventions include fistulography, computed tomography (CT), endoanal ultrasonography (EAUS), and perineal MRI.[11] However, the benefits of fistulography and CT are limited by their low accuracy.[12,13] Furthermore, CT exposes patients to ionizing radiation. The European Crohn's and Colitis Organisation Consensus Guidelines recommended contrast-enhanced high-resolution pelvic MRI as an initial and preferred diagnostic tool for the assessment of fistulizing CD.[14] Contrast-enhanced pelvic MRI can also be used to assess the rectal wall, anatomy of sphincters, pelvic lymph nodes, and abscess. In combination with examination under anesthesia (EUA), MRI can achieve an accuracy of 100% for the detection of perianal fistula and abscess.[15,16] Endoanal ultrasonography has been developed as an alternative imaging study for its low cost, high resolution, and real-time performance, which can be performed in those without rectal or anal stenosis.

Table 1
Classification of perianal fistulas

Category	Define	Diagnosis Modality	Therapy	Treatment Goal
Parks classification[10]				
Intersphincteric fistula	Lesions are confined to the intersphincteric space		a. Divide lower half of the internal sphincter b. Lay open track c. Adequate drainage d. Eradicate primary disease	
Transsphincteric fistula	Leave the intersphincteric space through the external anal sphincter		a. Open the fistula (uncomplicated type) b. Find and open the primary track (with a high blind track) c. Adequate drainage	
Suprasphincteric fistula	Pass through the intersphincteric space over the top of the puborectalis, track down the levator muscle before tracking and the skin		Modification of the lay open methods	
Extrasphincteric fistula	Pass from the perineal skin, and penetrate the levator muscle into the rectum		Temporary colostomy	

(continued on next page)

Table 1
(continued)

Category	Define	Diagnosis Modality	Therapy	Treatment Goal
AGA classification[1]				
Simple fistula	a. Low location b. Single external opening c. No evidence of perianal abscess, rectovaginal fistula, anorectal stricture	a. PE b. Rectosigmoid endoscopy c. EUA + EUS/MRI (when initial therapy fails)	a. Antibiotics b. Azathioprine, 6-mercaptopurine, infliximab c. Fistulotomy	Cure without suppressive maintenance therapy
Complex fistula	a. High location b. Multiple external openings c. Concomitant perianal abscess, rectovaginal fistula, anorectal stricture, and active rectal disease or not		a. Antibiotics b. Azathioprine, 6-mercaptopurine, infliximab c. Surgery	Typically fistula closure and suppression of recurrence
MRI classification[9]				
Simple linear intersphincteric fistula	a. Lesions are confined to sphincter complex b. Ischioanal and ischiorectal fossae are clear		Simple surgery or no surgery required	
Intersphincteric fistula with abscess or secondary track				
Transsphincteric fistula	Any track or abscess within the ischiorectal fossa or levator plate		Complex surgery and risk of incontinence and fecal diversion	
Transsphincteric fistula with abscess or secondary track within the ischiorectal fossa				
Supralevator and translevator disease				

Abbreviations: EUA, examination under anesthesia; EUS, endoscopic ultrasonography; MRI, magnetic resonance imaging; PE, physical examination.

Examination Under Anesthesia

Examination under anesthesia has been considered the most sensitive diagnostic modality for perianal disease, with a reported accuracy of 90%.[6,17] Examination under anesthesia is preferred to be performed by experienced colorectal surgeons.[14] Examination under anesthesia allows for delivery of concomitant therapy, such as placement of drainage catheter or seton. Persistent perianal pain with or without systemic symptoms, such as fever, night sweats, and chills, raises the possibility of an abscess. If an abscess is present or suspected, prompt diagnostic and potentially therapeutic EUA is recommended to reduce the risk for branching of fistula and formation of abscess or even pelvic sepsis.

EUA and MRI have complementary roles. MRI has an accuracy of 76% to 100% for the diagnosis of fistulas.[18,19] Pre-EUA pelvic MRI is preferable for all patients. However, in the absence of MRI, therapeutic EUA should not be delayed for those suspected of having an abscess. MRI may provide additional information for the surgical approach to fistulas (10%–20% of patients), and MRI may identify extension of t sinus tract, which cannot be assessed with EUA.[20–24] Findings of EUA may be used to guide medical therapy. In a clinical study of infliximab (IFX), a higher success rate and a lower recurrence rate were attained in patients undergoing EUA with abscess drainage and seton placement before starting antitumor necrosis factor (TNF) therapy.[25]

Endoanal Ultrasonography

Endoanal ultrasonography, also known as transrectal ultrasonography (TRUS),[26] may be performed with or without hydrogen peroxide for the diagnosis of CD-related perianal disease. The reported diagnostic accuracy of this approach ranged from 56% to 90%.[27] In contrast to MRI, EAUS may offer a less accurate delineation of sinus tracts, but a better detection of abscess or internal opening of a fistula. Endoanal ultrasonography may provide a better evaluation of the sphincter, especially in higher transducer frequencies.[28] Endoanal ultrasonography and MRI have been shown to have an excellent consistency in the diagnosis of perianal CD.[29,30] In experienced hands, endoanal ultrasonography may be superior to MRI for classifying transsphincteric and rectovaginal/anovulvar fistulas.[19,31] Hydrogen peroxide-enhanced 3-dimensional EAUS and endoanal MRI agreed in 88% (kappa = 0.45) for the primary fistula tract, in 90% (kappa = 0.83) for the location of the internal opening, in 78% (kappa = 0.62) for secondary tracts, and in 88% (kappa = 0.63) for fluid collections.[32]

Ultrasound fistula sign has been used to differentiate CD-related fistulae-in-ano from cryptogenic fistulae or abscesses, with positive and negative predictive values of 87% and 93%, respectively.[33] A recent prospective study compared the diagnostic accuracy of transperineal ultrasonography, transrectal ultrasonography, and MRI, with EUA, in 23 patients with active perianal CD and showed comparable overall diagnostic accuracy in the assessment of fistulas, abscesses, and rectal involvement.[34] However, a systematic review of the assessment of idiopathic and CD perianal fistulas showed that EAUS and MRI demonstrated comparable sensitivity. In contrast, the specificity of MRI was greater for than that of EAUS. The study suffered from a high degree of heterogeneity with regard to data sources.[35] Two studies comparing EAUS with MRI found that MRI was less effective in detecting abscesses.[29,31] However, a systematic review with a meta-analysis of 9 studies showed that transperineal ultrasonography had an overall sensitivity of 86%, and a positive predictive value of 90%, for the detection rate of perianal abscesses.[36] Endoanal ultrasonography has also been used for guiding medical and surgical therapy, such as monitoring of response to biological treatment[37] and drainage of perianal abscess.[38]

Endoanal ultrasonography is an inexpensive, noninvasive modality that effectively detects perianal disease in patients with CD. On the other hand, EAUS has limited depth of penetration (usually <5–6 cm), which compromises its ability in evaluation of deep lesions.[39–42]

NOVEL TREATMENT MODALITIES

Traditional surgical therapies for fistulae-in-ano include fistulotomy with sphincterotomy, seton placement, advancement flaps, and ligation of the intersphincteric fistula tract. The most important adverse effect associated with fistulotomy is fecal incontinence. Fistulotomy is therefore typically used for simple fistulas but not for complex fistulae-in-ano. Fistulotomy may be avoided in patients with complex fistulae-in-ano.

Laser Therapy

Fistula-tract laser closure (FiLaC, Biolitec, Germany) is a novel and promising technique for primary or secondary closure of perianal fistula tracts. This technique involves use of a radial emitting laser probe to destroy the epithelial layer of the fistula and simultaneously obliterate the fistula tract without damaging the sphincter. FiLaC has several advantages, including a lower risk for incontinence, a short learning curve, a short healing and operating time, and it allows for reapplication.[34,43–45] First reported by Wilhelm and colleagues, Treatment with FiLaC was successful in 9/11 patients in a median follow-up of 7.4 months.[45] Giamundo and colleagues reported that primary healing was observed in 25 (71.4%) patients with anal fistula using FiLaC.[44] Patients in this cohort who had been previously treated with a loose seton (19/24, 79%) achieved the best healing.[43] Eight (23%) procedures failed and 2 patients had recurrence. In a recent study of 103 patients, 41 (40%) with perianal fistulas had overall complete healing; 38 (37%) had persistent symptomatic drainage; 20 (19%) had mild drainage with minimal symptoms; and 4 (4%) had painful symptomatic drainage in a median follow-up of 28.3 months (range = 2.3–49.9 months).[46] Few studies were specifically focused on CD-related perianal fistulas. In the study by Wilhelm and colleague, the primary healing rate was 69.2% (9/13) for Crohn fistulas versus 63.5% (66/104) for cryptoglandular fistulas, and the secondary healing rate was 92.3% versus 85.5%, respectively. The results suggest that an underlying diagnosis of CD did not seem to have impact on either primary or secondary outcomes after FiLaC treatment.[47] Reported adverse effects of FiLaC included minor incontinence of mucus and gas, and late-onset abscess. However, no patients reported serious incontinence postoperatively. Therefore, laser therapy may be attempted in patients with CD- or non-CD-related perianal fistulas.

Topical Administration of Sealing Agents

Conservative topical techniques, such as biological glue and plugs, have been used in patients with previously well-drained fistulas or in the absence of associated abscesses.

Fibrin glue, a mixture of fibrinogen, calcium ions, and thrombin, injected into the fistula tract by way of a catheter within 60 seconds, is used to form a clot to fill the cavity and seal the fistula. The main advantage of this procedure is its ability to preserve anal sphincter function. A multicenter, open-label randomized controlled trial of fibrin glue was performed in patients with quiescent CD; half of the patients had a complex fistula. Clinical remission was observed in 13 of 34 patients (38%) in the fibrin glue group compared with 6 of 37 (16%) in the observation group at 8 weeks.[48] A similar healing rate (31%) was reported in a separate study.[49] However, early extravasation of the mixture from the fistula tract, or failure to identify branched fistulas, was shown to have a high recurrence rate. Studies by Cintron and colleagues showed that the use of either commercial fibrin adhesive or autologous blood admixed with fibrin adhesive achieved a recovery rate of 68% to 85% in patients with cryptoglandular fistula.[50–52] A study by Vitton and colleagues of 14 patients with CD and anal fistulas treated with fibrin glue injection showed completely dried fistulas in 10 (71%), decreased leakage in 1 (7%), and no observable improvement in the remaining 3 (21%) at 3-month follow-up.[53] More than half of the patients with CD had clinical remission within 2 years after treatment with fibrin glue. Adverse events, mainly abscess following injection with fibrin glue, were rare.

An anal fistula plug (AFP) is a cone-shaped plug synthesized from lyophilized porcine small intestinal submucosa. This material has inherent resistance to infection, producing no foreign-body or giant-cell reactions. Host cell tissue repopulates the AFP, promoting healing processes that permanently obliterate the fistula tract.[54–56] The technique of fistula plug deployment is similar to that of fibrin glue injection. Both modalities have a minimum risk for sphincter injury. The reported healing rate of the fistula plug ranged from 24% to 95% within the subsequent 3.5 to 12 months. In patients with complex fistulas, the healing rate was 35% to 87%.[57] The reported rate of plug protrusion, the primary cause of treatment failure in the early postoperative period (within 1 week), ranged from 4% to 41%.[57]

The reported efficacy of AFPs in patients with PFCD varied. Garg and colleagues reported clinical healing of fistulas in the anal tract in 29% to 86% of patients with CD.[57] A recent systematic review, including 12 studies of 84 patients with CD, showed that the total success rate of AFP, defined as closure of fistula tract, was in 49 patients (58.3%). Success in patients with recurrent anal fistulas was in 2 of 5 (40%). In 2 comparative studies, inferior overall success rates were found in patients who received preoperative concurrent immunomodulators than in those who did not (27.3% vs 73.9%).[58] Fistula plug has been applied for the treatment of rectovaginal and pouch-vaginal fistulas in patients with underlying inflammatory bowel disease (IBD). Chung and colleagues reported a healing rate of 75% at 12 weeks in 51 IBD patients, of whom 40 had underlying CD.[59] The healing rate of a special button plug was 58% (7/12) at 4 months in 1 series[60] and 88% (6/7) at 6 months in the other.[61] In a systematic review, O'Riordan and colleagues summarized the use of AFP for CD and non-CD perianal fistula, and reported that fistula closure was achieved in 54.8% of patients without CD and in 54.3% of those with CD at a follow-up of between 3 and 24 months. No changes in continence were found.[62] A recent randomized controlled trial that compared seton removal alone or with AFP insertion in 106 patients with CD showed that AFP was numerically more effective than seton removal alone in achieving fistula closure (31.5% vs 23.1%, $P = .19$).[56] Thus, AFPs may be attempted in patients with PFCD.

Endoscopic Therapy for Perianal Disease

Endoscopic balloon dilation and endoscopic stricturotomy with an insulated tip knife or a needle knife have been used in PFCD patients with concurrent anal or distal rectal stricture. Endoscopic fistulotomy has been used for the treatment of simple, superficial perianal fistula. In addition, endoscopic incision and drainage, and endoscopy-guided seton placement, have been described.[63–65]

Intralesional Antitumor Necrosis Factor Agents

Multiple studies have shown that systemic anti-TNF agents are effective in treating CD-related fistulas, for both fistula healing and maintaining fistula closure.[66,67] Topical application of anti-TNF agents in stricturing or fistulizing CD has been explored. Local injection of IFX was shown to be effective in 72.7% of patients, defined as decreased fistula drainage ≥50%. Complete cessation of drainage for a minimum of 4 weeks was achieved in 36.4% of patients. Of note, the study excluded patients who had previously received systemic treatment with IFX as well as patients with rectal or perianal complications, such as proctitis or abscess.[68] A separate study of 8 patients was conducted to evaluate combined repeated peri-fistula IFX injection and core-out fistulectomy as a treatment of refractory complex PFCD. Persistent closure was achieved in 7 (87.5%) patients 12 months after treatment, and in 5 (62.5%) patients at the end of median follow-up of 35 months (range = 19–43 months).[69] One recent review evaluated 6 case series (include 2 studies of adalimumab injection) with a total of 92 patients, and found that short-term efficacy (ie, complete or partial response) rate varied from 40% to 100%. No significant adverse events were reported.[70]

Local IFX therapy seems to be safe and may be effective. However, the reported outcomes are inconsistent because of small sample size, short follow-up, lack of controls, and the lack of standardization in outcome measures.

Hyperbaric Oxygen Therapy

The role of hypoxia as a modifying or causative factor in the genesis and maintenance of inflammation has been postulated. In vitro, as well as in vivo, studies have shown hypoxia to be an important trigger of inflammation.[71,72] Hyperbaric oxygen therapy (HBOT) involves the inhalation of pure oxygen in pressurized chambers at pressure greater than 1 atm. This technique may be used to optimize fibroblast proliferation and white blood cell activity. Hyperbaric oxygen therapy may also reduce the duration of hypoxia, by inducing changes in the secretion of interleukin-1 (IL-1), IL-6, IL-2, and TNF-α, and by stimulating angiogenesis.[73] Hyperbaric oxygen therapy has been shown to be effective in the treatment of steroid-refractory ulcerative colitis,[74] perineal disease, pyoderma gangrenosum, and persistent perineal sinus after proctectomy for IBD.[75–77] Brady and colleagues first reported using HBOT for severe perineal CD.[78] For patients with perineal or fistulizing CD who were treated with HBOT, 50% to 70% achieved a complete response, 9% to 41% had a partial response, and 12% to 20% showed no response.[79,80] One study reported that 9 patients achieved complete healing of fistulas by 6 to 28 weeks, and for a follow-up of 18 months by combining IFX, HBOT, and anti-MAP (*Mycobacterium avium* ss. *paratuberculosis*).[81] One systematic review of 40 IBD patients with perianal disease refractory to traditional therapy showed an overall response rate of 88% to HBOT.[82]

The adverse events associated with HBOT seem to be mild and are related to changes in barometric pressure and oxygen toxicity.[82] The most common complication is trauma to the middle ear or sinus.[83] Colombel and colleagues reported that 2 patients discontinued treatment after only a few sessions because of bilateral tympanic membrane perforation or mental intolerance.[79] Rare complications that were observed primarily in patients with underlying lung diseases included pneumothorax, air embolism, and temporary blurring of vision. Maturation of cataracts was reported after more than 150 treatments.[84,85]

Stem Cell Therapy

Stem cell therapy is speculated to reset the clock for immune response.[86,87] Mesenchymal stem cells (MSCs) (also called mesenchymal stromal cells) are initially isolated from bone marrow. Mesenchymal stem cells have the capacity to differentiate into various lineages, such as chondrocytes, tenocytes, and myoblasts.[88] Mesenchymal stem cells, including adipose tissue-derived MSCs (AD-MSCs) and bone marrow-derived MSCs, possess potent antiinflammatory and immunomodulatory properties. These cells suppress activation and proliferation of T cells, differentiation, maturation, and function of dendritic cells, activation of B cells, and proliferation of natural killer cells.[89] Mesenchymal stem cells have the capacity for self-renewal and may be maintained ex vivo for a long period of time. Of note, lymphocyte and dendritic cell activation, as well as natural killer cell proliferation, are contributing factors in the pathogenesis of fistula.[90,91] These findings provide the rationale for using MSCs in the treatment of perianal fistulizing CD.

The first clinical application of AD-MSCs was reported in 2003. One female patient with Crohn colitis, perianal suppurations, and rectovaginal fistula healed within 1 week and remained asymptomatic for 3 months after local injection of 9×10^6 AD-MSCs.[92] A phase I clinical trial including 9 fistulas in 4 patients was reported in 2005. Autologous cells from an adipose origin were used for treatment of patients with PFCD through local injection of MSCs. At week 8, 6 of 8 (75%) patients with fistulas achieved healing, with no adverse effects at the end of the follow-up period.[93] Other studies using cells from adipose tissue or bone marrow achieved high rates of fistula closure (75%–77%). Furthermore, those studies indicated that healing rates between CD and non-CD subgroups were similar.[94–96] To increase tolerance, investigators explored the injection of allogeneic MSCs. In an open-label study of administration of 20 to 60 million AD-MSCs in 24 patients, 28% of patients achieved closure of fistula tracts after 24 weeks.[97] A placebo-controlled, dose-ascending study in 21 patients with PFCD using 20 to 90 million bone marrow-derived MSCs showed a rate of closure of 33% to 80%, compared with 20% in the placebo group.[98] The first adequately powered randomized, placebo-controlled trial compared the efficacy of a single injection of 120 million allogeneic AD-MSCs compared with placebo in 212 patients.[99] Anti-TNF therapy had previously failed in greater than 78% of patients included in the study. At week 52, fistula closure was more common in patients treated with MSCs compared with controls (50% vs 34%; $P = .024$). The combined end point was met by 56.3% of patients treated with MSCs, compared with 38.6% of those who received placebo.

Results of long-awaited randomized controlled trials are available. A phase III ADMIRE trial was conducted on 212 patients with CD to assess the safety and efficacy of allogeneic AD-MSCs for treatment of complex perianal fistulas compared with placebo over a 24-week period and an extended follow-up period of up to 104 weeks. At week 24, combined remission had been achieved by a significantly higher percentage of treated patients, compared with those who received placebo (50% vs 34%).[99] The fistula rate of closure with intralesional or intravenous MSCs varied from 37% to 85%.[100] A recent systematic review and meta-analysis included 7 phase I studies, 3 phase II, and 1 phase III randomized clinical trials showed that MSCs were associated with improved healing compared with control subjects at primary end points of 6 to 24 weeks (odds ratio = 3.06) and 24 to 52 weeks (odds ratio = 2.37) without increasing adverse events or serious adverse events in patients with PFCD.[101] One series compared AD-MSC therapy with fibrin glue in the treatment of patients with CD and complex perianal fistula. The results showed that AD-MSCs were more effective than fibrin glue in patients with or without CD.[93,95,102]

Recently, a modified technique for delivering MSCs to the fistula tract by coating autologous MSCs on fistula plugs was tested in a phase I study. Twelve patients, who had failed anti-TNF therapy, with a single draining fistula for at least 3 months without proctitis, underwent intraoperative placement of the plug loaded with autologous MSCs. Complete fistula closure was achieved in 9 of 12 patients (75%) by 3 months, and in 10 of 12 patients (83.3%) at 6 months.[103] Another study combined

AD-MSCs, platelet-rich plasma, and endorectal advancement flaps for the therapy for refractory PFCD and showed a final healing rate of 91% (10/11) with a median follow-up period of 31 months.[104]

Mesenchymal stem cell therapy represents an effective intervention that has a low risk for adverse effects or for incontinence. The therapy may be particularly applicable in patients with CD who do not respond to conventional treatments. Stem cell treatment is ideally used for the treatment of patients with active perianal fistulizing disease, those with quiescent luminal disease that is naive to immunomodulators or anti-TNF therapy, or those with intolerance to systemic immunosuppression. There are limitations for stem cell therapy. First, the lack of a uniform protocol. Techniques for cell isolation, selection, expansion, and dosage are not identified and vary in different studies. Second, most published studies are not reliable owing to their small sample size and scant controlled data.[101] Third, no standard definition of fistula healing has been established, resulting in effective rates than vary broadly among studies.[105] Additional studies are necessary to overcome these limitations.

SUMMARY

The therapeutic targets of treatment of perianal disease/fistula in patients with CD have been maintenance of a well-drained tract and clinical remission without incontinence. With the development of novel diagnostic and therapeutic modalities, complete fistula healing may be achieved, resulting in improved QOL for the patient. Fistula in patients with CD should be managed by a multi-disciplinary team that includes a gastroenterologist, a colorectal surgeon, and a gastrointestinal radiologist. After primary diagnostic methods have been performed, a patient with complex fistulas should undergo further testing with MRI and EAUS. Novel treatment strategies, such as local sealing agent therapy, endoscopic therapy, HBOT, and stem cell therapy hold promise for treating patients with fistulas. However, current data are conflicting, and there is a paucity of randomized, controlled studies with large sample sizes. Any of the methods presented here may be combined with endoscopy to investigate the presence of inflammation in the rectosigmoid colon. Treatment of fistulas is unsuccessful without treatment of underlying, active disease.

ACKNOWLEDGMENTS

Dr. Xinying Wang is supported by National Natural Science Foundation of China (81572938); and Dr. Bo Shen is supported by the Ed and Joey Story Endowed Chair.

REFERENCES

1. Sandborn WJ, Fazio VW, Feagan BG, et al. AGA technical review on perianal Crohn's disease. Gastroenterology 2003;125:1508–30.
2. Schwartz DA, Ghazi LJ, Regueiro M, et al. Guidelines for the multidisciplinary management of Crohn's perianal fistulas: summary statement. Inflamm Bowel Dis 2015;21:723–30.
3. Cosnes J, Cattan S, Blain A, et al. Long-term evolution of disease behavior of Crohn's disease. Inflamm Bowel Dis 2002;8:244–50.
4. Lewis RT, Bleier JI. Surgical treatment of anorectal crohn disease. Clin Colon Rectal Surg 2013;26:90–9.
5. Roberts PL, Schoetz DJ Jr, Pricolo R, et al. Clinical course of Crohn's disease in older patients. A retrospective study. Dis Colon Rectum 1990;33:458–62.

6. Schwartz DA, Loftus EV Jr, Tremaine WJ, et al. The natural history of fistulizing Crohn's disease in Olmsted County, Minnesota. Gastroenterology 2002;122: 875–80.

7. Irvine EJ. Usual therapy improves perianal Crohn's disease as measured by a new disease activity index. McMaster IBD Study Group. J Clin Gastroenterol 1995;20:27–32.

8. Soltani A, Kaiser AM. Endorectal advancement flap for cryptoglandular or Crohn's fistula-in-ano. Dis Colon Rectum 2010;53:486–95.

9. Morris J, Spencer JA, Ambrose NS. MR imaging classification of perianal fistulas and its implications for patient management. Radiographics 2000;20: 623–35 [discussion: 635–7].

10. Parks AG, Gordon PH, Hardcastle JD. A classification of fistula-in-ano. Br J Surg 1976;63:1–12.

11. Halligan S, Stoker J. Imaging of fistula in ano. Radiology 2006;239:18–33.

12. Kuijpers HC, Schulpen T. Fistulography for fistula-in-ano. Is it useful? Dis Colon Rectum 1985;28:103–4.

13. Pomerri F, Dodi G, Pintacuda G, et al. Anal endosonography and fistulography for fistula-in-ano. Radiol Med 2010;115:771–83.

14. Gionchetti P, Dignass A, Danese S, et al. 3rd European evidence-based consensus on the diagnosis and management of Crohn's disease 2016: part 2: surgical management and special situations. J Crohns Colitis 2017;11: 135–49.

15. Maccioni F, Colaiacomo MC, Stasolla A, et al. Value of MRI performed with phased-array coil in the diagnosis and pre-operative classification of perianal and anal fistulas. Radiol Med 2002;104:58–67.

16. Tang LY, Rawsthorne P, Bernstein CN. Are perineal and luminal fistulas associated in Crohn's disease? A population-based study. Clin Gastroenterol Hepatol 2006;4:1130–4.

17. Haggett PJ, Moore NR, Shearman JD, et al. Pelvic and perineal complications of Crohn's disease: assessment using magnetic resonance imaging. Gut 1995;36: 407–10.

18. Lindsey I, Smilgin-Humphreys MM, Cunningham C, et al. A randomized, controlled trial of fibrin glue vs. conventional treatment for anal fistula. Dis Colon Rectum 2002;45:1608–15.

19. Orsoni P, Barthet M, Portier F, et al. Prospective comparison of endosonography, magnetic resonance imaging and surgical findings in anorectal fistula and abscess complicating Crohn's disease. Br J Surg 1999;86:360–4.

20. Buchanan GN, Halligan S, Bartram CI, et al. Clinical examination, endosonography, and MR imaging in preoperative assessment of fistula in ano: comparison with outcome-based reference standard. Radiology 2004;233:674–81.

21. Chapple KS, Spencer JA, Windsor AC, et al. Prognostic value of magnetic resonance imaging in the management of fistula-in-ano. Dis Colon Rectum 2000;43: 511–6.

22. deSouza NM, Hall AS, Puni R, et al. High resolution magnetic resonance imaging of the anal sphincter using a dedicated endoanal coil. Comparison of magnetic resonance imaging with surgical findings. Dis Colon Rectum 1996;39: 926–34.

23. Lunniss PJ, Barker PG, Sultan AH, et al. Magnetic resonance imaging of fistula-in-ano. Dis Colon Rectum 1994;37:708–18.

24. Schwartz DA, Wiersema MJ, Dudiak KM, et al. A comparison of endoscopic ultrasound, magnetic resonance imaging, and exam under anesthesia for evaluation of Crohn's perianal fistulas. Gastroenterology 2001;121:1064–72.

25. Regueiro M, Mardini H. Treatment of perianal fistulizing Crohn's disease with infliximab alone or as an adjunct to exam under anesthesia with seton placement. Inflamm Bowel Dis 2003;9:98–103.

26. Bezzio C, Bryant RV, Manes G, et al. New horizons in the imaging of perianal Crohn's disease: transperineal ultrasonography. Expert Rev Gastroenterol Hepatol 2017;11:523–30.

27. Sloots CE, Felt-Bersma RJ, Poen AC, et al. Assessment and classification of fistula-in-ano in patients with Crohn's disease by hydrogen peroxide enhanced transanal ultrasound. Int J Colorectal Dis 2001;16:292–7.

28. Frudinger A, Halligan S, Bartram CI, et al. Female anal sphincter: age-related differences in asymptomatic volunteers with high-frequency endoanal US. Radiology 2002;224:417–23.

29. Terracciano F, Scalisi G, Bossa F, et al. Transperineal ultrasonography: First level exam in IBD patients with perianal disease. Dig Liver Dis 2016;48:874–9.

30. Wedemeyer J, Kirchhoff T, Sellge G, et al. Transcutaneous perianal sonography: a sensitive method for the detection of perianal inflammatory lesions in Crohn's disease. World J Gastroenterol 2004;10:2859–63.

31. Maconi G, Tonolini M, Monteleone M, et al. Transperineal perineal ultrasound versus magnetic resonance imaging in the assessment of perianal Crohn's disease. Inflamm Bowel Dis 2013;19:2737–43.

32. West RL, Dwarkasing S, Felt-Bersma RJ, et al. Hydrogen peroxide-enhanced three-dimensional endoanal ultrasonography and endoanal magnetic resonance imaging in evaluating perianal fistulas: agreement and patient preference. Eur J Gastroenterol Hepatol 2004;16:1319–24.

33. Zawadzki A, Starck M, Bohe M, et al. A unique 3D endoanal ultrasound feature of perianal Crohn's fistula: the 'Crohn ultrasound fistula sign'. Colorectal Dis 2012;14:e608–11.

34. Ozturk E, Gulcu B. Laser ablation of fistula tract: a sphincter-preserving method for treating fistula-in-ano. Dis Colon Rectum 2014;57:360–4.

35. Siddiqui MR, Ashrafian H, Tozer P, et al. A diagnostic accuracy meta-analysis of endoanal ultrasound and MRI for perianal fistula assessment. Dis Colon Rectum 2012;55:576–85.

36. Maconi G, Greco MT, Asthana AK. Transperineal ultrasound for perianal fistulas and abscesses - a systematic review and meta-analysis. Ultraschall Med 2017; 38:265–72.

37. Chen CC, Wang SS, Lee FY, et al. Proinflammatory cytokines in early assessment of the prognosis of acute pancreatitis. Am J Gastroenterol 1999;94:213–8.

38. Lorentzen T, Nolsoe C, Skjoldbye B. Ultrasound-guided drainage of deep pelvic abscesses: experience with 33 cases. Ultrasound Med Biol 2011;37:723–8.

39. Domkundwar SV, Shinagare AB. Role of transcutaneous perianal ultrasonography in evaluation of fistulas in ano. J Ultrasound Med 2007;26:29–36.

40. Maconi G, Ardizzone S, Greco S, et al. Transperineal ultrasound in the detection of perianal and rectovaginal fistulae in Crohn's disease. Am J Gastroenterol 2007;102:2214–9.

41. Mallouhi A, Bonatti H, Peer S, et al. Detection and characterization of perianal inflammatory disease: accuracy of transperineal combined gray scale and color Doppler sonography. J Ultrasound Med 2004;23:19–27.

42. Zbar AP, Oyetunji RO, Gill R. Transperineal versus hydrogen peroxide-enhanced endoanal ultrasonography in never operated and recurrent crypto-genic fistula-in-ano: a pilot study. Tech Coloproctol 2006;10:297–302.
43. Giamundo P, Esercizio L, Geraci M, et al. Fistula-tract Laser Closure (FiLaC): long-term results and new operative strategies. Tech Coloproctol 2015;19: 449–53.
44. Giamundo P, Geraci M, Tibaldi L, et al. Closure of fistula-in-ano with laser–FiLaC: an effective novel sphincter-saving procedure for complex disease. Colorectal Dis 2014;16:110–5.
45. Wilhelm A. A new technique for sphincter-preserving anal fistula repair using a novel radial emitting laser probe. Tech Coloproctol 2011;15:445–9.
46. Terzi MC, Agalar C, Habip S, et al. Closing perianal fistulas using a laser: long-term results in 103 patients. Dis Colon Rectum 2018;61:599–603.
47. Wilhelm A, Fiebig A, Krawczak M. Five years of experience with the FiLaC laser for fistula-in-ano management: long-term follow-up from a single institution. Tech Coloproctol 2017;21:269–76.
48. Grimaud JC, Munoz-Bongrand N, Siproudhis L, et al. Fibrin glue is effective healing perianal fistulas in patients with Crohn's disease. Gastroenterology 2010;138:2275–81, 2281.e1.
49. Loungnarath R, Dietz DW, Mutch MG, et al. Fibrin glue treatment of complex anal fistulas has low success rate. Dis Colon Rectum 2004;47:432–6.
50. Cintron JR, Park JJ, Orsay CP, et al. Repair of fistulas-in-ano using autologous fibrin tissue adhesive. Dis Colon Rectum 1999;42:607–13.
51. Cintron JR, Park JJ, Orsay CP, et al. Repair of fistulas-in-ano using fibrin adhesive: long-term follow-up. Dis Colon Rectum 2000;43:944–9 [discussion: 949–50].
52. Park JJ, Cintron JR, Orsay CP, et al. Repair of chronic anorectal fistulae using commercial fibrin sealant. Arch Surg 2000;135:166–9.
53. Vitton V, Gasmi M, Barthet M, et al. Long-term healing of Crohn's anal fistulas with fibrin glue injection. Aliment Pharmacol Ther 2005;21:1453–7.
54. O'Connor L, Champagne BJ, Ferguson MA, et al. Efficacy of anal fistula plug in closure of Crohn's anorectal fistulas. Dis Colon Rectum 2006;49:1569–73.
55. Badylak S, Kokini K, Tullius B, et al. Morphologic study of small intestinal submu-cosa as a body wall repair device. J Surg Res 2002;103:190–202.
56. Senejoux A, Siproudhis L, Abramowitz L, et al. Fistula plug in fistulising ano-perineal Crohn's disease: a randomised controlled trial. J Crohns Colitis 2016; 10:141–8.
57. Garg P, Song J, Bhatia A, et al. The efficacy of anal fistula plug in fistula-in-ano: a systematic review. Colorectal Dis 2010;12:965–70.
58. Nasseri Y, Cassella L, Berns M, et al. The anal fistula plug in Crohn's disease patients with fistula-in-ano: a systematic review. Colorectal Dis 2016;18:351–6.
59. Chung W, Ko D, Sun C, et al. Outcomes of anal fistula surgery in patients with inflammatory bowel disease. Am J Surg 2010;199:609–13.
60. Gonsalves S, Sagar P, Lengyel J, et al. Assessment of the efficacy of the recto-vaginal button fistula plug for the treatment of ileal pouch-vaginal and rectova-ginal fistulas. Dis Colon Rectum 2009;52:1877–81.
61. Ellis CN. Outcomes after repair of rectovaginal fistulas using bioprosthetics. Dis Colon Rectum 2008;51:1084–8.
62. O'Riordan JM, Datta I, Johnston C, et al. A systematic review of the anal fistula plug for patients with Crohn's and non-Crohn's related fistula-in-ano. Dis Colon Rectum 2012;55:351–8.

63. Kochhar G, Shen B. Endoscopic fistulotomy in inflammatory bowel disease (with video). Gastrointest Endosc 2018;88:87–94.
64. Shen B. Exploring endoscopic therapy for the treatment of Crohn's disease-related fistula and abscess. Gastrointest Endosc 2017;85:1133–43.
65. Shen B, Kochhar G, Navaneethan U, et al. Role of interventional inflammatory bowel disease in the era of biological therapy: a position statement from the Global Interventional IBD Group. Gastrointest Endosc 2018;89(2):215–37.
66. Present DH, Rutgeerts P, Targan S, et al. Infliximab for the treatment of fistulas in patients with Crohn's disease. N Engl J Med 1999;340:1398–405.
67. Sands BE, Anderson FH, Bernstein CN, et al. Infliximab maintenance therapy for fistulizing Crohn's disease. N Engl J Med 2004;350:876–85.
68. Asteria CR, Ficari F, Bagnoli S, et al. Treatment of perianal fistulas in Crohn's disease by local injection of antibody to TNF-alpha accounts for a favourable clinical response in selected cases: a pilot study. Scand J Gastroenterol 2006;41: 1064–72.
69. Alessandroni L, Kohn A, Cosintino R, et al. Local injection of infliximab in severe fistulating perianal Crohn's disease: an open uncontrolled study. Tech Coloproctol 2011;15:407–12.
70. Adegbola SO, Sahnan K, Tozer PJ, et al. Review of local injection of anti-TNF for perianal fistulising Crohn's disease. Int J Colorectal Dis 2017;32:1539–44.
71. Gorgulu S, Yagci G, Kaymakcioglu N, et al. Hyperbaric oxygen enhances the efficiency of 5-aminosalicylic acid in acetic acid-induced colitis in rats. Dig Dis Sci 2006;51:480–7.
72. Vavricka SR, Rogler G, Biedermann L. High altitude journeys, flights and hypoxia: any role for disease flares in IBD patients? Dig Dis 2016;34:78–83.
73. Rossignol DA. Hyperbaric oxygen treatment for inflammatory bowel disease: a systematic review and analysis. Med Gas Res 2012;2:6.
74. Dulai PS, Buckey JC Jr, Raffals LE, et al. Hyperbaric oxygen therapy is well tolerated and effective for ulcerative colitis patients hospitalized for moderate-severe flares: a phase 2A pilot multi-center, randomized, double-blind, sham-controlled trial. Am J Gastroenterol 2018;113(10):1516–23.
75. Bekheit M, Baddour N, Katri K, et al. Hyperbaric oxygen therapy stimulates colonic stem cells and induces mucosal healing in patients with refractory ulcerative colitis: a prospective case series. BMJ Open Gastroenterol 2016;3: e000082.
76. Iezzi LE, Feitosa MR, Medeiros BA, et al. Crohn's disease and hyperbaric oxygen therapy. Acta Cir Bras 2011;26(Suppl 2):129–32.
77. Kranke P, Bennett MH, Martyn-St James M, et al. Hyperbaric oxygen therapy for chronic wounds. Cochrane Database Syst Rev 2012;(4):CD004123.
78. Brady CE 3rd, Cooley BJ, Davis JC. Healing of severe perineal and cutaneous Crohn's disease with hyperbaric oxygen. Gastroenterology 1989;97:756–60.
79. Colombel JF, Mathieu D, Bouault JM, et al. Hyperbaric oxygenation in severe perineal Crohn's disease. Dis Colon Rectum 1995;38:609–14.
80. Lavy A, Weisz G, Adir Y, et al. Hyperbaric oxygen for perianal Crohn's disease. J Clin Gastroenterol 1994;19:202–5.
81. Agrawal G, Borody T, Turner R, et al. Combining infliximab, anti-MAP and hyperbaric oxygen therapy for resistant fistulizing Crohn's disease. Future Sci OA 2015;1:Fso77.
82. Dulai PS, Gleeson MW, Taylor D, et al. Systematic review: the safety and efficacy of hyperbaric oxygen therapy for inflammatory bowel disease. Aliment Pharmacol Ther 2014;39:1266–75.

83. Grim PS, Gottlieb LJ, Boddie A, et al. Hyperbaric oxygen therapy. JAMA 1990; 263:2216–20.

84. Noyer CM, Brandt LJ. Hyperbaric oxygen therapy for perineal Crohn's disease. Am J Gastroenterol 1999;94:318–21.

85. Palmquist BM, Philipson B, Barr PO. Nuclear cataract and myopia during hyperbaric oxygen therapy. Br J Ophthalmol 1984;68:113–7.

86. Drakos PE, Nagler A, Or R. Case of Crohn's disease in bone marrow transplantation. Am J Hematol 1993;43:157–8.

87. Kashyap A, Forman SJ. Autologous bone marrow transplantation for non-Hodgkin's lymphoma resulting in long-term remission of coincidental Crohn's disease. Br J Haematol 1998;103:651–2.

88. Bernardo ME, Locatelli F, Fibbe WE. Mesenchymal stromal cells. Ann N Y Acad Sci 2009;1176:101–17.

89. Nauta AJ, Fibbe WE. Immunomodulatory properties of mesenchymal stromal cells. Blood 2007;110:3499–506.

90. Gonzalez-Rey E, Anderson P, Gonzalez MA, et al. Human adult stem cells derived from adipose tissue protect against experimental colitis and sepsis. Gut 2009;58:929–39.

91. Panes J, Ordas I, Ricart E. Stem cell treatment for Crohn's disease. Expert Rev Clin Immunol 2010;6:597–605.

92. Garcia-Olmo D, Garcia-Arranz M, Garcia LG, et al. Autologous stem cell transplantation for treatment of rectovaginal fistula in perianal Crohn's disease: a new cell-based therapy. Int J Colorectal Dis 2003;18:451–4.

93. Garcia-Olmo D, Garcia-Arranz M, Herreros D, et al. A phase I clinical trial of the treatment of Crohn's fistula by adipose mesenchymal stem cell transplantation. Dis Colon Rectum 2005;48:1416–23.

94. Ciccocioppo R, Bernardo ME, Sgarella A, et al. Autologous bone marrow-derived mesenchymal stromal cells in the treatment of fistulising Crohn's disease. Gut 2011;60:788–98.

95. Garcia-Olmo D, Herreros D, Pascual I, et al. Expanded adipose-derived stem cells for the treatment of complex perianal fistula: a phase II clinical trial. Dis Colon Rectum 2009;52:79–86.

96. Guadalajara H, Herreros D, De-La-Quintana P, et al. Long-term follow-up of patients undergoing adipose-derived adult stem cell administration to treat complex perianal fistulas. Int J Colorectal Dis 2012;27:595–600.

97. de la Portilla F, Alba F, Garcia-Olmo D, et al. Expanded allogeneic adipose-derived stem cells (eASCs) for the treatment of complex perianal fistula in Crohn's disease: results from a multicenter phase I/IIa clinical trial. Int J Colorectal Dis 2013;28:313–23.

98. Molendijk I, Bonsing BA, Roelofs H, et al. Allogeneic bone marrow-derived mesenchymal stromal cells promote healing of refractory perianal fistulas in patients with Crohn's disease. Gastroenterology 2015;149:918–27.e6.

99. Panes J, Garcia-Olmo D, Van Assche G, et al. Expanded allogeneic adipose-derived mesenchymal stem cells (Cx601) for complex perianal fistulas in Crohn's disease: a phase 3 randomised, double-blind controlled trial. Lancet 2016;388:1281–90.

100. Zalieckas JM. Treatment of perianal Crohn's disease. Semin Pediatr Surg 2017; 26:391–7.

101. Lightner AL, Wang Z, Zubair AC, et al. A systematic review and meta-analysis of mesenchymal stem cell injections for the treatment of perianal Crohn's disease: progress made and future directions. Dis Colon Rectum 2018;61:629–40.

102. Herreros MD, Garcia-Arranz M, Guadalajara H, et al. Autologous expanded adipose-derived stem cells for the treatment of complex cryptoglandular perianal fistulas: a phase III randomized clinical trial (FATT 1: fistula advanced therapy trial 1) and long-term evaluation. Dis Colon Rectum 2012;55:762–72.

103. Dietz AB, Dozois EJ, Fletcher JG, et al. Autologous mesenchymal stem cells, applied in a bioabsorbable matrix, for treatment of perianal fistulas in patients with Crohn's disease. Gastroenterology 2017;153:59–62.e2.

104. Wainstein C, Quera R, Fluxa D, et al. Stem cell therapy in refractory perineal Crohn's disease: long-term follow-up. Colorectal Dis 2018. [Epub ahead of print]. https://doi.org/10.1111/codi.14002.

105. Al-Maawali AK, Nguyen P, Phang PT. Modern treatments and stem cell therapies for perianal Crohn's fistulas. Can J Gastroenterol Hepatol 2016;2016:1651570.

Management of Inflammatory Bowel Disease–Associated Dysplasia in the Modern Era

Shailja C. Shah, MD[a], Steven H. Itzkowitz, MD[b],*

KEYWORDS

- Cancer early detection • Colorectal neoplasm
- Diagnostic techniques and procedures • Epidemiology • Prevention and control

KEY POINTS

- The optimal management of IBD-associated colorectal neoplasia is one that is individualized and considers patient-, disease-, and endoscopy-specific factors, in conjunction with the expertise of the treating gastroenterologists and advanced endoscopists.
- Although investigators continue to work in parallel for ways to definitively identify who will develop neoplastic complications of IBD and for ways to prevent the development of neoplasia from the outset (apart from simply controlling inflammation), we are at least in a dynamic era of expanding therapeutic endoscopic options for IBD-associated neoplasia when diagnosed.
- Hand-in-hand is an expanding body of literature on outcomes of nonoperative management of IBD-associated neoplasia to guide appropriate determination of patient and lesion candidacy for endoscopic resection and ongoing surveillance, as opposed to surgical management.
- However, with increasing access and availability of new technologies and techniques, clinicians need to take care to balance cost and resource utilization, and first and foremost ensure shared decision-making and appropriate counseling of risks versus benefits of endoscopic versus surgical management of IBD-associated neoplasia.

INTRODUCTION

Colorectal dysplasia and colorectal cancer (CRC) are among the most worrisome complications of inflammatory bowel disease (IBD) that affects the colon.[1–4] Although the incidence of colorectal neoplasia (CRN) in the IBD population seems

[a] Division of Gastroenterology, Hepatology and Nutrition, Department of Medicine, Vanderbilt University Medical Center, 2215 Garland Ave, Medical Building IV, Room 1030-C (mail), Nashville, TN 37232, USA; [b] Division of Gastroenterology, Department of Medicine, Icahn School of Medicine at Mount Sinai, Mount Sinai Hospital, 1468 Madison Avenue, Annenberg Building, Room 5-12, Box 1069, New York, NY, USA
* Corresponding author.
E-mail address: steven.itzkowitz@mountsinai.org

Gastrointest Endoscopy Clin N Am 29 (2019) 531–548
https://doi.org/10.1016/j.giec.2019.02.008
1052-5157/19/© 2019 Elsevier Inc. All rights reserved.

to be decreasing,[5,6] there is still an estimated two-fold higher risk of CRC compared with non-IBD populations in referral-based and population-based studies.[6] Higher rates depend on disease-related factors, including cumulative inflammatory burden and extent of disease, and patient-level risk factors, such as concomitant primary sclerosing cholangitis (PSC) and family history of CRC.[6–11] A recent meta-analysis reported a 2.6% and 6.6% cumulative risk of CRC at 10 to 20 years and more than 20 years of IBD duration, respectively, with 21% cumulative incidence after 20 years of extensive disease.[6]

In IBD, CRC develops from a progression that begins with inflammation followed, in some, by development of varying degrees of dysplasia before final malignant transformation to cancer. Despite considerable progress in the understanding of IBD pathogenesis and management, there is still no definitive way to predict who will develop neoplastic complications. Although extensive efforts have been invested in identifying noninvasive biomarkers to risk stratify patients and better predict who will most benefit from tight surveillance and more aggressive management, no molecular or genetic biomarkers have been identified that are reliably sufficient for clinical practice. Instead, risk stratification still hinges on clinical factors, such as PSC, prior dysplasia, and endoscopic and histologic disease activity, among others. Likewise, no chemopreventive agents have proven effective. Thus, CRC prevention relies on risk-reduction strategies that include enrollment in a CRN colonoscopic surveillance program, smoking cessation, and adherence to medical therapy to achieve deep remission. Adherence to routine surveillance colonoscopy, despite its limitations, cost, inconvenience for patients, and minimal but measurable procedural risk, remains the most effective way to diagnose, prevent, and in certain circumstances resect CRN, with continued surveillance thereafter.[12,13] The primary goal of dysplasia surveillance is the identification of early neoplasia with implementation of an appropriate treatment strategy if diagnosed. This has been consistently associated with reduced CRC-related mortality.[13–17] Years ago, dysplasia in the setting of IBD colitis was managed surgically with either colectomy or sometimes segmental resection in the case of limited Crohn's colitis. Such an aggressive approach is now less common, presumably because of enhanced endoscopic technology for dysplasia detection, and the ability to successfully manage IBD-associated dysplasia endoscopically, not to mention improved medical therapies to achieve disease remission.

This article first provides a brief overview of risk factors for CRN in IBD to concretize the approach to risk stratification, and then provides an up-to-date review of the diagnosis and management of dysplasia in IBD, which integrates new and emerging data in the field. This is particularly relevant in an era of increased attention to cost- and resource-containment from the health systems vantage point, coupled with a heightened prioritization of patient quality of life and shared decision-making. It ends with a brief discussion of the status of newer therapeutic techniques, namely, endoscopic submucosal dissection (ESD).

The most important takeaway point is that the decision to enter into a dysplasia surveillance program, as opposed to performing colectomy once dysplasia is detected, must be a joint decision between the patient and gastroenterologist that is informed by patient- and disease-specific factors. A successful surveillance program depends on open communication between both parties with routine office visits, colonoscopies, and most importantly, patient adherence with medical therapy and surveillance examinations.

RISK FACTORS FOR INFLAMMATORY BOWEL DISEASE–ASSOCIATED DYSPLASIA AND CANCER

The endoscopic and histologic characteristics of CRN, when diagnosed, are primary drivers for deciding therapeutic management. That said, it is important to adjunctively consider patient- and disease-specific factors, particularly when the decision between endoscopic resection versus surgery is not clear-cut. Generally speaking, risk factors for CRN in IBD are well-established and supported by increasingly robust epidemiologic literature (**Table 1**), although some discrepancies, such as male sex as a risk factor, do exist.[8,18,19] Disease-specific risk factors include disease duration, extent, and degree of inflammation, whereas patient-specific factors include concomitant PSC, prior history of CRN, family history of CRC in a first-degree relative, and possibly earlier age of disease onset.[20] Relative and absolute risks of each of these factors vary and most numbers are based on older data before the significant increase in use of biologic therapy and enhanced dysplasia detection techniques. Comparison across studies is also challenging because of heterogeneous populations and data sources, study designs and inclusion criteria, and unclear true population-prevalence of some risk factors, such as PSC.[21] Nonetheless, disease extent and duration, and concomitant PSC seem to confer the highest and most consistent disease-related risks for developing dysplasia or CRC in IBD. Pancolitis is associated with relative risk (RR) of 14.8 (95% confidence interval [CI], 11.4–18.9) compared with RR of 2.8 (95% CI, 1.6–4.4) in left-sided colitis and no increased risk with proctitis. PSC is associated with RR of 4.8 (95% CI, 3.9–6.4) starting at the time of diagnosis, but might even be higher. In PSC, lesions tend to be right-sided and risk of progression of low-grade dysplasia (LGD) to high-grade dysplasia (HGD) or CRC is nearly three-fold higher in patients with IBD colitis and concomitant PSC (8.4 per 100 patient-years) compared with those without PSC (2.0 per 100 patient-years; $P = .01$).[22] If there is a prior history of LGD, those with IBD and PSC have an even greater risk of subsequent advanced CRN, with one recent multicenter study estimating the rate of advanced CRN following an LGD diagnosis to be 2.8 times higher in patients with versus without PSC.[8] Ulcerative colitis (UC) disease duration of 10 years is associated with RR of 2.4 (95% CI, 0.6–6.0), whereas disease duration of 20 years is associated with RR of 2.8 (95% CI, 1.91–3.97) for developing colonic neoplasia, although estimates vary.[6,20] Active endoscopic (RR, 5.1; 95% CI, 2.7–11.1) or histologic (RR, 3.0; 95% CI, 1.4–6.3) disease also impacts risk of progression to CRN.[8,11] Having a first-degree relative with CRC younger than 50 years old confers an RR of 9.2 (95% CI, 3.7–23.0) compared with RR of 2.5 (95% CI, 1.4–4.4) if the first-degree relative is older than 50 years old.[20,23] Earlier age of IBD as a risk factor for CRC in IBD is

Table 1 Risk factors for IBD-associated colorectal neoplasia		
Patient-Specific Factors	**Disease-Specific Factors**	**Endoscopic Features**
Primary sclerosing cholangitis History of colorectal neoplasia Family history of colorectal cancer in first-degree relative Smoking (±) Early age of disease onset (±) Male sex	Disease duration Disease extent Cumulative inflammatory burden Active inflammation endoscopically or histologically	Stricture (ulcerative colitis, longer disease duration, proximal location, symptoms) Shortened tubular colon Pseudopolyps

See text for full details.

unsettled and there is likely at least some contribution of the non-IBD-related background risk of sporadic CRC after age 40 to 50 years.[3,24–27]

Structural alterations arising as a consequence of chronic inflammation, such as stricture, pseudopolyps, and shortened tubular colon, have long been considered important risk factors for CRC.[20,28–32] The literature regarding strictures in IBD and CRC risk is mixed, and it is likely that the neoplastic implications vary according to IBD type, symptoms, disease duration, and colonic location, with strictures in long-standing UC that are right-sided and symptomatic being the most concerning for harboring neoplasia (**Table 1**).[33] Earlier studies suggested that the risk of dysplasia or cancer associated with strictures ranged from 0% to 86%, with up to 40% of strictures themselves harboring cancer[28,29,33,34]; however, these studies were limited by small sample size and lack of detailed clinical and histologic details. A more recent study of 293 patients with colonic strictures (median disease duration at stricture diagnosis, 6–8 years) undergoing surgery for nonneoplastic diagnosis reported that 3.5% of strictures harbored previously undiagnosed neoplasia within the surgically resected stricture. As comparison, in one center included in this study, intrastricture neoplasia was the surgical indication in 0.6% of Crohn's disease (CD) colonic strictures and 2.5% of UC colonic strictures.[34] Among colonic strictures without diagnosed neoplasia preoperatively, those with underlying UC/IBD-U (n = 45) had LGD in 2%, HGD in 2%, and CRC in 5%, whereas those with CD (n = 245) had LGD in 1%, HGD in 0.4%, and CRC in 0.8%.[34] The only factor associated with neoplasia at the stricture site was lack of active disease at the time of surgery (odds ratio, 4.9; 1.1–21.3). This and other studies highlight that diagnosing neoplasia on stricture biopsies is imperfect, and there is still a measurable risk of neoplasia within the stricture.[35] The risk of malignant transformation from dysplasia to CRC in strictures is not known, but is generally thought to be low.[35] Risk factors for progression are similarly not well-described, but older age, right-sided location, change in stricture length or diameter over time, appearance of stricture later in the disease course, or symptoms (eg, obstruction, pain) should be considered higher risk and resection seriously considered.[33] In the absence of symptoms or high-risk personal or disease-related factors, nonneoplastic strictures particularly in patients with CD likely are safely managed with surveillance colonoscopy as long as the stricture is passable and the mucosal surface proximally and within the stricture itself can be comprehensively interrogated endoscopically and histologically.

Pseudopolyps, however, are probably not the high-risk factor that older literature had suggested, based on emerging data stemming from large cohort studies with more rigorous study designs and analyses that specifically control for inflammatory burden.[31] Rather, they should be considered a surrogate marker of more significant cumulative inflammatory burden, which is the driving risk factor. One study reported a low risk of neoplastic transformation of pseudopolyps,[31] supporting the current practice of not endoscopically removing pseudopolyps unless there is diagnostic uncertainty or other concerning features (eg, abnormal pit pattern by enhanced imaging techniques). So long as the mucosal surface is adequately visualized for neoplasia surveillance, pseudopolyps alone need not be considered a reason for shortened surveillance intervals, as some societal guidelines suggest.[36] If quality of surveillance is compromised because of impaired visualization from multiple pseudopolyps, colectomy should be considered.[20] Given the measurable risk of metachronous or synchronous neoplasia, the presence of several of the previously mentioned factors should lower threshold to recommend definitive total proctocolectomy when dysplasia that is otherwise resectable is diagnosed (discussed below).

PATHOPHYSIOLOGY OF COLORECTAL CANCER

The pathophysiology of CRC in IBD is distinct from sporadic CRC, although sporadic CRC can certainly occur in cases of IBD colitis. These differences are reflected in different molecular and phenotypic features. Generally speaking, the development of CRC in IBD colitis is thought to follow the inflammation-dysplasia-carcinoma sequence that is seen in other (luminal and nonluminal) gastrointestinal (GI) cancers, with cancers occurring in areas of active or prior inflammation and influenced by immune and inflammatory pathways.[20] At least in UC (and perhaps segmental Crohn's colitis), chronic inflammation of the colon creates a "field effect," whereby any part of the colon that is currently, or was previously, inflamed is at risk for neoplastic transformation,[11,28] thus justifying continued surveillance. Alterations in the microenvironment with dysregulated chemokine and cytokine pathways lead to direct DNA damage, immortalization of cells through proliferation, growth, and inhibited apoptosis; and also migration potential. Differences in the molecular and genetic features between IBD-associated and sporadic CRC have been described for decades. For example, IBD-associated CRCs less often have *APC* and *KRAS* mutations and more often have *TP53*, *IDH1*, and *MYC* mutations compared with sporadic tumors.[37,38] Additionally, although primary carcinogenic pathways appear conserved (eg, chromosomal instability and microsatellite instability), the timing and sequence of some pathways might be distinct (eg, early loss of *p53* in IBD-associated CRC).[39,40] To date, none of these differences have yet been successfully leveraged for personalization of therapeutic or surveillance options.

DYSPLASIA DIAGNOSIS AND SURVEILLANCE TECHNIQUE

Currently, there is no molecular biomarker or panel of biomarkers with adequate test characteristics for neoplasia surveillance and diagnosis in IBD, although some stool-based surveillance tests show preliminary promise in discriminating between IBD neoplasia and lack thereof.[41–43] Accordingly, neoplasia diagnosis still relies on a careful colonoscopic examination that meets adequate quality metrics. The interval for surveillance varies according to the GI society, with some recommending specific intervals based on risk stratification (high-, intermediate-, low-risk according to patient- and disease-related clinical characteristics),[36,44] whereas others (eg, the US societies) offer a nonstratified approach. A more comprehensive discussion of surveillance intervals in the absence of a neoplasia diagnosis is outside of the scope of this review, which is focused on the management of neoplasia once diagnosed.

A careful colonoscopic surveillance examination that meets adequate quality metrics and adheres to guideline recommendations[36,44–48] remains the gold standard for diagnosing early neoplasia and the only way to decrease CRC-related mortality. Quality metrics for colonoscopic surveillance in IBD mirror CRC screening/surveillance recommendations for the most part, with some nuances.[47] It is recommended that surveillance examinations be performed by a gastroenterologist experienced in IBD management, preferably at an IBD center, and when disease is in remission and the colon adequately prepped. Cecal (or neoterminal ileum) intubation is imperative, as is sufficient duration of withdrawal time. Active disease should not preclude performing the surveillance examination, but the extent and severity of disease activity should be clearly documented (especially if there are visible lesions) and the pathologist should be informed. Once medically optimized, consideration should be given to performing a repeat short-interval surveillance examination if in fact active inflammation made it difficult to discern neoplastic lesions. Even in quiescent disease, luminal abnormalities, such as pseudopolyps and scars, may compromise the dysplasia surveillance examination. If this is the case, or if there is an impassable stricture that precludes more proximal interrogation, colectomy should be discussed. Unfortunately, there is marked practice pattern variability and surprisingly low rates of adherence to recommended surveillance techniques.[49–52] Although multifactorial, this might explain, at least in part, why the rate of early or missed CRC following colonoscopy is 15% to 30% in patients with IBD, three- to six-fold higher than the general non-IBD population.[53,54]

Standard of care for surveillance includes high-definition white light colonoscopy (HD-WLE) with two to four nontargeted random biopsies taken every 10 cm from the cecum to the rectum (minimum of 32 biopsies), placed in separate jars, along with targeted biopsies as appropriate. For any lesion identified, biopsies should be taken from the surrounding "normal"-appearing mucosa and placed in a separate jar to evaluate for invisible dysplasia or inflammation. Nontargeted and targeted biopsies have been the recommended technique for decades and reflects an era when dysplasia was difficult to identify endoscopically with the unassisted eye, caused in large part by lower resolution optics. The therapeutic armamentarium was also more restricted in the pre-biologics era and, because mucosal healing was more difficult to achieve, the distinction between inflammation and dysplasia was often challenging.

Standard definition WLE is no longer acceptable for surveillance.[47,55] Over the past two decades, new technologies and image-enhancing techniques have emerged that collectively have greatly improved dysplasia detection. Most neoplasia is now accepted to be visible neoplasia.[56–58] Indeed, hand-in-hand with, and as a direct result of, these technological advancements, there has a been a paradigm shift in the definitions and classifications of dysplasia, which is now functionally described as "visible versus invisible" and "resectable versus nonresectable" in its most minimalistic form.

The main image-enhancing technique is dye chromoendoscopy (CE) with indigo carmine or methylene blue, which similarly necessitates adequate mucosal visualization (eg, adequate bowel preparation, minimal pseudopolyps) and endoscopically quiescent disease. CE is recommended by the Surveillance for Colorectal Endoscopic Neoplasia Detection and Management in IBD Patients: International Consensus (SCENIC) and is also considered standard of care for surveillance in IBD. However, the role of CE in the era of HD-WLE is unsettled and controversial, particularly because the procedural time for CE is often longer and superiority over HD-WLE not established.[59] Current evidence suggests that both HD-WLE and CE techniques are comparable, although CE might detect nonstatistically significantly more dysplasia versus HD-WLE.[47,55] A recent meta-analysis[60] of three RCTs and three observational studies, which included 1358 patients with IBD undergoing surveillance (670 CE, 688 HD-WLE) found that more dysplasia was found on CE versus HD-WLE (18.8% vs 9%; $P = .08$); a similar trend was reported on sensitivity analyses of just the three RCTs (242 CE, 151 HD-WLE; 12.4% vs 10.4%), and also parallels the findings of the SCENIC consensus.[47] There remain several unanswered questions regarding the optimal positioning of CE for surveillance from a practical and cost/resource utilization vantage point, including whether or not nontargeted biopsies are still beneficial, particularly given the additional cost implications. Despite high-definition colonoscopy, CE, and other enhanced detection modalities, 10% of dysplasia is still diagnosed on random biopsy and may relate to the less-experienced eye or suboptimal surveillance milieu. Data support random biopsies in CE for those at highest risk, including patients with PSC, personal history of neoplasia, or tubular-appearing colon (sign of cumulative inflammatory burden).[56] Updated surveillance guidelines should take into consideration

CE versus HD-WLE data, but further investigations are needed to identify which subgroups might benefit most from CE versus HD-WLE.

So-called virtual CE might bypass some of the shortcomings of CE, specifically those related to procedural time and cost. Virtual CE is an adjunct to HD-WLE and provides instant on-demand mucosal contrast enhancement without needing to spray dye as in CE. Some options include Fuji Intelligent Chromo Endoscopy (FICE, Fujinon, Wayne, NJ, USA) and iSCAN (Pentax, Pentax of America, Montvale, NJ, USA). Narrow band imaging has also been evaluated, but this does not increase the yield of dysplasia detection and is thus not currently recommended.[35,47,61,62] Virtual CE is a rapidly evolving and exciting area; however, data are still emerging and its role in CRC surveillance in IBD is not yet established. Furthermore, these technologies are not universally available in the United States. We certainly look forward to more data and head-to-head trials, especially because several of these technologies and others in the pipeline have the resolution and magnification to optically diagnose dysplasia without the need for biopsies.

DEFINITIONS OF DYSPLASIA AND CATEGORIZATION

The appropriate management of IBD-associated dysplasia is predicated on consistent definitions. The nomenclature and terminology used to describe dysplasia has transformed in parallel with improved endoscopic optics and CE. Terms such as dysplasia-associated lesion or mass and adenoma-associated lesion or mass, both of which are now obsolete, flat versus raised dysplasia, among others, are a source of confusion given their inconsistent definitions between the IBD and general endoscopy literature, and also within the IBD literature alone. For example, in the IBD literature, a "flat" lesion was historically used to describe any lesion not seen grossly, whereas in the general endoscopy literature a "flat" lesion refers to a slightly raised lesion (ie, less than 2.5 mm in height).[63]

To address this confusion and move toward standardization and simplification of nomenclature, the SCENIC consensus statement recommended broad categorization of dysplasia as "visible" (dysplastic lesion seen on endoscopy) versus "invisible" (dysplasia diagnosed histologically from random biopsies without an associated discrete lesion). Although most dysplasia is visible dysplasia in the modern era of HD-WLE and CE, an estimated 10% of dysplasia is invisible and is reflected in the iterative recommendation that segmental random biopsies still be performed even if CE is used, and targeted biopsies and biopsies from the mucosa surrounding a lesion be taken. It is likely that these recommendations may change as more contemporary data accumulate regarding the actual yield of biopsies from mucosa that appears grossly normal on HD-WLE. For example, a recent single-center study reported that among 302 polypoid lesions biopsied or resected from 131 patients with IBD in whom lesion-adjacent biopsies were obtained, the yield for invisible dysplasia was 0%.[64]

The newer nomenclature for visible dysplasia proposed by the SCENIC group is based on the Paris classification,[63] which has therapeutic and prognostic implications. At a minimum, descriptors of lesions should include size, morphology (polypoid vs nonpolypoid), border (distinct vs indistinct), and features that might be concerning for submucosal invasion and malignancy (eg, depression, ulceration, nonlifting of lesion with submucosal injection).[47] CE is an adjunct to HD-WLE that might better delineate lesion border. Polypoid lesions (pedunculated, sessile) are defined as those protruding at least 2.5 mm into the lumen, whereas nonpolypoid lesions (slightly elevated, flat, depressed) may range from superficially elevated (less than 2.5 mm) lesions to depressed lesions.[63] Gross and histologic characteristics of the surrounding mucosa should be noted. Appropriate reporting of these descriptors is critical for deciding whether lesions are amenable to endoscopic resection and, when endoscopic resection is performed, the likelihood that resection will be complete with low to negligible risk of recurrence at the site.

MANAGEMENT OF VISIBLE DYSPLASIA: ENDOSCOPIC VERSUS SURGICAL RESECTION

The management of visible dysplasia is multimodal and encompasses therapeutic resection (endoscopic vs surgical), ongoing medical management to achieve/maintain disease quiescence, risk factor modification where appropriate (eg, smoking cessation), and continued close interval colonoscopic surveillance in the absence of total proctocolectomy. Criteria for what constitutes endoscopically resectable lesions are not clearly delineated in published guidelines and depend largely on the comfort level and expertise of the individual endoscopist. Endoscopic resection includes endoscopic mucosal resection and ESD, although the latter is not yet a viable option in the United States (discussed later). The goal of endoscopic resection is en bloc resection, with negative lateral and vertical margins. If this cannot be reliably achieved or is not confirmed following endoscopic resection, then surgery is indicated. Compared with patients without IBD, en bloc resection is uniquely challenging because recurrent cycles of inflammation and healing increase the likelihood of submucosal fibrosis, and, consequently, higher risk of incomplete resection and complications such as perforation, bleeding, recurrence. Because ESD dissects through the submucosal plane, it is tempting as an option that allows full en bloc resection of dysplastic lesions in carefully selected patients with IBD. CD might present additional challenges for endoscopic resection because of the potential for transmural involvement and more frequent fibrosis.[65]

Patient Selection: Patient Preference and Lesion Characteristics

First and foremost, the decision of endoscopic resection versus surgical resection must follow a comprehensive and realistic discussion with the patient that specifically includes discussion of (1) risks of endoscopic resection, (2) risk of incomplete resection and need for surgery anyway, (3) risk of missed synchronous lesion, and (4) ongoing need for continued aggressive colonoscopic surveillance (± future therapeutic intervention) because of a high risk of metachronous lesions. This latter point is an important nuance for IBD dysplasia compared with sporadic polyps/neoplasia in patients without IBD, and needs to be highlighted for its potential cost and patient convenience/quality of life implications. If the patient does not accept these risks or is unable to commit to continued surveillance, then she or he should be referred for surgery. Patients with PSC, history of CRC, severe pseudopolyposis or stricture limiting adequate quality surveillance, multifocal dysplasia (some exceptions), or first-degree relative with early CRC should be referred for surgery. Although early CRC without submucosal invasion (T1) arising in patients without IBD is increasingly being removed by ESD in experienced centers, particularly in the East, the data for patients with IBD are limited[66–68] and is not recommended in the United States.

Generally speaking, the assessment of endoscopic resectability of visible lesions should follow the same considerations in patients with IBD as in patients without IBD, with some additional key considerations. Well-demarcated, nonmultifocal lesions without features suggestive of invasion should be completely resected by an endoscopist with appropriate expertise regardless of grade of dysplasia. The absence of dysplasia in the surrounding mucosa must be ruled out before endoscopic resection. If dysplasia is identified, the lesion is considered unresectable and the patient should be referred for surgery. Ideally, the surrounding mucosa should be endoscopically/histologically quiescent, although the impact of active inflammation on outcomes of endoscopic resection in this population is not quantified. The activity of the surrounding mucosa might also impact the assessment for submucosal invasion, because areas of active inflammation might have a positive nonlifting sign and overlying ulceration. In patients without IBD, lesions with depression, ulcerations, irregular contours, deformity, mass-like appearance, or nonlifting sign raise concern for the presence of invasive malignancy. But, these features are more difficult to assess in patients with IBD particularly in the face of active disease, and thus do not necessarily carry the same tenacious association with malignant transformation. Whether the lesion was found in a background of quiescent disease, active colitis, or other mucosal abnormalities such pseudopolyposis should be noted in the procedure report.

For well-demarcated lesions distinction should be made between polypoid and nonpolypoid lesions, not only because methods for endoscopic resection and postresection surveillance vary, but because the risk of progression to cancer is higher in the latter.[69,70] Whether the more benign course of polypoid lesions reflects the underlying biology of the lesions, or that polypoid lesions are generally more amenable to en bloc removal with less risk of piecemeal and incomplete resection, remains to be clarified, but it is likely a combination of these factors. Although a larger proportion of nonpolypoid lesions are being detected as a result of improved technology, this may also represent a true shift in natural history of dysplasia in IBD.

Polypoid, well-circumscribed lesions, in principle, should be amenable to en bloc resection by standard snare polypectomy or mucosectomy. The mucosa surrounding the polyp should be biopsied and a tattoo should be placed one to two folds distal to the resection site. Although there is no set size threshold for endoscopic resection of polypoid lesions, 1 to 2 cm is often cited for purposes of guiding subsequent surveillance recommendations and reflects the threshold above which piecemeal resection is often needed. If both the resection margins from the lesion and the surrounding mucosa are negative and no additional dysplasia is detected in the colon, then continued endoscopic surveillance according to a modified schedule may be adequate. For lesions removed piecemeal or lesions greater than 1 cm, there is a significantly higher risk of retained neoplastic tissue and recurrence. Thus, SCENIC recommendations are that surveillance colonoscopy should be performed within 3 to 6 months (earlier threshold if endoscopist-specific concerns) with biopsies at the site of the resection and, if negative, annual surveillance with adherence to quality metrics continued thereafter. For patients with en bloc resection of polypoid lesions less than 1 cm and confirmed negative margins, surveillance colonoscopy is recommended at 12 months.[47] If incomplete resection or recurrence is confirmed histologically, then surgical referral is indicated. These surveillance intervals are based on pooled analyses by the SCENIC international group, who reported a 6% (2%–13%) incidence of CRC on follow-up between 36 and 82 months. A meta-analysis by Wander and colleagues[69] underscored the importance of ongoing surveillance, because the risk of subsequent dysplasia following endoscopic resection of polypoid dysplasia is high at 65 cases per 1000 patient-years; however, the clinical implications are unclear because the risk of CRC was low at 5.3 per 1000 patient years. Histologic grade of the resected neoplastic lesion and also focality (unifocal vs multifocal) impacts prognosis. Recent studies reporting longer term follow-up of completely resected unifocal LGD are reassuring, because low rates of progression following complete resection were reported even up to 3 years.[22,71–73] In a study of 18 patients with resected multifocal LGD, 50% were subsequently diagnosed with HGD or CRC at median 32 months.[74] The management following complete resection of a visible lesion confirmed to be HGD is controversial, and the decision of continuing shorter interval surveillance versus colectomy should be individualized.[47,48,75] The safety of lengthening the interval after consecutive colonoscopies with quiescent disease confirmed histologically where no dysplasia is identified is not known, but emerging data suggest that it might be safe to lengthen the interval in the absence of other high-risk features, such as PSC and family history of CRC, but more data are certainly needed before any recommendation is made for this high-risk group.[76]

Nonpolypoid lesions are more challenging and multiple patient-, provider-, and lesion-specific factors must be considered when determining optimal course of management. Patient-specific factors are those already discussed, which relate to the probability of synchronous or metachronous neoplasia, patient preference, comorbidities, or presence of an additional surgical indication (eg, medically refractory disease, impassable stricture). Provider factors relate to level of experience and comfort, and nonpolypoid lesions should be managed by advanced endoscopists with appropriate expertise. For lesions located within strictures, poorly circumscribed, with irregular surface, indistinct borders, or endoscopically inaccessible, endoscopic resection should be deferred in favor of referring for surgery. As compared with polypoid lesions, the natural history of nonpolypoid lesions following endoscopic resection is not as well-defined and a lower threshold for surgical referral is warranted particularly given the higher risk of incomplete resection, the higher rate of recurrence, and more than eight-fold higher rate of progression of LGD to HGD/CRC compared with polypoid lesions.[77] As with all endoscopically resected lesions, a tattoo should be placed one to two folds distally and the resection site/surrounding mucosa biopsied adequately on subsequent surveillance examinations. For nonpolypoid lesions with confirmed complete removal, surveillance recommendations are based on expert opinion and mirror those for polypoid lesions greater than 1 cm or removed piecemeal.

Endoscopic Submucosal Dissection: Is the West There Yet?

The primary goal of endoscopic resection for dysplasia in patients with IBD is to minimize the risk of recurrence or progression to cancer and avoid the need for surgery. If this cannot be reliably achieved, then surgical referral is recommended. Borrowing from the non-IBD literature, in appropriately selected patients, appropriately selected lesions, and appropriate provider expertise, endoscopic mucosal resection is safe and effective if en bloc resection is achieved.[78,79] However, incomplete resection and recurrence are major considerations if en bloc resection cannot be achieved with endoscopic mucosal resection, because this is necessary to evaluate for curative resection. En bloc resection is often difficult if not impossible for larger lesions (typically ≥20 mm) and also for lesions in areas of chronic intestinal inflammation where there might be submucosal fibrosis in the absence of invasive dysplasia. Piecemeal resection is associated with high local recurrence rates (10%–25%) and potentially inaccurate histopathologic assessment.[80] If HGD and most certainly carcinoma are identified, surgical resection is recommended. At least in patients without IBD, ESD of colonic neoplasia is a major advance and allows for higher rates of en bloc resection for larger lesions when performed in experienced hands. ESD involves direct visualization and dissection through the submucosal plane using a special electrocautery knife. ESD was born initially in East Asia in the early mid-1990s as a noninvasive technique to remove early gastric neoplasia. Screening and surveillance programs in some East Asian countries (eg, Japan, Korea) enabled detection of gastric cancer in the early stage before submucosal invasion and where resection via ESD could be curative. With continued refinement of ESD techniques and instruments since its introduction, ESD is now commonly performed for non-IBD-associated CRN in East Asia. Colonic ESD is more technically difficult than gastric ESD because of the significantly thinner lining of the colonic mucosa and colonoscope maneuverability, both of which are particularly problematic for right-sided lesions. A recent meta-analysis of 97 studies (71 from Asia) with 17,483 patients (none with a mention of IBD) reported an overall 91% en bloc resection rate (82.9% negative vertical and horizontal margins, "R0"), which was significantly lower in non-Asian (71.3% R0; 81.2% en bloc) versus Asian (85.6% R0; 93% en bloc) countries for the standard ESD technique[81]; the frequency of ESD-related adverse events was nearly four-fold higher in non-Asian versus Asian countries (3.1% vs 0.8%). Hybrid ESD, which combines a snaring technique, was associated with poorer outcomes, including higher complication rate.[81] Only 2 of the 26 studies from Western countries originated from the United States, and even these were limited to abstracts,[82,83] since no full text studies from the United States were identified.

However, endoscopic resection in patients with IBD presents several unique challenges, including the downstream effect of relapsing and remitting inflammation on mucosal and submucosal remodeling caused by fibrosis and scarring. Unfortunately, the data regarding safety and long-term outcomes of ESD for colonic neoplasia in patients with IBD are limited to three case-series with 65 patients total (Japan, United Kingdom, Italy).[66–68] All patients among these studies were in clinical remission and had a single lesion that was well-demarcated with favorable histology. Even though all lesions were removed by an identified expert in ESD, en bloc resection ranged from 60% to 100%, with noncurative resection in 21% to 30%. With respect to complications, bleeding ranged from 0%[67] to 10%,[66] whereas perforation rate ranged from 0%[66,68] to 4%.[67] The first US experience was only recently published as a brief letter, and reported on a total of seven patients with IBD (71% UC, 29% CD) who had colonic ESD performed between 2014 and 2017 at a single center by a single endoscopist.[84] En bloc resection was achieved in 86%, because one patient needed colectomy caused by inadequate lifting of a polyp. No patients had clinically significant perforation or bleeding that required hospitalization. The final resected pathology specimen confirmed HGD in 43% (three of seven), LGD in 43% (three of seven), and no dysplasia in 14.2% (one of seven, sessile serrated adenoma).[84] The authors reported that on surveillance colonoscopy at 6-month follow-up, there was no dysplasia.

ESD is certainly an attractive option for a select group of patients, but the need for advanced endoscopists with adequate training and adequate case volume is a major barrier to the safe introduction of ESD in the armamentarium of therapeutic options for IBD-associated colonic neoplasia. Also limiting its primetime appearance are reimbursement considerations, and overall cost-effectiveness when considering the likely longer procedure time and the higher rate of complications and recurrence that might necessitate surgery regardless. Indeed, it is premature to extrapolate the promising safety profile reported in the Eastern experience to the West and, more specifically, the United States. We certainly welcome and support the enthusiasm for developing training programs in ESD for GI neoplasia in the West and look forward to additional safety and outcomes data to help guide positioning of ESD for the management of CRN in IBD.

MANAGEMENT OF ENDOSCOPICALLY "INVISIBLE" DYSPLASIA

Most dysplasia is seen on endoscopy in the current era of HD-WLE and/or CE. One-third of dysplasia initially considered to be "invisible" is actually visible and may be amenable to endoscopic resection.[85] If dysplasia is identified by random biopsies (presumably invisible dysplasia), the pathologic diagnosis of dysplasia should first be confirmed by an expert pathologist with particular expertise in IBD. If confirmed, a repeat colonoscopy with enhanced detection capabilities (eg, high definition, CE) should be performed by a gastroenterologist with adequate experience in IBD dysplasia surveillance examinations. If no lesions are identified despite careful examination and adequate mucosal visualization, random biopsies should be again taken every 10 cm and placed in separate jars. If invisible dysplasia is again confirmed, subsequent management should also take into consideration the individual patient and disease-related risk factors for CRC as described previously. If LGD is detected on random biopsy, the surveillance interval should be shortened to every 3 to 6 months. The idea of colectomy should be discussed with the patient, and documentation of their understanding that although biopsies revealed LGD, they are at significant risk of progressing to HGD and cancer, and may even harbor such pathology currently.[77] If HGD is detected on random biopsy the histologic interpretation should be confirmed by an expert GI pathologist. If confirmed, a repeat colonoscopy in expert hands using enhanced imaging techniques should see whether there may have in fact been a visible lesion that could be endoscopically resected. If that is not the case, colectomy should be very strongly considered.

In UC, the presence of dysplasia is assumed to be a field defect placing the entire colon at risk of harboring neoplasia, thus justifying total colectomy; whether this is true in the segmentally affected Crohn's colon remains to be clarified. The safest approach is total proctocolectomy, but this should be thoroughly discussed with the patient and referral to an experienced IBD gastroenterologist and surgeon with review of all pathology by an expert is recommended. It remains to be clarified, however, whether patients with segmental Crohn's colitis found to have HGD (or cancer) in the affected colitis segment have similar outcomes if they undergo segmental resection for localized CRN, as opposed to total colectomy. Current data favor total proctocolectomy in these patients because of the high risk of synchronous dysplasia or even cancer, and later development of metachronous neoplasia.[86] A retrospective study of 75 patients with CD and localized colon cancer undergoing segmental resection or subtotal colectomy found that 39% had at least one metachronous cancer despite most having annual screening colonoscopy; the mean time to new dysplasia and cancer was 5 and 6.8 years, respectively.[86]

SUMMARY

The optimal management of IBD-associated CRN is one that is individualized and considers patient-, disease-, and endoscopy-specific factors, in conjunction with the expertise of the treating gastroenterologists and advanced endoscopists. Although investigators continue to work in parallel for ways to definitively identify who will develop neoplastic complications of IBD and for ways to prevent the development of neoplasia from the outset (apart from simply controlling inflammation), we are at least in a dynamic era of expanding therapeutic endoscopic options for IBD-associated neoplasia when diagnosed. Hand-in-hand is an expanding body of literature on outcomes of nonoperative management of IBD-associated neoplasia to guide appropriate determination of patient and lesion candidacy for endoscopic resection and ongoing surveillance, as opposed to surgical management. However, with increasing access and availability of new technologies and techniques, we need to take care to balance cost and resource utilization, and first and foremost ensure shared decision making and appropriate counseling of risks versus benefits of endoscopic versus surgical management of IBD-associated neoplasia.

REFERENCES

1. Karlén P, Löfberg R, Broström O, et al. Increased risk of cancer in ulcerative colitis: a population-based cohort study. Am J Gastroenterol 1999;94:1047–52.
2. Bernstein CN, Blanchard JF, Kliewer E, et al. Cancer risk in patients with inflammatory bowel disease: a population-based study. Cancer 2001;91:854–62.
3. Ekbom A, Helmick C, Zack M, et al. Ulcerative colitis and colorectal cancer. A population-based study. N Engl J Med 1990;323:1228–33.
4. Gillen CD, Walmsley RS, Prior P, et al. Ulcerative colitis and Crohn's disease: a comparison of the colorectal cancer risk in extensive colitis. Gut 1994;35:1590–2.
5. Söderlund S, Brandt L, Lapidus A, et al. Decreasing time-trends of colorectal cancer in a large cohort of patients with inflammatory bowel disease. Gastroenterology 2009;136:1561–7 [quiz: 1818].
6. Lutgens MWMD, van Oijen MGH, van der Heijden GJMG, et al. Declining risk of colorectal cancer in inflammatory bowel disease: an updated meta-analysis of population-based cohort studies. Inflamm Bowel Dis 2013;19:789–99.
7. Samadder NJ, Valentine JF, Guthery S, et al. Family history is associated with increased risk of colorectal cancer in patients with inflammatory bowel diseases. Clin Gastroenterol Hepatol 2018. https://doi.org/10.1016/j.cgh.2018.09.038.
8. Shah SC, Ten Hove JR, Castaneda D, et al. High risk of advanced colorectal neoplasia in patients with primary sclerosing cholangitis associated with inflammatory bowel disease. Clin Gastroenterol Hepatol 2018;16:1106–13.e3.
9. Nieminen U, Jussila A, Nordling S, et al. Inflammation and disease duration have a cumulative effect on the risk of dysplasia and carcinoma in IBD: a case-control observational study based on registry data. Int J Cancer 2014;134:189–96.
10. Ullman TA, Itzkowitz SH. Intestinal inflammation and cancer. Gastroenterology 2011;140:1807–16.
11. Gupta RB, Harpaz N, Itzkowitz S, et al. Histologic inflammation is a risk factor for progression to colorectal neoplasia in ulcerative colitis: a cohort study. Gastroenterology 2007;133:1099–105 [quiz: 1340].
12. Velayos FS, Loftus EV, Jess T, et al. Predictive and protective factors associated with colorectal cancer in ulcerative colitis: a case-control study. Gastroenterology 2006;130:1941–9.
13. Karlén P, Kornfeld D, Broström O, et al. Is colonoscopic surveillance reducing colorectal cancer mortality in ulcerative colitis? A population based case control study. Gut 1998;42:711–4.
14. Choi C-HR, Rutter MD, Askari A, et al. Forty-Year analysis of colonoscopic surveillance program for neoplasia in ulcerative colitis: an updated overview. Am J Gastroenterol 2015;110:1022–34.
15. Ananthakrishnan AN, Cagan A, Cai T, et al. Colonoscopy is associated with a reduced risk for colon cancer and mortality in patients with inflammatory bowel diseases. Clin Gastroenterol Hepatol 2015;13:322–9.e1.
16. Löfberg R, Broström O, Karlén P, et al. Colonoscopic surveillance in longstanding total ulcerative colitis: a 15-year follow-up study. Gastroenterology 1990;99:1021–31.

17. Eaden J, Abrams K, Ekbom A, et al. Colorectal cancer prevention in ulcerative colitis: a case-control study. Aliment Pharmacol Ther 2000;14:145–53.

18. Ullman TA. Inflammatory bowel disease-associated cancers: does gender change incidence? Gastroenterology 2010;138:1658–60.

19. Söderlund S, Granath F, Broström O, et al. Inflammatory bowel disease confers a lower risk of colorectal cancer to females than to males. Gastroenterology 2010; 138:1697–703.

20. Farraye FA, Odze RD, Eaden J, et al. AGA technical review on the diagnosis and management of colorectal neoplasia in inflammatory bowel disease. Gastroenterology 2010;138:746–74, 774.e1.

21. Lunder AK, Hov JR, Borthne A, et al. Prevalence of sclerosing cholangitis detected by magnetic resonance cholangiography in patients with long-term inflammatory bowel disease. Gastroenterology 2016;151:660–9.e4.

22. Pekow JR, Hetzel JT, Rothe JA, et al. Outcome after surveillance of low-grade and indefinite dysplasia in patients with ulcerative colitis. Inflamm Bowel Dis 2010;16: 1352–6.

23. Askling J, Dickman PW, Karlén P, et al. Family history as a risk factor for colorectal cancer in inflammatory bowel disease. Gastroenterology 2001;120:1356–62.

24. Friedman S, Rubin PH, Bodian C, et al. Screening and surveillance colonoscopy in chronic Crohn's colitis: results of a surveillance program spanning 25 years. Clin Gastroenterol Hepatol 2008;6:993–8 [quiz: 953].

25. Greenstein AJ, Sachar DB, Smith H, et al. Cancer in universal and left-sided ulcerative colitis: factors determining risk. Gastroenterology 1979;77:290–4.

26. Markowitz J, McKinley M, Kahn E, et al. Endoscopic screening for dysplasia and mucosal aneuploidy in adolescents and young adults with childhood onset colitis. Am J Gastroenterol 1997;92:2001–6.

27. Gyde SN, Prior P, Allan RN, et al. Colorectal cancer in ulcerative colitis: a cohort study of primary referrals from three centres. Gut 1988;29:206–17.

28. Rutter MD, Saunders BP, Wilkinson KH, et al. Cancer surveillance in longstanding ulcerative colitis: endoscopic appearances help predict cancer risk. Gut 2004; 53:1813–6.

29. Lashner BA, Turner BC, Bostwick DG, et al. Dysplasia and cancer complicating strictures in ulcerative colitis. Dig Dis Sci 1990;35:349–52.

30. Reiser JR, Waye JD, Janowitz HD, et al. Adenocarcinoma in strictures of ulcerative colitis without antecedent dysplasia by colonoscopy. Am J Gastroenterol 1994;89:119–22.

31. Mahmoud R, Shah S, Ten Hove J, et al. Su1882 - post-inflammatory polyps do not predict colorectal neoplasia in patients with inflammatory bowel disease: a multinational retrospective cohort study. Gastroenterology 2018;154. S-618-S-619.

32. De Dombal FT, Watts JM, Watkinson G, et al. Local complications of ulcerative colitis: stricture, pseudopolyposis, and carcinoma of colon and rectum. Br Med J 1966;1:1442–7.

33. Gumaste V, Sachar DB, Greenstein AJ. Benign and malignant colorectal strictures in ulcerative colitis. Gut 1992;33:938–41.

34. Fumery M, Pineton de Chambrun G, Stefanescu C, et al. Detection of dysplasia or cancer in 3.5% of patients with inflammatory bowel disease and colonic strictures. Clin Gastroenterol Hepatol 2015;13:1770–5.

35. Ignjatovic A, Tozer P, Grant K, et al. Outcome of benign strictures in ulcerative colitis. Gut 2011;60:A221–2.

36. Eaden JA, Mayberry JF. British Society for Gastroenterology, Association of Coloproctology for Great Britain and Ireland. Guidelines for screening and

surveillance of asymptomatic colorectal cancer in patients with inflammatory bowel disease. Gut 2002;51(Suppl 5):V10-2.

37. Yaeger R, Shah MA, Miller VA, et al. Genomic alterations observed in colitis-associated cancers are distinct from those found in sporadic colorectal cancers and vary by type of inflammatory bowel disease. Gastroenterology 2016;151: 278-87.e6.

38. Vogelstein B, Fearon ER, Hamilton SR, et al. Genetic alterations during colorectal-tumor development. N Engl J Med 1988;319:525-32.

39. Itzkowitz SH. Inflammatory bowel disease and cancer. Gastroenterol Clin North Am 1997;26:129-39.

40. Hussain SP, Amstad P, Raja K, et al. Increased p53 mutation load in noncancerous colon tissue from ulcerative colitis: a cancer-prone chronic inflammatory disease. Cancer Res 2000;60:3333-7.

41. Kisiel JB, Ahlquist DA. Stool DNA testing for cancer surveillance in inflammatory bowel disease: an early view. Therap Adv Gastroenterol 2013;6:371-80.

42. Azuara D, Rodriguez-Moranta F, de Oca J, et al. Novel methylation panel for the early detection of neoplasia in high-risk ulcerative colitis and Crohn's colitis patients. Inflamm Bowel Dis 2013;19:165-73.

43. Klepp P, Kisiel JB, Småstuen MC, et al. Multi-target stool DNA test in the surveillance of inflammatory bowel disease: a cross-sectional cohort study. Scand J Gastroenterol 2018;53:273-8.

44. Harbord M, Eliakim R, Bettenworth D, et al. Corrigendum: third European evidence-based consensus on diagnosis and management of ulcerative colitis. Part 2: current management. J Crohns Colitis 2017;11:1512.

45. Kornbluth A, Sachar DB, Practice Parameters Committee of the American College of Gastroenterology. Ulcerative colitis practice guidelines in adults: American College of Gastroenterology, Practice Parameters Committee. Am J Gastroenterol 2010;105:501-23 [quiz: 524].

46. American Society for Gastrointestinal Endoscopy Standards of Practice Committee, Shergill AK, Lightdale JR, et al. The role of endoscopy in inflammatory bowel disease. Gastrointest Endosc 2015;81:1101-11021.e1.

47. Laine L, Kaltenbach T, Barkun A, et al. SCENIC international consensus statement on surveillance and management of dysplasia in inflammatory bowel disease. Gastrointest Endosc 2015;81:489-501.e26.

48. Annese V, Beaugerie L, Egan L, et al. European evidence-based consensus: inflammatory bowel disease and malignancies. J Crohns Colitis 2015;9:945-65.

49. Gearry RB, Wakeman CJ, Barclay ML, et al. Surveillance for dysplasia in patients with inflammatory bowel disease: a national survey of colonoscopic practice in New Zealand. Dis Colon Rectum 2004;47:314-22.

50. Kaplan GG, Heitman SJ, Hilsden RJ, et al. Population-based analysis of practices and costs of surveillance for colonic dysplasia in patients with primary sclerosing cholangitis and colitis. Inflamm Bowel Dis 2007;13:1401-7.

51. Eaden JA, Ward BA, Mayberry JF. How gastroenterologists screen for colonic cancer in ulcerative colitis: an analysis of performance. Gastrointest Endosc 2000;51:123-8.

52. van Rijn AF, Fockens P, Siersema PD, et al. Adherence to surveillance guidelines for dysplasia and colorectal carcinoma in ulcerative and Crohn's colitis patients in the Netherlands. World J Gastroenterol 2009;15:226.

53. Wang YR, Cangemi JR, Loftus EV, et al. Rate of early/missed colorectal cancers after colonoscopy in older patients with or without inflammatory bowel disease in the United States. Am J Gastroenterol 2013;108:444-9.

54. Mooiweer E, van der Meulen-de Jong AE, Ponsioen CY, et al. Incidence of interval colorectal cancer among inflammatory bowel disease patients undergoing regular colonoscopic surveillance. Clin Gastroenterol Hepatol 2015;13:1656–61.

55. Iannone A, Ruospo M, Wong G, et al. Chromoendoscopy for surveillance in ulcerative colitis and Crohn's disease: a systematic review of randomized trials. Clin Gastroenterol Hepatol 2017;15:1684–97.e11.

56. Moussata D, Allez M, Cazals-Hatem D, et al. Are random biopsies still useful for the detection of neoplasia in patients with IBD undergoing surveillance colonoscopy with chromoendoscopy? Gut 2018;67:616–24.

57. van den Broek FJC, Stokkers PCF, Reitsma JB, et al. Random biopsies taken during colonoscopic surveillance of patients with longstanding ulcerative colitis: low yield and absence of clinical consequences. Am J Gastroenterol 2014;109:715–22.

58. Rubin DT, Rothe JA, Hetzel JT, et al. Are dysplasia and colorectal cancer endoscopically visible in patients with ulcerative colitis? Gastrointest Endosc 2007;65:998–1004.

59. Mohammed N, Kant P, Abid F, et al. 446 high definition white light endoscopy (HDWLE) versus high definition with chromoendoscopy (HDCE) in the detection of dysplasia in long standing ulcerative colitis: a randomized controlled trial. Gastrointest Endosc 2015;81:AB148.

60. Jegadeesan R, Desai M, Sundararajan T, et al. P172 chromoendoscopy versus high definition white light endoscopy for dysplasia detection in patients with inflammatory bowel disease: a systematic review and meta-analysis. Gastroenterology 2018;154:S93.

61. Dekker E, van den Broek FJ, Reitsma JB, et al. Narrow-band imaging compared with conventional colonoscopy for the detection of dysplasia in patients with longstanding ulcerative colitis. Endoscopy 2007;39:216–21.

62. Pellisé M, López-Cerón M, Rodríguez de Miguel C, et al. Narrow-band imaging as an alternative to chromoendoscopy for the detection of dysplasia in longstanding inflammatory bowel disease: a prospective, randomized, crossover study. Gastrointest Endosc 2011;74:840–8.

63. Endoscopic Classification Review Group. Update on the Paris classification of superficial neoplastic lesions in the digestive tract. Endoscopy 2005;37:570–8.

64. Lahiff C, Mun Wang L, Travis SPL, et al. Diagnostic yield of dysplasia in polyp-adjacent biopsies for patients with inflammatory bowel disease: a cross-sectional study. J Crohns Colitis 2018;12:670–6.

65. Iacucci M, Uraoka T, Fort Gasia M, et al. Novel diagnostic and therapeutic techniques for surveillance of dysplasia in patients with inflammatory bowel disease. Can J Gastroenterol Hepatol 2014;28:361–70.

66. Iacopini F, Saito Y, Yamada M, et al. Curative endoscopic submucosal dissection of large nonpolypoid superficial neoplasms in ulcerative colitis (with videos). Gastrointest Endosc 2015;82:734–8.

67. Kinoshita S, Uraoka T, Nishizawa T, et al. The role of colorectal endoscopic submucosal dissection in patients with ulcerative colitis. Gastrointest Endosc 2018;87:1079–84.

68. Suzuki N, Toyonaga T, East JE. Endoscopic submucosal dissection of colitis-related dysplasia. Endoscopy 2017;49:1237–42.

69. Wanders LK, Dekker E, Pullens B, et al. Cancer risk after resection of polypoid dysplasia in patients with longstanding ulcerative colitis: a meta-analysis. Clin Gastroenterol Hepatol 2014;12:756–64.

70. Voorham QJM, Rondagh EJA, Knol DL, et al. Tracking the molecular features of nonpolypoid colorectal neoplasms: a systematic review and meta-analysis. Am J Gastroenterol 2013;108:1042–56.

71. Navaneethan U, Jegadeesan R, Gutierrez NG, et al. Progression of low-grade dysplasia to advanced neoplasia based on the location and morphology of dysplasia in ulcerative colitis patients with extensive colitis under colonoscopic surveillance. J Crohns Colitis 2013;7:e684–91.

72. Zisman TL, Bronner MP, Rulyak S, et al. Prospective study of the progression of low-grade dysplasia in ulcerative colitis using current cancer surveillance guidelines. Inflamm Bowel Dis 2012;18:2240–6.

73. Ten Hove JR, Mooiweer E, van der Meulen de Jong AE, et al. Clinical implications of low grade dysplasia found during inflammatory bowel disease surveillance: a retrospective study comparing chromoendoscopy and white-light endoscopy. Endoscopy 2017;49:161–8.

74. Ullman TA, Loftus EV, Kakar S, et al. The fate of low grade dysplasia in ulcerative colitis. Am J Gastroenterol 2002;97:922–7.

75. ASGE Standards of Practice Committee, Evans JA, Chandrasekhara V, Chathadi KV, et al. The role of endoscopy in the management of premalignant and malignant conditions of the stomach. Gastrointest Endosc 2015; 82:1–8.

76. Ten Hove JR, Shah SC, Shaffer SR, et al. Consecutive negative findings on colonoscopy during surveillance predict a low risk of advanced neoplasia in patients with inflammatory bowel disease with long-standing colitis: results of a 15-year multicentre, multinational cohort study. Gut 2018. https://doi.org/10.1136/gutjnl-2017-315440.

77. Choi CR, Ignjatovic-Wilson A, Askari A, et al. Low-grade dysplasia in ulcerative colitis: risk factors for developing high-grade dysplasia or colorectal cancer. Am J Gastroenterol 2015;110:1461–71 [quiz: 1472].

78. Panteris V, Haringsma J, Kuipers EJ. Colonoscopy perforation rate, mechanisms and outcome: from diagnostic to therapeutic colonoscopy. Endoscopy 2009;41: 941–51.

79. Arora G, Mannalithara A, Singh G, et al. Risk of perforation from a colonoscopy in adults: a large population-based study. Gastrointest Endosc 2009; 69:654–64.

80. Hong SN. Endoscopic therapeutic approach for dysplasia in inflammatory bowel disease. Clin Endosc 2017;50:437–45.

81. Fuccio L, Hassan C, Ponchon T, et al. Clinical outcomes after endoscopic submucosal dissection for colorectal neoplasia: a systematic review and meta-analysis. Gastrointest Endosc 2017;86:74–86.e17.

82. Karr JR, Decker CH, Margolin D a, et al. Tu1438 modified needle knives in endoscopic submucosal dissection of large sessile and flat colorectal lesions: the largest US experience. Gastrointest Endosc 2013;77:AB540.

83. Antillon MR, Pais WP, Diaz-Arias AA, et al. Effectiveness of endoscopic submucosal dissection as an alternative to traditional surgery for large lateral spreading polyps and early malignancies of the colon and rectum in the united states. Gastrointest Endosc 2009;69:AB279.

84. Kochhar G, Steele S, Sanaka M, et al. Endoscopic submucosal dissection for flat colonic polyps in patients with inflammatory bowel disease, a single-center experience. Inflamm Bowel Dis 2018;24:e14–5.

85. Kaltenbach T, McQuaid KR, Soetikno R, et al. Improving detection of colorectal dysplasia in inflammatory bowel disease surveillance. Gastrointest Endosc 2016;83:1013–4.

86. Maser EA, Sachar DB, Kruse D, et al. High rates of metachronous colon cancer or dysplasia after segmental resection or subtotal colectomy in Crohn's colitis. Inflamm Bowel Dis 2013;19:1827–32.

Strictures in Crohn's Disease and Ulcerative Colitis

Is There a Role for the Gastroenterologist or Do We Always Need a Surgeon?

Jason Reinglas, MD, Talat Bessissow, MDCM*

KEYWORDS

- Endoscopic balloon dilatation • Stricture • Crohn's disease • Ulcerative colitis

KEY POINTS

- Symptomatic strictures occur more often in Crohn's disease (CD) than in ulcerative colitis (UC).
- Strictures in UC are more often malignant and treated surgically, whereas strictures in CD are more often fibrotic and treated with endoscopic balloon dilation (EBD).
- EBD should be considered as first line therapy for straight ileal fibrotic strictures under 5 cm, if the goal is to delay surgical resection.
- Serious complications occur in less than 3% of procedures. Risk factors for perforation include inflammation, corticosteroid use, and dilation of ileorectal or ileosigmoid anastomotic strictures.
- The focus of this chapter is on EBD of CD strictures. Adjuvant techniques, such as intralesional injection, stricturotomy, and stent insertion, are briefly discussed.

INTRODUCTION

Persistent tissue inflammation leads to chronic tissue damage and repair resulting in the development of fibrosis and strictures in ulcerative colitis (UC) and Crohn's disease (CD).[1,2] Although the pathophysiology of intestinal strictures is generally similar among patients with UC and patients with CD, their characteristics and prevalence are markedly different in comparison.[1,2] In CD, one-third of the patient population develops a stricture within 10 years of disease onset.[3] Factors that predict fibrostenotic stricture formation are found in **Box 1**. CD strictures are classified into inflammatory, fibrotic, or mixed leading to luminal narrowing.[3,4] Infrequently, CD strictures may harbor or be the result of malignancy.[4] Patients frequently complain of progressive

Division of Gastroenterology, McGill University Health Centre, Montreal General Hospital, 1650 Ave. Cedar, D16.173.1, Montreal, QC, H3G 1A4, Canada
* Corresponding author.
E-mail address: talat.bessissow@mcgill.ca

Gastrointest Endoscopy Clin N Am 29 (2019) 549–562
https://doi.org/10.1016/j.giec.2019.02.009
1052-5157/19/© 2019 Elsevier Inc. All rights reserved.

Box 1
Predictors of fibrostenotic disease

Serologic

Anti-*Saccharomyces cerevisiae* antibodies IgA in Asians

Anti-Cbir1 (antibacterial flagellin CBir1 antibody)

ACCA (antichitobioside carbohydrate antibody)

Anti-OmpC (anti-*Escherichia coli* outer membrane protein C antibody)

Anti-I2 (anti-*Pseudomonas*-associated sequence I2 antibody)

Anti-L (antilaminarin carbohydrate antibody)

Genetic

NOD2/CARD15 mutations on both chromosomes

TNF superfamily 15 (TNFSF15) in Asians

5T5T in the MMP3 gene

Nucleotide oligomerization domain 2 (NOD2) variants

Janus-associated kinase 2 (JAK2)

Caspase-recruitment domain 15 (CARD15)

IL12-B

SOCS3

Jak-Tyk2-STAT3

Smad7

Smad3

Endoscopic

Extensive and deep mucosal ulceration

Clinical

Use of steroids during first exacerbation

Age at diagnosis less than 40 years

Perianal disease at diagnosis

Prior appendectomy

Environmental

Smoking

Adapted from Rieder F, Lawrance IC, Leite A, Sans M. Predictors of fibrostenotic Crohn's disease. Inflamm Bowel Dis 2011;17:2000–7 [PMID: 21308880 DOI: https://doi.org/10.1002/ibd.21627]; and Ko JZ, Abraham JP, Shih DQ. Pathogenesis of Crohn's Disease- and Ulcerative Colitis-Related Strictures [Internet]. In: Interventional Inflammatory Bowel Disease: Endoscopic Management and Treatment of Complications. Elsevier; 2018 [cited 2018 Nov 7]. page 35–41.

---

post-prandial abdominal pain, bloating, nausea, vomiting, and weight loss. The diagnosis of intestinal strictures usually coincides with a spiraling decline in quality of life in the absence of effective therapy. Stricturing disease is currently a main indication for surgery in CD.[3,5] In fact, 75% of affected individuals undergo surgery in their lifetime.[2] Disease recurrence at the site of anastomosis is common, which may lead to recurrence of luminal strictures.[6] As a result, patients with CD are exposed to short- and long-term risks of postoperative complications, such as short bowel syndrome, loss of gut functionality, and high risk of stricture recurrence (up to 50%).[3] Given the previously mentioned risks, endoscopic balloon dilatation (EBD) has emerged as an appealing alternative therapeutic procedure.[7] Most strictures are located in the colon or ileum, therefore accessible by using the colonoscope or balloon-assisted enteroscope.[8–11]

Strictures in patients with UC are rare but more often associated with malignancy. Gumaste and colleagues[12] retrospectively reviewed 1156 patients with UC admitted to their institution from 1959 to 1983 and identified intestinal strictures in 5% of their cohort. Of these 70 strictures, 17 (24%) were malignant and only four were candidates for resection. UC strictures found proximal to the sigmoid colon, associated with bowel obstruction, or diagnosed after 20 years of disease onset were independently associated with increased risk for malignancy. In contrast, the most common site for a benign stricture was found to be the rectum.[12]

This article presents current data on the endoscopic management of intestinal strictures in CD. Emphasis is placed on EBD given its firm establishment in practice. Novel endoscopic interventions, such as sphincterotomy, intralesional injections, and stenting, are briefly reviewed. The management of strictures related to UC is not further discussed given the sparse data available as a result of their infrequent symptomatic occurrence.

PATHOGENESIS OF INTESTINAL STRICTURES

Central to the development of fibrosis in CD is the activation of mesenchymal cells via a dysregulated immune response to gut flora.[3,13,14] Chronic neutrophil infiltration of the lamina propria leads to the continuous release of profibrotic cytokines resulting in mesenchymal cell activation and transformation into myofibroblasts, which secrete extracellular matrix proteins resulting in pathologic fibrosis. This disordered repair process is further impaired through a reduction in the secretion of extracellular matrix-degrading matrix metalloproteinases and increased secretion of tissue inhibitors of matrix metalloproteinases.[15] There may also exist a point where inflammation is no longer required to trigger fibrosis. As extracellular matrix is deposited during chronic inflammation, the bowel wall becomes stiffer.[16] Bowel wall stiffness acts independently as a mesenchymal cell activator. As the baseline release of profibrotic cytokines increases over time, luminal narrowing progresses to a critical point resulting in fistulization, bowel obstruction, and potential intestinal perforation.

The pathophysiology of stricture development in UC is likely similar to CD; however, the fibrosis and scar formation in UC is limited to the mucosa as opposed to the muscle layer in CD.[1] As a result, strictures often take a considerable amount of time to become clinically apparent in UC and may include additional mechanisms. T-helper cell type 2 cytokines, namely interleukin-4 and interleukin-13, have been found to be elevated in fibrostenotic disease and promote fibroblast activation, proliferation, and collagen synthesis.[17] Because it is hypothesized that UC is driven by a T-helper cell type 2 response, these cytokines may be important mediators for the development of strictures in UC.[1,14] Many other important mediators for fibrosis in CD and UC, such as transforming growth factor-β and beta-fibroblast growth factor, have been identified but their clinical relevance remains to be elucidated.[18]

APPROACH TO LUMINAL STRICTURES

CD strictures are usually a combination of inflammatory and fibrotic components. Medical therapy is effective for the inflammatory but not the fibrotic component of strictures. Therefore, determining the predominant constituent of the stricture is critical to deciding which therapeutic modality best suits the patient.[19,20] Because the mechanism of stricture formation in anastomotic and native strictures differ, it is speculated that their compositions differ. Despite the differences, the approach to evaluating all strictures is the same.[21] Patient history, physical examination, biochemical markers of inflammation (eg, elevated fecal calprotectin and C-reactive protein), imaging, and endoscopic and histologic findings should all be used in unison to best estimate the degree of inflammation of the stricture because it is often not clearly apparent (**Fig. 1**).[22] If a considerable inflammatory component exists, optimization of medical management should be sought first before endoscopic therapeutic interventions are undertaken because poorly controlled inflammation is a risk factor for endoscopic procedural complications.[23] Computed tomography and magnetic resonance enterography are important tools for evaluating the burden of luminal and extraluminal disease, including ruling out complications associated with strictures, such as perforations, abscesses, fistulization, and malignancy. All patients with suspected strictures should undergo imaging before any interventions.

Candidacy for EBD in fibrostenotic disease depends on patient factors, provider experience, and resources available. Therapeutic endoscopy should not be performed in an emergency setting, such as in unstable patients or acute bowel obstruction, coagulopathy, and in patients who are poor candidates for rescue surgical therapy.[24] Endoscopic therapy has not been demonstrated to prevent surgical intervention; rather, it has been demonstrated to delay or act as a bridge to surgery while nutritional status and medical therapy are optimized.[25] Based on current evidence, the best supported endoscopic intervention is balloon dilation.[19,25,26] Alternate modalities that have less evidence for their use include stricturotomy, stenting, and intralesional injections.

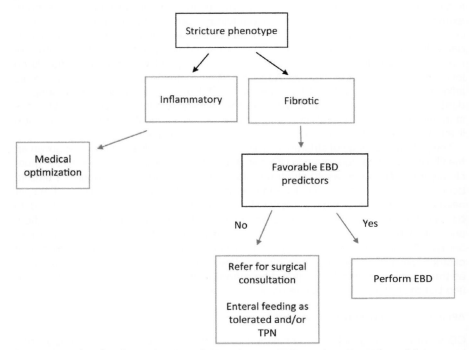

Fig. 1. Algorithm for the evaluation of CD strictures. TPN, total parenteral nutrition.

EFFICACY OF ENDOSCOPIC BALLOON DILATATION

The lack of medical therapy available to treat intestinal fibrosis makes EBD a good bowel conservation alternative. EBD has become an accepted modality for the treatment of bowel strictures in patients with CD. Most CD strictures are short and located at the ileocolonic anastomosis.[24,26,27] Most of the published data on outcomes of EBD are from observational studies, which are cluttered with their inherent design limitations. Despite that, the role of EBD is well established with excellent short-term efficacy and moderate long-term efficacy in the management of CD strictures.[23,25]

Short-term efficacy has been loosely defined as the technical success of the procedure or the ability to traverse the dilated area freely with the endoscope immediately after dilatation.[28,29] Long-term efficacy has been described as the time elapsed until another intervention (either surgical or endoscopic) is required.[3,28,29] Morar and colleagues[26] performed a meta-analysis involving 1089 patients (2664 EBDs) across 25 studies and documented the technical success to be greater than that of the symptomatic improvement (92% vs 70%, respectively). Following 2 years, 58% of patients had required repeat EBD. At 5 years, most patients required recurrent dilations (80%) and/or surgical interventions (75%). Similarly, in a large pooled analysis of 12 studies evaluating 3213 EBD procedures in 1463 patients with CD with predominantly short ileal anastomotic strictures, Bettenworth and colleagues[27] also found the technical success of stricture dilation to be greater than that of the symptomatic improvement of patients postdilation (89% vs 81%, respectively). Following 2 years, the symptomatic recurrence rate was also high. Repeat EBD was performed in 74% and surgical intervention was required in 43% of their cohort. The poor association between technical success and symptomatic relief is a common finding in many studies.[25] This may have occurred as a result of another process contributing to patient symptoms (eg, small intestinal bacterial overgrowth, active inflammation, irritable bowel syndrome) or because of a lack of a standardized definition for technical and clinical efficacy. In general, 80% of patients have their first bowel resection 10 years following their diagnosis of CD.[3]

Whether EBD is more efficacious in anastomotic or native CD strictures is still a controversial topic. In the aforementioned large systematic reviews, long-term outcomes did not differ between the two types of strictures. Although Bettenworth and colleagues[27] found technical success to be better in patients with native strictures, Morar and colleagues[26] did not reciprocate this finding. Similarly, in one of the largest prospective cohort studies involving 128 patients who underwent 430 EBD procedures over a follow-up period of 33 months, no difference was found between primary or anastomotic strictures with respect to the need for surgery (34.1% vs 29.6%; $P = .53$), redilation (59.1% vs 58%; $P = .89$), or total interventions (surgery and redilations, 71.6% vs 72.8%; $P = .86$).[30] Smaller studies have found better long-term outcomes in anastomotic as compared with native strictures. Mueller and colleagues[31] retrospectively evaluated a cohort of 55 patients who had underwent 93 EBD for 74 strictures over a 44-month observation period and found similar technical success rates but poor long-term outcomes in patients with native strictures. Nearly half of the patients with native strictures required surgery about 2 months following their EBD as opposed to zero patients in the anastomotic stricture group. Of note, patients with anastomotic strictures had significantly shorter strictures as compared with patients with native strictures (2.5 cm vs 7.5 cm, respectively). Similarly, another small study evaluating the performance of 47 EBD procedures in 30 patients with 17 anastomotic and 30 native strictures reported a greater surgical-free survival and complication rate with anastomotic as opposed to native strictures.[32]

The efficacy of balloon-assisted enteroscopy for dilating small bowel strictures has been evaluated in only a few studies but with favorable results. Nishida and colleagues[33] retrospectively evaluated 37 patients with CD who had undergone 72 EBD with double balloon enteroscopy sessions and 112 procedures between 2006 and 2015. Although this therapeutic modality was considered successful in this study, the presence of multiple strictures increased the risk for requiring surgical intervention (adjusted hazard ratio [HR], 14.94; 95% confidence interval [CI], 1.91–117.12). One patient (6.7%) required surgery among 15 who had single strictures compared with 17 (77.3%) among 22 patients with multiple strictures. Therefore, caution should be used in the setting of multiple strictures given the difficulty associated with intervening on the clinically significant stricture.

Factors Predicting the Outcomes of Endoscopic Balloon Dilatation

Successful EBD of fibrostenotic strictures depends on the characteristics of the stricture and presence of stricture-related complications, technical expertise, size of dilation, and comorbidities (**Box 2**). Factors associated with efficacious short-term EBD outcomes include technical success, stricture less than or equal to 5 cm, greater maximal dilation diameter of at least 1.5 cm (odds ratio [OR], 1.4; $P<.001$), native strictures (OR, 2.3; $P<.001$), absence of smoking, and ulcers in the stricture.[34–36] Technical success is facilitated when both ends of the stricture are appreciated. Thus, EBD

Box 2
Predictors of success and risk factors for complications of EBD

Predictors favoring successful dilation

De novo stricture

First dilation

Symptomatic predominantly fibrotic stricture

Short (≤5 cm) stricture

Single straight stricture

Stricture distal to the duodenum

Lack of a superimposed process contributing to symptoms (eg, small intestine bacterial overgrowth or irritable bowel syndrome)

Risk factors for complications

Predominantly inflammatory stricture

Stricture greater than 5 cm

Multiple small bowel strictures

Fistulization within 5 cm of the area to be dilated

Adjacent intra-abdominal collection

Complete small bowel obstruction

Unable to visualize proximal and distal stricture ends

Duodenal, ileosigmoid, or ileorectal stricture

Strictures caused by extrinsic compression (eg, adhesions)

High probability for surgical resection

Data from Refs.[1–6]

performed in patients with short straight strictures in-line with the bowel lumen are associated with better outcomes.[23,37] In the absence of direct visualization, fluoroscopic guidance should be used. There are no predictors for successful long-term outcomes.[23] Markers of disease severity, such as C-reactive protein, endoscopic disease activity, and medical treatment post-EBD, have not been influential in preventing reintervention.[38]

Factors related to poor short-term outcomes leading to complications or the need for reintervention include size of the dilation, upper gastrointestinal stricture location, use of steroids, adjacent fistulization and collections, and the length and diameter of the dilation. Strictures located in the duodenum compared with those located in the jejunum/ileum or colon have been associated with a nearly five times increased hazard for shorter time to surgery (HR, 4.7; $P<.038$; HR, 5.6; $P<.03$, respectively).[23] Every 1-cm increase in the length of the stricture greater than 5 cm was associated with an 8% increase in the risk for surgical intervention.[23] Although a larger diameter of dilation has been associated with better outcomes, dilations greater than 25 mm have been associated with a complication rate of near 9.3% (20 of 216 EBD procedures) in one large prospective study.[39] In contrast, dilations smaller than 14 mm have been associated with the need for salvage surgical intervention (HR, 2.88; 95% CI, 1.10–7.53).[40] Healing of enteroenteric fistulas proximal to a small bowel stricture may be facilitated by reducing the luminal pressure at its orifice by successfully performing EBD of the associated stricture distal to it. However, the orifice of the fistula should be at least 5 cm from the dilation site because of the risk of disrupting the tract and causing perforation.[41] The risk for perforation is increased in patients taking steroids (OR, 7.68; 95% CI, 1.48–39.81), active inflammation (OR, 3.82; 95% CI, 1.03–15.24), and when dilating ileorectal or ileosigmoid strictures.[35,42] Late risk factors that increase the risk for requiring surgical intervention were reported by the Cleveland Clinic group to be upfront surgery for ileocolonic anastomosis strictures (HR, 0.49; 95% CI, 0.32–0.76), a longer time from diagnosis to inception (HR, 0.96; 95% CI, 0.93–0.99), a shorter interval from the last surgery to inception (HR, 1.05; 95% CI, 1.01–1.09), only one previous resection (HR, 0.41; 95% CI, 0.26–0.66), and the absence of concurrent strictures (HR, 1.68; 95% CI, 0.97–2.9).[37]

SAFETY OF ENDOSCOPIC DILATATION

Albeit rare, bleeding, bowel perforation, and missed malignancy have been well reported in the literature as potential serious adverse events.[23,26,37,43] In the aforementioned review performed by Bettenworth and colleagues,[27] major complications resulting in hospital admissions occurred in 2.8% of reviewed patients. Another large review reported similar low rates of complications. In 1163 patients with CD who had undergone EBD, iatrogenic perforation, bleeding, and infection occurred in 3% to 4% of patients. Although inflammatory bowel disease is an independent risk factor for perforation during colonoscopy, EBD carries an independent and comparable risk for perforation in patients with inflammatory bowel disease and patients without inflammatory bowel disease (OR, 6.63; 95% CI, 3.95–11.11).[44,45] Despite these serious adverse events, no deaths as a result of EBD have been reported. In comparison with surgical intervention, the postoperative complication rate (eg, anastomotic leaks, perforation, and intra-abdominal sepsis) is 8.8%.[37]

Delayed consequences of EBD may include missing malignancy or increasing the risk for postoperative complications. In the absence of extraintestinal symptoms of malignancy, benign and malignant CD strictures cannot be accurately determined on imaging.[20] Consequentially, bowel length–preserving procedures harbor the risk of missing malignancy, which should otherwise be excised. Fortunately, the risk of malignant transformation of CD strictures is exceedingly low. A recent systematic review and meta-analysis of patients with CD undergoing strictureplasties reported a rate of 0.21% to 0.34%.[43] As a result, obtaining biopsies of all strictures before any endoscopic intervention is supported.[46] There exists no evidence to suggest that performing biopsies of a fibrotic CD stricture before dilation increases the risk for perforation. The risks of salvage surgery following the failure of EBD to alleviate obstruction was reported in a prospective study by Li and colleagues,[47] which included 194 patients who underwent surgery (58.8% without prior EBD). In multivariate analysis, EBD was independently associated with surgical site infection (OR, 3.16; 95% CI, 1.01–9.84) and stoma diversion (OR, 3.33; 95% CI, 1.14–9.78), although it is difficult to ascertain whether the patients' poorly controlled disease was the main culprit for these findings as opposed to the EBD contributing.

ADJUVANT TECHNIQUES
Endoscopic Intralesional Injection

The efficacy and safety of intralesional steroid injection has been supported for peptic, corrosive, anastomotic, and postradiotherapy fibrotic strictures but not yet in CD.[48–50] Rather, the American College of Gastroenterology and British Society of Gastroenterology position statements suggest not considering this as a therapeutic option given the lack of evidence and potential for harm.[51,52] One small randomized controlled trial evaluating 13 patients with CD with anastomotic strictures was stopped early because of a trend toward harm.[53] Five of the seven patients in the intervention group required redilation and one patient developed a complication. In contrast, only one patient in the placebo saline injection group required redilation without complication.[53] Lack of efficacy was also reported in a subgroup analysis of a large systematic review evaluating the management of anastomotic and de novo strictures.[54]

Intralesional injection of anti–tumor necrosis factor has been evaluated in several studies and is still considered controversial given concerns related to the development of immunogenicity but early reports suggest possible benefit. Two small case series investigated the use of infliximab intralesional injections into the strictures of nine patients and reported improvements in patients symptoms and simple endoscopic score-CD scores.[55,56] A larger randomized controlled trial evaluating the long-term efficacy of stricture dilation following adalimumab intralesional injection is ongoing.[57]

Endoscopic Stricturotomy

Endoscopic stricturotomy uses electrocautery delivered by either a needle-knife or isolated-tip knife to disrupt fibrotic tissue.[58] This procedure is still in its infancy and more often performed on biliary strictures as opposed to CD strictures. To date, reports discussing its efficacy and safety are largely anecdotal. Lan and Shen[59] reported 100% technical success in their cohort of 85 patients undergoing endoscopic stricturotomy. Although 60% of their patients required repeat intervention over a 1-year follow-up period, serious adverse events occurred in only 3.7% of 272 stricturotomies (one perforation and nine delayed bleeding). The greatest barrier to this method is technical expertise and experience given the level of skill required to perform this procedure in a safe and controlled fashion.[58]

Endoscopic Stenting

Endoscopic self-expanding stents have been suggested as a potential minimally invasive alternative to EBD and surgery. Self-expanding metal stents have good technical success but carry a high risk of stent impaction or migration in addition to the similar risks of perforation, bleeding, and missed malignancy as compared with the aforementioned options.[60,61] To avoid stent impaction, some studies suggest removing the stent 1 month following its deployment.[62–64] Loras and colleagues[64] evaluated the use of metal stents in 17 patients refractory to medical or endoscopic therapy and reported efficacy was maintained in 65% of patients at 60 weeks. Five patients with stent impactions had technically difficult endoscopic extractions of the stents and one patient required surgical extraction as a result. Additionally, a small prospective cohort study concluded the risk to be too high to advocate for the use of metal stents in colonic CD strictures.[62] Their potential use as a palliative modality of therapy for anastomotic leaks and colovaginal fistulas has been reported to be promising, although the risks need be discussed thoroughly with the patient.[65] Biodegradable stents have been reported to demonstrate good technical success but poor efficacy.[66,67] In a case series performed by Rejchrt and coworkers,[67] 4 of the 11 biodegradable stents had failed over the first few days following deployment and the remainder of the stents had failed at 4 months.

PERFORMING ENDOSCOPIC BALLOON DILATION

Two different EBD catheters are used for intestinal strictures in CD: through-the-scope and over-the-wire. Both are comprised of inflatable thermoplastic polymers, which enable them to have a reproducible and uniform expansion of the balloon. Because of their simplicity and safety profile, single-use through-the-scope balloon catheters are most commonly used.[29] The maximum diameter of the radially

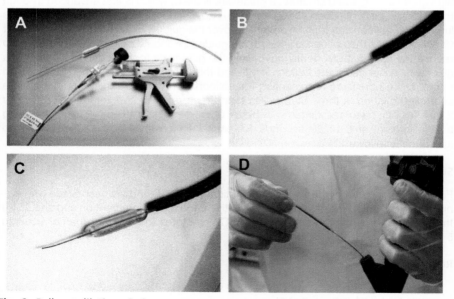

Fig. 2. Balloon dilation. Syringe gun, manometer, and balloon (*A*). Through-the-scope balloon (*B*), and following inflation (*C*). Through-the-scope balloon is inserted into the operating channel (*D*).

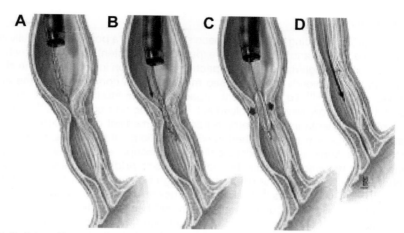

Fig. 3. Balloon dilatation. Through-the-scope balloon inserted into the endoscopic lumen (*A*). Through-the-scope balloon passed through the stricture (*B*). Insufflation of balloon to dilate stricture (*C*). Dilated stricture (*D*). TTS, through-the-scope.

expanding balloons varies widely; however, an acceptable safe maximum range is 18 to 20 mm.[39] Most balloons allow for sequential radial expansion via pressure injection of water or radiopaque contrast by using a handle accessory device (**Fig. 2**). Throughout the dilation, the hydraulic pressure of the balloon is monitored manometrically to ensure the amount of radially expanding force applied to the intestinal wall is not too great.[68]

Once the stenotic bowel is in direct view, the size of the dilator to be used is estimated. The dilation is carried out with or without a guidewire. In the setting of a high grade or angulated stricture, a guidewire is used, which is first advanced through the stenosis. Lack of resistance as the wire is advanced suggests the wire is within the lumen. The balloon can then be advanced over the guidewire and inflated under direct visualization. As the balloon is inflated, the guidewire should be pulled back slightly to reduce the risk of inadvertently advancing the guidewire forward during inflation. If a guidewire is not used, the balloon is passed through the stenotic lumen and inflated to the desired pressure representing the balloon diameter (**Fig. 3**). To induce a more controlled dilation, a three-step inflation is often preferred.[68] A total dilation time of 2 minutes has been associated with better outcomes.[26] Some authors suggest using a time interval of 5 to 20 seconds for each inflation time if a graded three-step approach is followed.[41]

SUMMARY

Fibrostenotic strictures are common complications of CD and are associated with significant symptoms. EBD is a safe and effective endoscopic intervention and should be the preferred treatment of simple straight CD strictures that are less than or equal to 5 cm in length.

REFERENCES

1. Rogler G. Pathogenesis of strictures in ulcerative colitis: a field to explore. Digestion 2011;84:10–1.
2. Cosnes J, Cattan S, Blain A, et al. Long-term evolution of disease behavior of Crohn's disease. Inflamm Bowel Dis 2002;8:244–50.

3. Rieder F, Zimmermann EM, Remzi FH, et al. Crohn's disease complicated by strictures: a systematic review. Gut 2013;62:1072–84.

4. Bettenworth D, Nowacki TM, Cordes F, et al. Assessment of stricturing Crohn's disease: current clinical practice and future avenues. World J Gastroenterol 2016;22:1008–16.

5. Oberhuber G, Stangl PC, Vogelsang H, et al. Significant association of strictures and internal fistula formation in Crohn's disease. Virchows Arch 2000;437:293–7.

6. Rutgeerts P, Geboes K, Vantrappen G, et al. Predictability of the postoperative course of Crohn's disease. Gastroenterology 1990;99:956–63.

7. Saunders BP, Brown GJ, Lemann M, et al. Balloon dilation of ileocolonic strictures in Crohn's disease. Endoscopy 2004;36:1001–7.

8. Louis E, Collard A, Oger AF, et al. Behaviour of Crohn's disease according to the Vienna classification: changing pattern over the course of the disease. Gut 2001; 49:777–82.

9. Despott EJ, Gupta A, Burling D, et al. Effective dilation of small-bowel strictures by double-balloon enteroscopy in patients with symptomatic Crohn's disease (with video). Gastrointest Endosc 2009;70:1030–6.

10. Karstensen JG, Hendel J, Vilmann P. Endoscopic balloon dilatation for Crohn's strictures of the gastrointestinal tract is feasible. Dan Med J 2012;59:A4471.

11. Neufeld DM, Shemesh EI, Kodner IJ, et al. Endoscopic management of anastomotic colon strictures with electrocautery and balloon dilation. Gastrointest Endosc 1987;33:24–6.

12. Gumaste V, Sachar DB, Greenstein AJ. Benign and malignant colorectal strictures in ulcerative colitis. Gut 1992;33:938–41.

13. Fiocchi C, Lund PK. Themes in fibrosis and gastrointestinal inflammation. Am J Physiol Gastrointest Liver Physiol 2011;300:G677–83.

14. Ko JZ, Abraham JP, Shih DQ. Pathogenesis of Crohn's disease- and ulcerative colitis-related strictures. In: Shen B, editor. Interventional inflammatory bowel disease: endoscopic management and treatment of complications. London: Academic Press, Elsevier; 2018. p. 35–41. Available at: https://linkinghub.elsevier.com/retrieve/pii/B9780128113882000038. Accessed November 7, 2018.

15. Meijer MJ. Role of matrix metalloproteinase, tissue inhibitor of metalloproteinase and tumor necrosis factor-α single nucleotide gene polymorphisms in inflammatory bowel disease. World J Gastroenterol 2007;13:2960.

16. Wells RG. The role of matrix stiffness in regulating cell behavior. Hepatology 2008;47:1394–400.

17. Wynn TA. Fibrotic disease and the T(H)1/T(H)2 paradigm. Nat Rev Immunol 2004; 4:583–94.

18. Zhang Z, Li C, Zhao X, et al. Anti-*Saccharomyces cerevisiae* antibodies associate with phenotypes and higher risk for surgery in Crohn's disease: a meta-analysis. Dig Dis Sci 2012;57:2944–54.

19. Gionchetti P, Dignass A, Danese S, et al, ECCO. 3rd European evidence-based consensus on the diagnosis and management of Crohn's disease 2016: part 2: surgical management and special situations. J Crohns Colitis 2017;11:135–49.

20. Bruining DH, Zimmermann EM, Loftus EV, et al, Society of Abdominal Radiology Crohn's Disease-Focused Panel. Consensus recommendations for evaluation, interpretation, and utilization of computed tomography and magnetic resonance enterography in patients with small bowel Crohn's disease. Radiology 2018;286: 776–99.

21. Bharadwaj S, Fleshner P, Shen B. Therapeutic armamentarium for stricturing Crohn's disease: medical versus endoscopic versus surgical approaches. Inflamm Bowel Dis 2015;21:2194–213.

22. Peyrin-Biroulet L, Sandborn W, Sands BE, et al. Selecting therapeutic targets in inflammatory bowel disease (STRIDE): determining therapeutic goals for treat-to-target. Am J Gastroenterol 2015;110:1324–38.

23. Bettenworth D, Rieder F. Medical therapy of stricturing Crohn's disease: what the gut can learn from other organs. A systematic review. Fibrogenesis Tissue Repair 2014;7:5.

24. Shen B. Multidisciplinary approach to stricturing Crohn's disease. In: Shen B, editor. Interventional inflammatory bowel disease: endoscopic management and treatment of complications. London: Academic Press, Elsevier; 2018. p. 249–60. Available at: https://linkinghub.elsevier.com/retrieve/pii/B9780128113882000221. Accessed November 7, 2018.

25. Bessissow T, Reinglas J, Aruljothy A, et al. Endoscopic management of Crohn's strictures. World J Gastroenterol 2018;24:1859–67.

26. Morar PS, Faiz O, Warusavitarne J, et al, Crohn's Stricture Study (CroSS) Group. Systematic review with meta-analysis: endoscopic balloon dilatation for Crohn's disease strictures. Aliment Pharmacol Ther 2015;42:1137–48.

27. Bettenworth D, Gustavsson A, Atreja A, et al. A pooled analysis of efficacy, safety, and long-term outcome of endoscopic balloon dilation therapy for patients with stricturing Crohn's disease. Inflamm Bowel Dis 2017;23:133–42.

28. Klag T, Wehkamp J, Goetz M. Endoscopic balloon dilation for Crohn's disease-associated strictures. Clin Endosc 2017;50:429–36.

29. Hirai F. Current status of endoscopic balloon dilation for Crohn's disease. Intest Res 2017;15:166–73.

30. Atreja A, Aggarwal A, Dwivedi S, et al. Safety and efficacy of endoscopic dilation for primary and anastomotic Crohn's disease strictures. J Crohns Colitis 2014;8:392–400.

31. Mueller T, Rieder B, Bechtner G, et al. The response of Crohn's strictures to endoscopic balloon dilation. Aliment Pharmacol Ther 2010;31:634–9.

32. Endo K, Takahashi S, Shiga H, et al. Short and long-term outcomes of endoscopic balloon dilatation for Crohn's disease strictures. World J Gastroenterol 2013;19:86–91.

33. Nishida Y, Hosomi S, Yamagami H, et al. Analysis of the risk factors of surgery after endoscopic balloon dilation for small intestinal strictures in Crohn's disease using double-balloon endoscopy. Intern Med 2017;56:2245–52.

34. Hirai F, Andoh A, Ueno F, et al. Efficacy of endoscopic balloon dilation for small bowel strictures in patients with Crohn's disease: a nationwide, multi-centre, open-label, prospective cohort study. J Crohns Colitis 2018;12:394–401.

35. Couckuyt H, Gevers AM, Coremans G, et al. Efficacy and safety of hydrostatic balloon dilatation of ileocolonic Crohn's strictures: a prospective longterm analysis. Gut 1995;36:577–80.

36. Hoffmann JC, Heller F, Faiss S, et al. Through the endoscope balloon dilation of ileocolonic strictures: prognostic factors, complications, and effectiveness. Int J Colorectal Dis 2008;23:689–96.

37. Lian L, Stocchi L, Remzi FH, et al. Comparison of endoscopic dilation vs surgery for anastomotic stricture in patients with Crohn's disease following ileocolonic resection. Clin Gastroenterol Hepatol 2017;15:1226–31.

38. Thienpont C, D'Hoore A, Vermeire S, et al. Long-term outcome of endoscopic dilatation in patients with Crohn's disease is not affected by disease activity or medical therapy. Gut 2010;59:320–4.

39. Gustavsson A, Magnuson A, Blomberg B, et al. Endoscopic dilation is an efficacious and safe treatment of intestinal strictures in Crohn's disease. Aliment Pharmacol Ther 2012;36:151–8.

40. Reutemann BA, Turkeltaub JA, Al-Hawary M, et al. Endoscopic balloon dilation size and avoidance of surgery in stricturing Crohn's disease. Inflamm Bowel Dis 2017;23:1803–9.

41. Chen M, Shen B. Endoscopic therapy in Crohn's disease: principle, preparation, and technique. Inflamm Bowel Dis 2015;21:2222–40.

42. Navaneethan U, Kochhar G, Phull H, et al. Severe disease on endoscopy and steroid use increase the risk for bowel perforation during colonoscopy in inflammatory bowel disease patients. J Crohns Colitis 2012;6:470–5.

43. Campbell L, Ambe R, Weaver J, et al. Comparison of conventional and nonconventional strictureplasties in Crohn's disease: a systematic review and meta-analysis. Dis Colon Rectum 2012;55:714–26.

44. Mukewar S, Costedio M, Wu X, et al. Severe adverse outcomes of endoscopic perforations in patients with and without IBD. Inflamm Bowel Dis 2014;20: 2056–66.

45. Chen M, Shen B. Comparable short- and long-term outcomes of colonoscopic balloon dilation of Crohn's disease and benign non-Crohn's disease strictures. Inflamm Bowel Dis 2014;20:1739–46.

46. Rieder F, Latella G, Magro F, et al. European Crohn's and colitis organisation topical review on prediction, diagnosis and management of fibrostenosing Crohn's disease. J Crohns Colitis 2016;10:873–85.

47. Li Y, Stocchi L, Shen B, et al. Salvage surgery after failure of endoscopic balloon dilatation versus surgery first for ileocolonic anastomotic stricture due to recurrent Crohn's disease. Br J Surg 2015;102:1418–25 [discussion: 1425].

48. Hanaoka N, Ishihara R, Motoori M, et al. Endoscopic balloon dilation followed by intralesional steroid injection for anastomotic strictures after esophagectomy: a randomized controlled trial. Am J Gastroenterol 2018;113:1468–74.

49. Nelson RS, Hernandez AJ, Goldstein HM, et al. Treatment of irradiation esophagitis. Value of hydrocortisone injection. Am J Gastroenterol 1979;71:17–23.

50. Takahashi H, Arimura Y, Okahara S, et al. A randomized controlled trial of endoscopic steroid injection for prophylaxis of esophageal stenoses after extensive endoscopic submucosal dissection. BMC Gastroenterol 2015;15. https://doi.org/10.1186/s12876-014-0226-6. Available at: http://bmcgastroenterol.biomedcentral.com/articles/10.1186/s12876-014-0226-6. Accessed November 10, 2018.

51. Lichtenstein GR, Hanauer SB, Sandborn WJ. Practice Parameters Committee of American College of Gastroenterology. Management of Crohn's disease in adults. Am J Gastroenterol 2009;104:465–83 [quiz: 464, 484].

52. Carter MJ, Lobo AJ, Travis SPL, IBD Section, British Society of Gastroenterology. Guidelines for the management of inflammatory bowel disease in adults. Gut 2004;53(Suppl 5):V1–16.

53. East JE, Brooker JC, Rutter MD, et al. A pilot study of intrastricture steroid versus placebo injection after balloon dilatation of Crohn's strictures. Clin Gastroenterol Hepatol 2007;5:1065–9.

54. Bevan R, Rees CJ, Rutter MD, et al. Review of the use of intralesional steroid injections in the management of ileocolonic Crohn's strictures. Frontline Gastroenterol 2013;4:238–43.

55. Hendel J, Karstensen JG, Vilmann P. Serial intralesional injections of infliximab in small bowel Crohn's strictures are feasible and might lower inflammation. United European Gastroenterol J 2014;2:406–12.

56. Swaminath A, Lichtiger S. Dilation of colonic strictures by intralesional injection of infliximab in patients with Crohn's colitis. Inflamm Bowel Dis 2008;14:213–6.

57. A randomized, double-blinded, placebo-controlled study on the effects of adalimumab intralesional intestinal strictures of Crohn's disease patients. Available at: Clinicaltrials.gov https://clinicaltrials.gov/ct2/show/study/NCT01986127 Clinical Trials.gov. Accessed November 10, 2018.

58. Shen B. Endoscopic stricturotomy. In: Shen B, editor. Interventional inflammatory bowel disease: endoscopic management and treatment of complications. London: Academic Press, Elsevier; 2018. p. 171–80. Available at: https://linkinghub.elsevier.com/retrieve/pii/B9780128113882000142. Accessed November 10, 2018.

59. Lan N, Shen B. Endoscopic stricturotomy with needle knife in the treatment of strictures from inflammatory bowel disease. Inflamm Bowel Dis 2017;23:502–13. https://doi.org/10.1097/MIB.0000000000001044.

60. Ali S, Navaneethan U. Endoscopic stent treatment for Crohn's disease. In: Shen B, editor. Interventional inflammatory bowel disease: endoscopic management and treatment of complications. London: Academic Press, Elsevier; 2018. p. 181–6. Available at: https://linkinghub.elsevier.com/retrieve/pii/B9780128113882000154. Accessed November 10, 2018.

61. Levine RA, Wasvary H, Kadro O. Endoprosthetic management of refractory ileocolonic anastomotic strictures after resection for Crohn's disease: report of nine-year follow-up and review of the literature. Inflamm Bowel Dis 2012;18:506–12.

62. Attar A, Maunoury V, Vahedi K, et al, GETAID. Safety and efficacy of extractible self-expandable metal stents in the treatment of Crohn's disease intestinal strictures: a prospective pilot study. Inflamm Bowel Dis 2012;18:1849–54.

63. Branche J, Attar A, Vernier-Massouille G, et al. Extractible self-expandable metal stent in the treatment of Crohn's disease anastomotic strictures. Endoscopy 2012;44(Suppl 2 UCTN):E325–6.

64. Loras C, Pérez-Roldan F, Gornals JB, et al. Endoscopic treatment with self-expanding metal stents for Crohn's disease strictures. Aliment Pharmacol Ther 2012;36:833–9.

65. Lamazza A, Fiori E, Schillaci A, et al. Treatment of rectovaginal fistula after colorectal resection with endoscopic stenting: long-term results. Colorectal Dis 2015;17:356–60.

66. Karstensen JG, Christensen KR, Brynskov J, et al. Biodegradable stents for the treatment of bowel strictures in Crohn's disease: technical results and challenges. Endosc Int Open 2016;4:E296–300.

67. Rejchrt S, Kopacova M, Brozik J, et al. Biodegradable stents for the treatment of benign stenoses of the small and large intestines. Endoscopy 2011;43:911–7.

68. ASGE Technology Committee, Siddiqui UD, Banerjee S, Barth B, et al. Tools for endoscopic stricture dilation. Gastrointest Endosc 2013;78:391–404.

The Role of Laparoscopic, Robotic, and Open Surgery in Uncomplicated and Complicated Inflammatory Bowel Disease

David M. Schwartzberg, MD, Feza H. Remzi, MD*

KEYWORDS

- Crohn's disease • Ulcerative colitis • Redo pouch • Minimally invasive surgery
- Open surgery

KEY POINTS

- The incidence of inflammatory bowel disease is increasing in the United States.
- Even with recent advancements of medical therapy, 80% of patients with Crohn's disease and 30% of patients with ulcerative colitis will require surgery.
- Minimally invasive procedures have given operative advancements with decreases in pain, narcotic requirement, length of stay, and overall postoperative morbidity.
- Complicated Crohn's disease may require a hybrid laparoscopic approach or an open operation.
- Proctectomy and ileal pouch anal anastomosis have unique challenges because of the bony confines of the pelvis, and minimally invasive surgery has led to increasing rates of pouch failure and patients who need redo pouch procedures.

INTRODUCTION

Inflammatory bowel disease (IBD), amalgamated by Crohn's disease (CD), ulcerative colitis (UC), and indeterminant colitis, are defined as autoimmune intestinal diseases associated with extraintestinal manifestations. IBD is a result of complex interactions between genetic predispositions, the microbiota, and environmental factors.[1] Although results vary, population-based studies have shown an increase in IBD in industrialized countries with the incidence of UC and CD in North America at 19.2 and 20.2 per 100,000, respectively, and a combined IBD incidence of 249 per

Department of Surgery, Inflammatory Bowel Disease Center, New York University Langone Health, 240 East 38th Street, 23rd Floor, New York, NY 20016, USA
* Corresponding author.
E-mail address: Feza.Remzi@NYULangone.Org

Gastrointest Endoscopy Clin N Am 29 (2019) 563–576
https://doi.org/10.1016/j.giec.2019.02.012
1052-5157/19/© 2019 Elsevier Inc. All rights reserved.

100,000 in North America.[2,3] Although the rates of IBD are increasing, optimal treatments involving the complex relationship between gastroenterology and surgery, medical and surgical therapy, biologics and steroids, minimally invasive and open operations, and the timing of these various modalities continues to be paramount. In fact, despite optimal treatment involving multidisciplinary teams and medical therapy, 80% of patients with CD or 30% of patients with UC will require operative intervention during their lifetime.[4,5] A recent review by Abelson et al[6] and Gu et al[7] showed that since infliximab was approved to treat UC, patients with UC have not only continued to require surgery, but in the postinfliximab era, have suffered greater postoperative morbidity and more staged procedures, hypothesizing a sicker population.

In a population that typically requires 1 or more operations during their lifetime, the IBD population represents a challenging cohort of patients with specific operative concerns. The patient with IBD has multiple operative risk factors and can be young or elderly, often times anemic and hypoalbuminemic in a catabolic state, and possess intraabdominal phlegmons, fistulae, abscesses, and adhesions from previous operations. Furthermore, in young populations, there are specific concerns for fertility; autonomic nerve preservation for bowel, urinary, and sexual function; and psychosocial body awareness as a result of stoma creation and abdominal scars.[8]

Open surgery remained the cornerstone for surgery in the IBD population because of its many advantages in reoperative surgery, specifically redo pelvic pouch procedures, but also in vessel ligation in friable Crohn's mesentery, tactile assessment of healthy bowel free from active disease, and pelvic nerve preservation in the UC population. However, recently laparoscopic and robotic surgery have been proven to positively affect patients undergoing surgery with decreased levels of pain and narcotic requirements, less adhesion formation, early return of bowel function, and a shorter length of stay.[9] Laparoscopy has evolved so far as to permit single incision surgery for UC with pelvic pouch formation, and robotics may offer minimally invasive benefits for patients whose surgeons may be fluent robotically but not have a sufficient laparoscopic skill set. With these advancements, proper patient selection and clinical acumen for minimally invasive techniques must be balanced with effective and safe open operative interventions, especially in the complex IBD and redo pouch cohort. This text highlights some minimally invasive advancements in treating the IBD population while clarifying the role of open surgery in complex, reoperative surgery our group uses to best serve our patients and provide them with an improved quality of life.

CROHN'S DISEASE: LAPAROSCOPIC, ROBOTIC, AND OPEN OPERATIVE CONSIDERATIONS

Since the 1990s, laparoscopic surgery has been attempted in the field of colorectal surgery; early studies were designed to assess its feasibility and safety.[10,11] Laparoscopic surgery trials for IBD began in 1993, which saw an almost 20% conversion rate to open during the early years of adoption.[10] Casillas and colleagues[12] demonstrated that, with appropriate case selection, converting to an open procedure remained beneficial to the patient, and thus minimally invasive surgery persisted and over the next years conversion rates decreased and are now reported at between 9% and 11%. Stocchi and colleagues[13] analyzed a prospective cohort of laparoscopic versus open ileocolectomy for more than 10 years and concluded that laparoscopic outcomes were comparable with those from open procedures. This finding was also reflected in a study by Lowney and colleagues[14] on the median time to recurrence and medication requirements of 113 patients with a 63-month follow-up. Their results showed that there was no difference between laparoscopic and open cases. Duepree and colleagues[11] concluded that laparoscopically treated ileocecal disease did not only result in a shorter length of stay, but also showed significant cost savings. Furthermore, because laparoscopy was gaining popularity, Aytac and colleagues[15] showed that attempting laparoscopic surgery for disease recurrence after an initial laparotomy was feasible, and further endorsed laparoscopic IBD surgery. Eshuis and colleagues[16] found that cosmesis was significantly improved with laparoscopic (vs open) ileocolic resection and recurrence rates and quality of life between the two were comparable.

Since that time, the vast advantages of minimally invasive surgery via a laparoscopic platform has established itself as the standard of care for many indications in CD. With that being said, patients presenting for surgery have vastly different indications within the same patient cohort; some present with uncomplicated ileocolic structuring disease, whereas others present in extremis secondary to perforation or hemorrhage, or can present with multiple fistulae, phlegmons, abscesses, or multifocal disease. Thus, the differences in pathology must dictate the operative planning and patient selection for laparoscopic surgery.

Patients with CD are candidates for minimally invasive surgery because they often have a low body mass index (measured in kg/m^2), commonly young, frequently require repeat operations, and do not require anatomic oncologic operations, which itself increases the risk of damaging adjacent organs and autonomic nerves.[17] In many ways, patients with uncomplicated CD are the ideal laparoscopic candidates and can benefit the most from laparoscopy (decreased pain, narcotic requirements, length of stay, early time to bowel function, hasten time to daily activities, and decreased intraabdominal adhesions).[17,18] Juxtapose to this ideal candidate are patients with complicated disease, such as fistulae (enteroentero, ileal-sigmoid/rectal, ileal-duodenal, ileal-vesicle), abscess (pelvic, psoas), phlegmon, multifocal disease, ileus leading to decreased visualization with laparoscopy, and adhesions from previous intraabdominal operation. Those stigmata of advanced disease may still permit laparoscopy for some defined elements of the operation; however, a hybrid approach is frequently used. A hybrid laparoscopic/open approach is helpful in certain circumstances where a total laparoscopic procedure maybe unsafe, so elements of the procedure are undertaken safely laparoscopically, while possibility limiting the size of the incision (ie, mobilizing the hepatic flexure and dividing the omentum off the transverse colon laparoscopically before focusing on the complicated terminal ileal disease). Once those portions of the procedures are completed, the remaining portions of the procedure are undertaken in an open fashion. However, in certain patients, although a hybrid approach should be considered, the patient is best served with an open operation early to avoid inadequate resections, missed enterotomies from adhesiolysis, high intraoperative blood loss, and sever postoperative complications. Regardless of whether there is straightforward or complex disease, each patient demands an individualized surgical approach formatted to each patients' specific pathology.

DIFFERENCES IN SURGICAL APPROACH TO UNCOMPLICATED AND COMPLICATED DISEASE

Ileocolic disease is the most common disease in Crohn's and, therefore, ileocolic resections are commonly performed.[16] The majority of data of laparoscopy CD surgery use ileocolic resections as a litmus test for feasibility. As stated, ileocolic disease can vary greatly and operations must be tailed to each patients' disease.

Uncomplicated stricturing ileocolic disease can be approached a number of ways, but typically an optical trocar is inserted periumbilically with two 5-mm ports in the left hemiabdomen. Single incision laparoscopic surgery has been attempted for noncomplicated disease with success, but large trials are lacking.[19] An assessment of the thickened mesentery is crucial to decide if the procedure can continue laparoscopically. With minimally inflamed mesentery, a medial-to-lateral approach can be safely undertaken with subsequent ligation of the ileocolic artery, followed by lateral mobilization and hepatic flexure mobilization. Once the right colon and small bowel are mobilized from the retroperitoneum, a chosen extraction site is used to exteriorize the bowel. With minimally inflamed mesentery, a vessel sealer can be used to efficiently divide the mesentery. The small and large bowel are resected to soft, pliable bowel and a stapled or hand-sewn anastomosis created with or without temporary protective stoma. An advantage of robotic ileocolic resections in uncomplicated ileocolic disease is the ability to perform an intraabdominal/intracorporeal stapled or handsewn anastomosis without having to extract the bowel to perform the anastomosis.[20] An intracorporeal anastomosis is helpful in 2 ways: it can limit the size of the extraction incision and subsequent incisional hernia rates, and less colonic mobilization is required because the bowel does not need to be eviscerated. Further efforts to decrease the size on extraction sites has led to alternative types of specimen extraction. Eshuis and colleagues[21] published on 8 patients who underwent successful transcolonic specimen extraction; however, large studies are not available and these investigators concluded there may be an association with intraabdominal infections.

Complicated disease can range from thickened mesentery with intramesenteric abscess to phelgmons and complex fistulizing disease involving multiple target fistulas or multicentric disease. An assessment of the feasibility of laparoscopic management must ensue before either aborting or proceeding laparoscopically. To address each pathology, stricturing disease with inflamed, friable mesentery or phlegmons in the pelvis may be able to be addressed laparoscopically before converting to an open procedure by proceeding laparoscopically to circumvent the diseased bowel. Mobilizing the hepatic flexure laparoscopically and caudal along the white line of Toldt can be accomplished safely and, by doing so, limit the cephalad extent of the incision. After colonic mobilization of the right colon, the inflamed, thickening, friable Crohn's mesentery should be mobilized and ligated in an open fashion with suture-ligatures with #1 chromic sutures between overlapping Kocher clamps through a lower midline incision. If there are enteroentero fistulas present, they are best finger fractured after eviscerating the bowel, so it is important to determine which target fistulas demand segmental resection versus debridement and oversewing (**Fig. 1**). For multifocal disease, lateral mobilization and hepatic flexure mobilization can be attempted; however, for multisegment stricureplasties or resections, an appropriate midline incision should be made. One report by Tou and colleagues[22] on a robotic strictureplasty was described; however, further research is needed on the efficacy of the technique. In patients with ileosigmoid fistulas, the sigmoid fistula is tackled after separating the small bowel and colon intraperitoneally with blunt and sharp dissection. The vast majority of these fistulas are present on the antemesenteric sigmoid bowel and, therefore, require a nonanatomic, segmental resection; the minority, being antimesenteric fistulas, can be debrided and oversewn. The colocolonic anastomosis can be completed with an end-to-end stapled or hand-sewn anastomosis. For combined ileocolic and ileosigmoid/segmental colon resections, a protective stoma is advocated. Adhesions from previous surgery are the most common reason for conversation to open or from a lack of working space from chronic partial bowel obstructions leading to dilation and a thin bowel (**Fig. 2**). Thick, dense, vascularized adhesions should prompt a

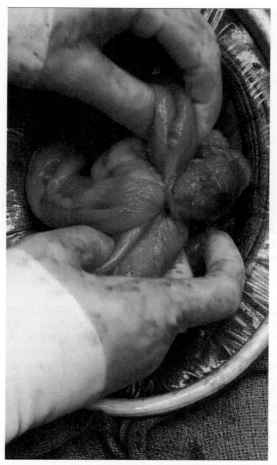

Fig. 1. Multiple fistulae at the site of a previous ileocolic resection. A hybrid laparoscopic resection of neoterminal ileum for recurrent stricturing disease. Laparoscopic mobilization of the right colon and hepatic flexure was performed, before making a lower midline incision to safely resection the diseased bowel and repair the target fistulae.

midline incision; however, laparoscopic adhesiolysis can be attempted with softer adhesions, as long as the surgeon continues to make progress. Re-resection of symptomatic ileocolic disease is also possible and beneficial to the patient.[21] Holubar and colleagues[23] showed that, in 40 patients with recurrent ileocolic disease requiring operative intervention, successful completion of the operation laparoscopically occurred in 75% of the patients and resulted in short-term benefits.

ULCERATIVE COLITIS: LAPAROSCOPIC, ROBOTIC, AND OPEN OPERATIVE CONSIDERATIONS

Restorative proctocolectomy with ileal anal pouch anastomosis (IPAA) is the standard of care for patients with UC. Differing from CD, UC can be cured with removing the colon and rectum with staged procedures (1, 2, modified 2-stage, or 3-stage procedures) in the development of a pelvic pouch formation with success rates exceeding

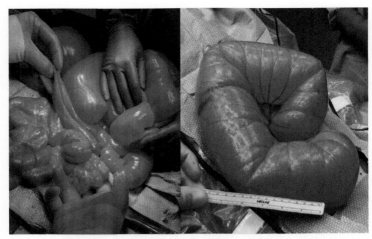

Fig. 2. Stricture terminal ileal CD causing a chronic partial small bowel obstruction. The case was started laparoscopically; however, without any visibility owing to the severely dilated small bowel, it converted to an open procedure with ileocolic resection.

95% at 10 years.[24] Although the procedures are staged, they are unlikely to need repeat operations (like recurrent ileocolic CD), so in a largely young population, the adoption of minimally invasive techniques were promising because all of the positive effects of laparoscopy could be applied to the UC patient population. In addition, the deep pelvic dissection during proctectomy involves dissection near the pelvic nerves and the female reproductive organs, and the reduced inflammation and adhesion formation is thought to benefit women who wish to become pregnant. In UC, the roles of minimally invasive surgery are divided into abdominal and pelvic operations. Therefore, the use of minimally invasive platforms has been evaluated differently. In addition, minimally invasive surgery for UC can be further divided into indications for intraabdominal colectomy, as classified as emergent, secondary to toxic colitis with hemorrhage, perforation, or megacolon, or elective, with disease progression through medical management or dysplasia. Minimally invasive techniques also need to be applied for the succeeding staged procedures, such as proctectomy with IPAA.

To address minimally invasive abdominal colectomies, Telem and colleagues[25] published a retrospective review of 90 patients with medically refractory UC treated at their institution with a subtotal colectomy and end ileostomy. Twenty-nine were treated by laparoscopy and 61 by an open approach, and the results showed less intraoperative blood loss and a shorter length of stay for the patients undergoing laparoscopic subtotal colectomy. During that same time period, laparoscopic surgery for UC was being performed throughout the country, and eventually the American College of Surgeons National Surgical Quality Improvement Program database was queried by Causey and colleagues,[26] with results demonstrating that laparoscopy was becoming increasing common throughout the United States and patients undergoing laparoscopic surgery for UC (subtotal colectomy, proctocolectomy with ileostomy, proctocolectomy with IPAA) had a lower morbidity and mortality than those undergoing open procedures. Larson and colleagues[27] operated on 4 patients with UC who successfully had total proctocolectomies with a transperineal extraction site. Robotic surgery has also been proven to be safe for emergent subtotal colectomy for patients with UC. Five patients underwent robotic subtotal colectomy for toxic colitis in UC at our institution (Alexis Grucela, MD, unpublished data, 2018). The case-matched control to the laparoscopic cohort showed that, in the robotic group, there was no conversion to open and no significant difference in operative blood loss or operative time. Laparoscopic and robotic surgery have proven to be safe in colorectal surgery and in the UC population undergoing emergent surgery, with the additional benefits in decreased adhesions for subsequent proctectomy and IPAA creation.[28] For example, McLemore and colleagues[29] were successful in conducting robotic proctectomy with IPAA in UC after all their patients previously underwent a laparoscopic subtotal colectomy.

Laparoscopic surgery showed significant advances compared with open in the proper indications and improved fertility (defined as the ability for a women to conceive) in patients who underwent a laparoscopic proctectomy with IPAA.[30] Larson and colleagues[31] published an article in 2006 comparing 100 laparoscopic IPAA versus 200 open IPAA operations, and the result was equivalency of the 2 safety and feasibility. Robotic-assisted laparoscopic surgery aimed to further provide the benefits of a minimally invasive platform, which maybe especially advantageous in the pelvis with improved, 3-dimensional visualization, articulating wristed instruments, a stable camera, and the use of a third retracting arm (**Fig. 3**). A case-matched control study by Miller and colleagues[32] compared the outcomes of laparoscopic and robotic completion proctectomy with IPAA formation. They found that there was no significant difference between operative time, postoperative complications, or bowel and sexual function. Grucela and colleagues showed that robotic proctectomy with IPAA was safe without any morbidity and a short length of stay (compared with laparoscopic) in 15 patients (Alexis Grucela, MD, unpublished data, 2018). As stated, McLemore had 3 successful completion proctectomies without any fecal incontinence, nocturnal seepage, or sexual dysfunction after the initial laparoscopic subtotal colectomy.[29] They did cite their concerns for the lack of a standardized method of distal rectal transection, trying both open and endoscopic linear staplers, and/or everting the rectum transanally. For their minimally invasive approach, they still formed the IPAA via a suprapubic incision. This concern

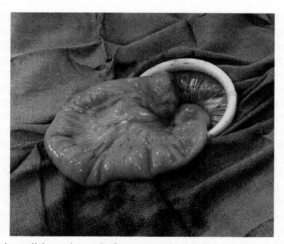

Fig. 3. Eviscerated small bowel just before J-pouch construction in a robotic completion proctectomy with IPAA, after a robotic stage 1 colectomy with end ileostomy. The ileostomy site functions as the stoma aperture, specimen extraction site, and pouch creation site. (*Courtesy of* Alexis Grucela, MD, New York, unpublished data, 2018.)

was echoed by Mark-Christensen and colleagues[33] in their series observing the short-term outcomes of robotic IPAA. The ability to comfortably transect the rectum during minimally invasive surgery remains a concern; however, Lightner and colleagues[34] has chosen to use 2 or 3 firings of the da Vinci Endo Wrist 45-mm stapler to transect the rectum just above the anal canal and levator complex during the completion proctectomy with IPAA creation. They also have not elected to use a suprapubic or Pfannenstiel incision, but rather use the ileostomy site for J-pouch creation and proctectomy specimen extraction, therefore eliminating any incision larger than the standard robotic ports and the stoma site itself. A major concern is the number of overlapping staple lines to complete the anorectal transection, because increasing staple lines have been associated with anastomotic leaks.[35,36] A risk-benefit relationship of incision size and postoperative outcomes must accompany the decision to use minimally invasive techniques because different equipment is offered for each platform and, therefore, has consequential results for the patient. Of utmost importance is to not make any sacrifice to the long-term postoperative outcomes to simply save incision length. Pedraza and colleagues[37] have shown that, in elective procedures, such as for dysplasia, a total abdominal colectomy with proctectomy and IPAA creation is safe, without conversation to open, and free of any postoperative complications in 5 patients.

DIFFERENCES IN SURGICAL APPROACH TO TOTAL ABDOMINAL COLECTOMY, PROCTECTOMY, AND ILEAL POUCH ANAL ANASTOMOSIS

A recent report from Abelson and colleagues[6] analyzed more than 7000 patients who underwent surgical therapy for UC. The cohorts were divided into 2 groups, one group that underwent operation from 1995 to 2005 and the other between 2005 and 2013. The major difference during that specific time period was the introduction of biologic therapy. The results demonstrate that, since 2005, patients are more likely to require multiple operations and have worse postoperative morbidity in both the index hospitalization, and up to 1 year of follow-up. The increase of staged procedures along with higher morbidity postoperatively is indicative of a sicker patient population. The major difference in this time period is also that a total proctocolectomy with IPAA and temporary diverting stoma (2-staged procedure) (or a 1-stage without protective stoma) was replaced with a total colectomy with end ileostomy, leaving the proctectomy and IPAA creation for a future procedure. The decrease in 1- or 2- staged procedures necessitates repeat intraabdominal operations, so the obvious choice was to expand the indications for minimally invasive surgery to the population of patients with UC requiring surgery to mitigate intraabdominal adhesion formation. Laparoscopic subtotal colectomy has been proven safe and, as surgeons became more adept and comfortable with robotic-assisted surgery, so too did the attempts at robotic subtotal colectomy with end ileostomy, even applying robotic surgery to nonelective patients and, therefore, a sicker patient population. One characteristic of robotic surgery has been longer operating times and, therefore, a longer time period the patient is maintained in awkward positioning like extreme Trendelenburg (head down).[38] Positioning with extreme head down/Trendelenburg has physiologic consequences like decreased venous return and bradycardia, with subsequent hypotension.[39] Therefore, when a patient is in extremis requiring emergent surgery for toxic colitis, the best option for the patient is not always a minimally invasive surgery because it can be associated with longer operating times. These longer operating times and increased costs may limit the widespread adoption of robotic surgery for a total colectomy with end ileostomy, and laparoscopic colectomy may remain the standard.[40]

Robotic proctectomy has been described to be superior to laparoscopy because it offers a stable platform, wristed instruments, and increased magnification in the bony confines of the pelvis.[37] However, with all the benefits minimally invasive surgery can theoretically offer, its role in proctectomy and IPAA has not been fully solidified, from our viewpoint as a quaternary referral medical center and redo pouch center. An issue with minimally invasive advancements is their ability to compromise on existing techniques without any advantage to the patient. The learning curve for laparoscopic IPAA showed that, during the learning curve, pelvic sepsis was the most consistent and relevant complication from a 2017 article by Rencuzogullari and colleagues.[41] Although reports on the major advantages of minimally invasive surgery have been published, our experience has been that a majority of patients needing a redo pelvic pouch had initially underwent a minimally invasive IPAA (laparoscopic/robotic; **Fig. 4**). Minimally invasive pouches have, therefore, been responsible for a number of mechanical defects, such as retained rectums, ischemic strictures, and/or pouch twists that ultimately require operative correction in a very complicated and staged procedures, with 9 months of having an ileostomy, 3 operations, and many additional tests and procedures. In a study by Remzi and colleagues[42] of more than 500 redo pouches, these patients retain a high quality of life after redo pouch; in the interim, however, these mechanical problems caused prolonged suffering, narcotic administration, and many treatment for a presumptive diagnosis of CD of the pouch, which has its own harmful side effect profile.

Advocates for robotic surgery have produced studies described various stapling techniques to achieve an adequate and proper proctectomy with transection of the rectum at the anorectal junction. And although some of the instrumentation may lend itself to pelvic surgery, the deep pelvic space prohibits the ability of an endoscopic stapler to successfully fire a single stapler-fire to perform a double-stapled technique. The crisscrossing of multiple staple lines can contribute to an anastomotic

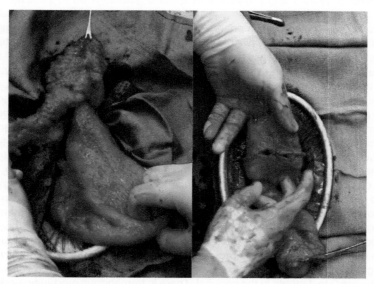

Fig. 4. Two patients who were referred as having CD of the pouch after minimally invasive IPAA with intraoperative findings consistent with mechanical pathology. *Left,* retained rectum (Babcock clamp on retained rectum). *Right,* anastomotic leak causing ongoing sepsis and a pseudotwist of the pouch.

leak at the ileal pouch–anal anastomosis with ongoing pelvic sepsis.[36] Or, to achieve a single staple fire, the proper level of transection is sacrificed to a more proximal level, which then leads to retained rectum and ongoing inflammation from the presence of ongoing proctitis, both being a significant source of morbidity to the patient and a reason patients with mechanical pouch failures are often misdiagnosed as having CD of the pouch.[43] Pouch twists are also commonly found after minimally invasive procedures. To correctly orient the pouch to the anal canal, the optimal view is to follow the cut edge of the small bowel mesentery from the superior mesenteric artery, which has been mobilized to under the duodenum, and follow it into the deep pelvis to ensure that no bowel is trapped under the pouch and to ensure that no pouch twist is present. This view is often limited with minimally invasive platforms because the small bowel obscures the view or, when sweeping the bowel to allow visualization, the perspective is lost and there is misbelief in the proper orientation. In addition, being able to mobilize the bowel mesentery under the duodenum and perform mesenteric lengthening procedures to the peritoneal surface of the mesentery can be dangerous and costly because it can sacrifice the blood supply to the pouch and prevent IPAA.[44] In minimally invasive scenarios where mobilizing to the duodenum and mesenteric lengthening procedures are needed to achieve a tension-free anastomosis, surgeons may shy away from these risky maneuvers because of limitations, comfortably performing them laparoscopically or robotically but to avoid converting to an open procedure. The lack of these needed maneuvers may result in a pouch under tension and, therefore, can lead to an ischemic stricture at the anal–anastomotic site, causing obstructive defecation and pouch dysfunction.

When these patients develop pouch failure, they are often presented with the overwhelming odds that they will need to live with a permanent end ileostomy. Patients who cannot accept that fate often seek out to have a redo pouch procedure. Redo pouches consist of multiple staged procedures and extensive workup. Beginning with a thorough history and physical with specific questions on to the exact timing of pelvic symptoms needed (within 1 year is highly suggestive of a mechanical problem), followed by a gastrografin enema, pelvic MRI to assess for fistulas, strictures, and retained rectum or pouch twist is completed. An abdominopelvic MR enterography is also completed to assess for Crohn's-like lesions in the remaining small bowel. This is followed up with an examination under anesthesia and pouchoscopy. Some patients are also candidates for anal manometry and pelvic floor biofeedback. During the workup, patients are usually suffering from more than 20 bowel movements per day and are on high-dose pain medication, leading to social, diet, sexual, and work restrictions and an overall low quality of life. Eventually, if the patient is deemed to have a correctable mechanical problem with their pouch and is a candidate for a redo pouch, they then undergo a laparoscopic or open diverting ileostomy with intra-abdominal assessment of the small bowel and pelvic pouch to assess for twist, reach, or other complications. This stoma is in place for approximately 6 months while any sepsis is resolved and any pouch elongation from obstructive defecation can settle. The redo pouch procedure includes an epidural, arterial line, ureteric stents and exploratory laparotomy with pouch augmentation, new pouch formation, or, in rare cases, pouch excision. A pelvic drain is left in place and a more proximal diverting stoma is created for 3 months to protect the pouch. Barring any postoperative leak, a gastrografin enema confirms no pouch leak or twist and the stoma is reversed, typically spending 2 to 4 nights in the hospital. There is tremendous morbidity, both physical and emotional, to the patient; sadly, for many of the reasons, these patients have to undergo these steps to correct an avoidable mechanical issue from their index pouch operation.

Last, the creation of a J-shaped IPAA at the start of the procedure and before assessing the full reach of the bowel to the pelvis may limit the ability to perform an anastomosis because of reach issues and leave the patient with an end-ileostomy, citing reach issues from prohibiting pelvic pouch formation. This finding is further echoed because a small number of patients will need an S-, reverse lower-case H- or W-pouch based on bowel length, which is often times not known until the proctectomy has been completed, and well after the stapler has already been fired to create the J-pouch.

Our group's unique perspective is confounded by referral bias and the current surgical environment, because more minimally invasive operations are taking place and, therefore, contribute to a higher percentage of pouch failures needing redo procedures. Regardless, often the platform and technique advancements may allow for procedural omissions that are standard practice in traditional techniques.[45] As an example, the debate between mucosectomy and double-stapled anastomotic techniques was driven by the fear that stapling the distal rectum would lead to retained rectums, whereas a mucosectomy ensured complete proctectomy. Ultimately, ensuring a safe, durable, reproducible procedure for patients with UC to have intestinal continuity while minimizing morbidity is the goal of all IBD surgeons and platform should not affect that.

SUMMARY

The incidence of IBD is increasing in the United States and, despite advancements in medical therapy, patients continue to require operations for complications of IBD. Minimally invasive surgical options have dramatically impacted postoperative morbidity, with decreasing rates of length of stay, opioid use, pain scores, and intra-abdominal adhesion formation.[17] The IBD population is typically a younger cohort of patients, who are concerned with both successful operative therapy, ability to return to their lifestyle, and cosmesis. Additionally, as a group they may undergo multiple operations and therefore, collectively, can benefit most from laparoscopic and robotic surgery. Laparoscopic surgery for CD has proven to benefit patients with ileocolic or colonic disease and complicated disease with fistulae, phlegmon, abscess, or multicentric disease is best served with a hybrid approach consisting of elements of laparoscopy and open surgery. UC has seen advancements in 3-staged procedures with a minimally invasive subtotal colectomy with end ileostomy. Although minimally invasive proctectomy with IPAA has been reported to be safe with minimal morbidity and good functional outcomes, pouch failure seems to be associated with minimally invasive platforms with retained rectums, pouch twists, and anastomotic leaks requiring a redo pouch. The benefits of minimally invasive surgery must be balanced with reproducible and durable outcomes, and ultimately, regardless of the platform, the success of the patient is paramount.

REFERENCES

1. Olivera P, Danese S, Jay N, et al. Big data in IBD: a look into the future. Nat Rev Gastroenterol Hepatol 2019. https://doi.org/10.1038/s41575-019-0102-5.
2. Molodecky NA, Soon IS, Rabi DM, et al. Increasing incidence and prevalence of the inflammatory bowel diseases with time, based on systematic review. Gastroenterology 2012;142(1):46–54.e42 [quiz: e30].
3. Gajendran M, Loganathan P, Catinella AP, et al. A comprehensive review and update on Crohn's disease. Dis Mon 2018;64(2):20–57.

4. Neumann PA, Rijcken E. Minimally invasive surgery for inflammatory bowel disease: review of current developments and future perspectives. World J Gastrointest Pharmacol Ther 2016;7(2):217–26.
5. Marceau C, Alves A, Ouaissi M, et al. Laparoscopic subtotal colectomy for acute or severe colitis complicating inflammatory bowel disease: a case-matched study in 88 patients. Surgery 2007;141(5):640–4.
6. Abelson JS, Michelassi F, Mao J, et al. Higher surgical morbidity for ulcerative colitis patients in the era of biologics. Ann Surg 2018;268(2):311–7.
7. Gu J, Stocchi L, Ashburn J, et al. Total abdominal colectomy vs. restorative total proctocolectomy as the initial approach to medically refractory ulcerative colitis. Int J Colorectal Dis 2017;32(8):1215–22.
8. Gaidos JKJ, Kane SV. Sexuality, fertility, and pregnancy in Crohn's disease. Gastroenterol Clin North Am 2017;46(3):531–46.
9. Holder-Murray J, Marsicovetere P, Holubar SD. Minimally invasive surgery for inflammatory bowel disease. Inflamm Bowel Dis 2015;21(6):1443–58.
10. Casillas S, Delaney CP, Senagore AJ, et al. Does conversion of a laparoscopic colectomy adversely affect patient outcome? Dis Colon Rectum 2004;47(10): 1680–5.
11. Duepree HJ, Senagore AJ, Delaney CP, et al. Advantages of laparoscopic resection for ileocecal Crohn's disease. Dis Colon Rectum 2002;45(5):605–10.
12. Maggiori L, Panis Y. Surgical management of IBD–from an open to a laparoscopic approach. Nat Rev Gastroenterol Hepatol 2013;10(5):297–306.
13. Stocchi L, Milsom JW, Fazio VW. Long-term outcomes of laparoscopic versus open ileocolic resection for Crohn's disease: follow-up of a prospective randomized trial. Surgery 2008;144(4):622–7 [discussion: 7–8].
14. Lowney JK, Dietz DW, Birnbaum EH, et al. Is there any difference in recurrence rates in laparoscopic ileocolic resection for Crohn's disease compared with conventional surgery? A long-term, follow-up study. Dis Colon Rectum 2006;49(1): 58–63.
15. Aytac E, Stocchi L, Remzi FH, et al. Is laparoscopic surgery for recurrent Crohn's disease beneficial in patients with previous primary resection through midline laparotomy? A case-matched study. Surg Endosc 2012;26(12):3552–6.
16. Eshuis EJ, Polle SW, Slors JF, et al. Long-term surgical recurrence, morbidity, quality of life, and body image of laparoscopic-assisted vs. open ileocolic resection for Crohn's disease: a comparative study. Dis Colon Rectum 2008;51(6): 858–67.
17. Kessler H, Mudter J, Hohenberger W. Recent results of laparoscopic surgery in inflammatory bowel disease. World J Gastroenterol 2011;17(9):1116–25.
18. Lesperance K, Martin MJ, Lehmann R, et al. National trends and outcomes for the surgical therapy of ileocolonic Crohn's disease: a population-based analysis of laparoscopic vs. open approaches. J Gastrointest Surg 2009;13(7):1251–9.
19. Moftah M, Burke J, Narendra A, et al. Single-access laparoscopic surgery for ileal disease. Minim Invasive Surg 2012;2012:697142.
20. Lujan HJ, Plasencia G, Rivera BX, et al. Advantages of robotic right colectomy with intracorporeal anastomosis. Surg Laparosc Endosc Percutan Tech 2018; 28(1):36–41.
21. Eshuis EJ, Voermans RP, Stokkers PC, et al. Laparoscopic resection with transcolonic specimen extraction for ileocaecal Crohn's disease. Br J Surg 2010; 97(4):569–74.
22. Tou S, Pavesi E, Nasser A, et al. Robotic-assisted strictureplasty for Crohn's disease. Tech Coloproctol 2015;19(4):253–4.

23. Holubar SD, Dozois EJ, Privitera A, et al. Laparoscopic surgery for recurrent ileo-colic Crohn's disease. Inflamm Bowel Dis 2010;16(8):1382–6.
24. Remzi FH, Lavryk OA, Ashburn JH, et al. Restorative proctocolectomy: an example of how surgery evolves in response to paradigm shifts in care. Colorectal Dis 2017;19(11):1003–12.
25. Telem DA, Vine AJ, Swain G, et al. Laparoscopic subtotal colectomy for medically refractory ulcerative colitis: the time has come. Surg Endosc 2010;24(7):1616–20.
26. Causey MW, Stoddard D, Johnson EK, et al. Laparoscopy impacts outcomes favorably following colectomy for ulcerative colitis: a critical analysis of the ACS-NSQIP database. Surg Endosc 2013;27(2):603–9.
27. Larson DW, Dozois E, Sandborn WJ, et al. Total laparoscopic proctocolectomy with Brooke ileostomy: a novel incisionless surgical treatment for patients with ulcerative colitis. Surg Endosc 2005;19(9):1284–7.
28. Trinh BB, Jackson NR, Hauch AT, et al. Robotic versus laparoscopic colorectal surgery. JSLS 2014;18(4) [pii:e2014.00187].
29. McLemore EC, Cullen J, Horgan S, et al. Robotic-assisted laparoscopic stage II restorative proctectomy for toxic ulcerative colitis. Int J Med Robot 2012;8(2):178–83.
30. Bartels SA, D'Hoore A, Cuesta MA, et al. Significantly increased pregnancy rates after laparoscopic restorative proctocolectomy: a cross-sectional study. Ann Surg 2012;256(6):1045–8.
31. Larson DW, Cima RR, Dozois EJ, et al. Safety, feasibility, and short-term outcomes of laparoscopic ileal-pouch-anal anastomosis: a single institutional case-matched experience. Ann Surg 2006;243(5):667–70 [discussion: 70–2].
32. Miller AT, Berian JR, Rubin M, et al. Robotic-assisted proctectomy for inflammatory bowel disease: a case-matched comparison of laparoscopic and robotic technique. J Gastrointest Surg 2012;16(3):587–94.
33. Mark-Christensen A, Pachler FR, Norager CB, et al. Short-term outcome of robot-assisted and open IPAA: an observational single-center study. Dis Colon Rectum 2016;59(3):201–7.
34. Lightner AL, Kelley SR, Larson DW. Robotic platform for an IPAA. Dis Colon Rectum 2018;61(7):869–74.
35. Saurabh B, Chang SC, Ke TW, et al. Natural orifice specimen extraction with single stapling colorectal anastomosis for laparoscopic anterior resection: feasibility, outcomes, and technical considerations. Dis Colon Rectum 2017;60(1):43–50.
36. Lee S, Ahn B, Lee S. The relationship between the number of intersections of staple lines and anastomotic leakage after the use of a double stapling technique in laparoscopic colorectal surgery. Surg Laparosc Endosc Percutan Tech 2017;27(4):273–81.
37. Pedraza R, Patel CB, Ramos-Valadez DI, et al. Robotic-assisted laparoscopic surgery for restorative proctocolectomy with ileal J pouch-anal anastomosis. Minim Invasive Ther Allied Technol 2011;20(4):234–9.
38. Bhama AR, Obias V, Welch KB, et al. A comparison of laparoscopic and robotic colorectal surgery outcomes using the American College of Surgeons National Surgical Quality Improvement Program (ACS NSQIP) database. Surg Endosc 2016;30(4):1576–84.
39. Raimondi F, Colombo R, Costantini E, et al. Effects of laparoscopic radical prostatectomy on intraoperative autonomic nervous system control of hemodynamics. Minerva Anestesiol 2017;83(12):1265–73.
40. Rawlings AL, Woodland JH, Vegunta RK, et al. Robotic versus laparoscopic colectomy. Surg Endosc 2007;21(10):1701–8.

41. Rencuzogullari A, Stocchi L, Costedio M, et al. Characteristics of learning curve in minimally invasive ileal pouch-anal anastomosis in a single institution. Surg Endosc 2017;31(3):1083–92.
42. Remzi FH, Aytac E, Ashburn J, et al. Transabdominal redo ileal pouch surgery for failed restorative proctocolectomy: lessons learned over 500 patients. Ann Surg 2015;262(4):675–82.
43. Garrett KA, Remzi FH, Kirat HT, et al. Outcome of salvage surgery for ileal pouches referred with a diagnosis of Crohn's disease. Dis Colon Rectum 2009; 52(12):1967–74.
44. Baig MK, Weiss EG, Nogueras JJ, et al. Lengthening of small bowel mesentery: stepladder incision technique. Am J Surg 2006;191(5):715–7.
45. Parks AG, Nicholls RJ. Proctocolectomy without ileostomy for ulcerative colitis. Br Med J 1978;2(6130):85–8.

Moving?

Make sure your subscription moves with you!

To notify us of your new address, find your **Clinics Account Number** (located on your mailing label above your name), and contact customer service at:

Email: journalscustomerservice-usa@elsevier.com

800-654-2452 (subscribers in the U.S. & Canada)
314-447-8871 (subscribers outside of the U.S. & Canada)

Fax number: 314-447-8029

Elsevier Health Sciences Division
Subscription Customer Service
3251 Riverport Lane
Maryland Heights, MO 63043

*To ensure uninterrupted delivery of your subscription, please notify us at least 4 weeks in advance of move.

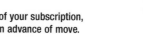

Printed and bound by CPI Group (UK) Ltd, Croydon, CR0 4YY

08/05/2025

01864745-0001